COLLABORATIVE TREATMENT
OF TRAUMATIZED CHILDREN AND TEENS

Collaborative Treatment of Traumatized Children and Teens

THE TRAUMA SYSTEMS THERAPY APPROACH

Glenn N. Saxe
B. Heidi Ellis
Julie B. Kaplow

THE GUILFORD PRESS
New York   London

© 2007 The Guilford Press
A Division of Guilford Publications, Inc.
72 Spring Street, New York, NY 10012
www.guilford.com

Printed in the United States of America

This book is printed on acid-free paper.

Last digit is print number: 9 8 7 6 5 4

Library of Congress Cataloging-in-Publication Data
Saxe, Glenn N.
   Collaborative treatment of traumatized children and teens: the trauma systems
therapy approach / by Glenn N. Saxe, Heidi B. Ellis, Julie B. Kaplow.
      p. cm.
   Includes bibliographical references and index.
   ISBN: 978-1-60623-349-8 (paperback)   ISBN: 978-1-59385-315-0 (hardcover)
   1. Post-traumatic stress disorder in children—Treatment.   2. Post-traumatic stress
disorder in adolescence—Treatment.   3. Psychic trauma in children—
Treatment.   4. Psychic trauma in adolescence—Treatment.   5. Child
psychotherapy.   6. Adolescent psychotherapy.   I. Ellis, Heidi B.   II. Kaplow, Julie B.,
1974–   III. Title.
   RJ506.P55S39 2006
   618.92′8521—dc22
                                                                    2006006044

To the memory of Roslyn Sheps Saxe (1936–2005),
who, in her 69 years of life, blazed a path from survival
to transcendence, and in so doing, inspired her son to develop
an intervention for traumatized children,
so that they could follow in her path

About the Authors

Glenn N. Saxe, MD, Associate Chief of Psychiatry for Research and Development at Children's Hospital in Boston and Harvard Medical School. He leads a program devoted to finding and building mental health program models that will be helpful for inner-city children and families with severe and complex social, psychological, and medical problems. Trauma systems therapy was developed over nearly a decade of effort, and is now used in many different clinics and agencies across the United States. Dr. Saxe also leads the Center for Children at Risk of the National Child Traumatic Stress Network (NCTSN) and has been a member of the Steering Committee of this important organization since its founding.

B. Heidi Ellis, PhD, is a clinical psychologist and Assistant Professor of Psychiatry at Boston University School of Medicine and Boston Medical Center, with joint appointments in Psychology and Pediatrics. Her primary area of interest is in developing interventions for traumatized youth. In particular, Dr. Ellis seeks to build interventions that work for families who typically do not access mental health care. As associate director of the Center for Children at Risk of the NCTSN, she has dedicated her efforts to making mental health care more relevant and accessible cross-culturally, with a specific focus on helping refugee children.

Julie B. Kaplow, PhD, is a licensed clinical psychologist and Assistant Professor in the Department of Psychiatry at New Jersey Medical School. Her primary research interest is the psychological consequences of childhood trauma, with a focus on identifying effective coping strategies that can help to inform interventions for traumatized youth. Dr. Kaplow has conducted research and clinical work with various populations of traumatized children, including those suffering from sexual abuse, traumatic injuries, and bereavement. She has served on the Traumatic Grief Task Force of the NCTSN and has been involved in educating health service personnel on the assessment and treatment of childhood traumatic grief.

Preface

Welcome to the world of trauma systems therapy (TST). As you will read, TST is designed for children and families for whom trauma is not only part of the past, but an ongoing part of present, everyday life. TST is designed for children and families facing such ongoing stress as poverty, family and community violence, and parental mental illness and substance abuse. Frequently, these children receive care in services systems that are frayed and fragmented.

You will soon be introduced to children such as Gerald, Denise, and Robert and the approach to their treatment. As you read, you will learn that this treatment always addresses two things: (1) a traumatized child who is not able to regulate emotional states; and (2) a social environment and/or a system of care that is not sufficiently able to help the child to regulate these emotional states.

These two things define what we call a trauma system, and that is why we have called this treatment trauma systems therapy. To address the trauma system that Gerald, Denise, and Robert inhabit requires the engagement of a lot of people: parents, guardians, relatives, friends, teachers, social service workers, therapists, psychopharmacologists, advocates, and home- and community-based clinicians. TST offers these inhabitants of the trauma system a highly focused and integrative treatment approach.

This book, and TST, may be of interest to you if you are:

- A psychotherapist who wants to learn about the fundamentals of traumatic stress care and how to build integrated treatment approaches within the organization where you work.
- A psychopharmacologist who wants to learn how psychopharmacology fits synergistically with the other interventions that traumatized children receive, and have the tools to connect your practice with other elements of the services system.
- A teacher who wants to learn about the manifestations of traumatic stress in the classroom and how to integrate the educational program with the mental health interventions your children receive.
- A social service worker who wants to build skills in safety assessment and learn how child protection work is a critical part of traumatic stress care.
- A home- or community-based clinician who wants to improve home-based interventions and connect these interventions to the other services traumatized children and families receive.
- A lawyer or other professional advocate who wants to learn how focused advocacy for services to which children and families are entitled are a critical part of traumatic stress care and can be integrated with this care.
- An administrator of a mental health organization who wants to learn how services for traumatized children in your agency can be more focused, integrated, and effective.
- An administrator of any program in the child services system who wants to learn how your services can be better integrated with effective mental health services.
- A public policymaker who wants ideas about how to improve the services system for traumatized children.
- A student or trainee in social work, psychology, psychiatry, pediatrics, or law who wants to understand the fundamentals about traumatic stress and its treatment.
- A parent or guardian who wants to understand the problems that your children are coping with and interventions that can make a difference in their lives.
- A teenager who has experienced trauma and wants to understand the problems you are coping with and how you can be helped.

TST treatment can involve such interventions as emotional regulation skill building, home- and community-based treatment, advocacy, and psychopharmacology; and when these varied intervention approaches together address the trauma system, treatment becomes tightly focused, synergistic, and most important, effective. As you will also read, the process of getting the people necessary to fix the trauma system together (the people mentioned above) involves the critical process of collaboration. Often providers work in different agencies and have never talked to each other. Often providers have never sat down together with the child and family to really understand what is most important to them. Collaboration is critical, and doable.

TST has been in development for about 8 years. This development has involved a long process of trying new things, evaluating whether they worked, and improving TST based on this evaluation. Although the book you have in your hands is the first published book on the TST treatment model, versions of this book, as a treatment manual, have been used by clinical teams for almost a decade.

We have designed TST to be adaptable without too much difficulty in a wide variety of settings. TST is being used in mental health clinics, schools, child welfare agencies, residential programs, and pediatric intensive care units. It has been adapted for adolescents with substance abuse, for refugees, and for children with injuries and illnesses, in addition to its original development for children who have experienced maltreatment and family and community violence. TST is now being successfully used by many agencies across the nation.

TST is meant to be *adapted*. We understand there are a great many variables at play within any given organization that will determine whether a new intervention can work within that agency. These variables include cost, access to services, administrative support, politics, and the reimbursement model within any given county or state. Every organization is different and is contending with a unique array of these variables. Therefore, for any new treatment to be adapted, it must be flexible enough so that these unique organizational variables do not become insurmountable barriers to adaptation. As you will read, TST has a lot of structure and focus; but this structure and focus contains flexibility to make it work within a great many diverse organizations. The services contained within TST, for example, can be paid for via third-party reimbursement in most states. The challenge is to form the right collaborations to make the treatment work.

TST is public property. It is designed to be used and is owned by its users. If you use TST, we consider you part of our innovation community and hope that you will use your skill and creativity to adapt it to best suit your needs, and more important, to the needs of the children and families whom you serve. If you make a useful adaptation to TST based on what will work in your organization, that is great and we hope you will share your innovation with us. It is our sincere hope that these innovations will continually work to create an ever improved TST, and a model that users can feel they own.

The process of treating children with traumatic stress, like the process of developing a treatment model for these children, is, in a way, never ending. What, really, is the finished product? We quote from the final chapter of this book here:

> We do not believe in finished products. The work of helping traumatized children requires, on the part of everyone, a continual struggle to make things better and better. This book is the result of an 8-year effort to develop a treatment that will work. We hope, however, that our book is only the first version of a process that is continually improved in response to people's experiences. Similarly, when we leave a traumatized child at what we call the end of therapy, we do not really believe he/she is "better" or "cured" or whichever professional term is used to make us feel better. The best we can hope for is to leave the child and the family with tools they will use to meet their challenges thoughout their lives. (p. 301)

So, welcome to the world of TST. You are now a member of a community of innovators. Use it. Change it. Make it better and do your best with the Geralds, Denises, and Roberts in your practice and in your lives.

Acknowledgments

This book, and the treatment model upon which it is based, could not have been developed without the hard work of the many families, clinicians, and providers who have been part of the team along the way.

We give particular thanks to Carolyn MacDuffee Chapman, Theresa Cain, Kendra Johnson, Joel Goldstein, and Tom Faxon from the Home for Little Wanderers in Boston; to David Barlow and Liza Suarez from the Department of Psychology at Boston University; to Pamela Tames, Ellen Lawton, and Amanda Sonis from the Division of Pediatrics at Boston Medical Center; and to Susan Hanson, Cheryl Quamar, Marshall Beckman, Barbara Sorkin, and Glenn Decker from the Ulster County, New York, Departments of Mental Health and Social Services for their help adapting and implementing some of the ideas in this book. In addition, many members of the Boston Medical Center Child Psychiatry Clinic and Treatment Development Team have contributed to the success of trauma systems therapy (TST). In particular, we thank Robert Casey, Michelle Bosquet, Jason Fogler, Stephen Luippold, Kassie Goforth, Helen MacDonald, Jill Harper, and Peter Rempelakis. We also thank the following experts who gave important advice in the development and writing of TST: Bessel van der Kolk, Terence Keane, Barry Zuckerman, Frank Putnam, and Lisa Amaya-Jackson; and Wanda Grant-Knight, who helped to build the foundation of TST through both her work with the conceptual model and her efforts to develop a training program devoted to caring for the children of Boston using the principles of TST.

We thank our editors at The Guilford Press—Kitty Moore, Sarah Lavender Smith, and Laura Specht Patchkofsky—for their invaluable comments, criticisms, and edits of this book. Their work has made TST immeasurably more accessible to readers.

We are particularly grateful to our friends and families who have supported us throughout the years of development of TST (and even before). We thank Joanna Bures-Saxe for her great, critical reads of the manuscript and for bringing her psychoanalytic expertise to the process of developing a useful psychotherapy treatment manual, and especially for the invaluable "signals of care" she devoted to her husband through the process of this book's development. Thanks to Ryan and Benjamin Saxe for patiently waiting for their dad to come home while he was writing this book.

We also thank Chris Bogan for the support and encouragement he provided throughout the development and writing of this book, and Eva Bogan, who waited until after the manuscript was completed to make her appearance.

We are grateful to Alan Prossin for his unwavering support and clinical insights, and to Robert and Lois Kaplow, who have always demonstrated the importance of using one's skills and knowledge to make a difference in others' lives.

We also give thanks to the National Child Traumatic Stress Network of the Substance Abuse and Mental Health Services Administration, the State Street Bank, and the Boston Foundation for providing the funding to make this possible.

And finally, we especially thank the families of Boston Medical Center, who have taught us much about the human capacity for resilience and the power of hope.

Contents

Introduction

Trauma Systems Therapy
for Child Traumatic Stress

LEARNING OBJECTIVES

- To introduce Trauma Systems Therapy for child traumatic stress
- To outline the four goals of this intervention approach
- To provide a guide for the rest of this book

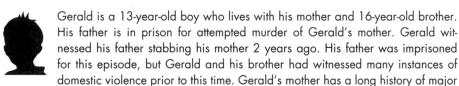 Gerald is a 13-year-old boy who lives with his mother and 16-year-old brother. His father is in prison for attempted murder of Gerald's mother. Gerald witnessed his father stabbing his mother 2 years ago. His father was imprisoned for this episode, but Gerald and his brother had witnessed many instances of domestic violence prior to this time. Gerald's mother has a long history of major depression and is currently quite depressed, staying in bed throughout most of the day. His brother has been arrested numerous times for assault and car theft. Gerald's brother has also severely assaulted his mother on two occasions. Gerald's mother is terrified to set a limit on her older son's behavior for fear of being assaulted. Gerald and his brother do not get along. There are frequent arguments at home that have escalated to fist fights. Gerald has been knocked unconscious by his brother and is perpetually in fear that his brother will "lose it" again. Gerald has frequent intrusive memories of witnessing domestic violence, he is vigilant about being assaulted, and has an exaggerated startle response. He has poor sleep with frequent nightmares and very poor concentration. He failed the sixth grade because he found it hard to focus on schoolwork. He is at risk for failing the sixth grade again this year and has told his therapist that if that happens, he intends to kill himself.

What do you do? What do you say? Where do you begin? If you are like most mental health clinicians in the United States, you work out of your office or a mental health clinic. The story of Gerald is probably very familiar to you. In your caseload there are probably five Geralds. You see him for his first intake appointment. Perhaps you see him again for a follow-up visit. If you end up treating Gerald, you notice quickly that his attendance is spotty. He shows up for a few sessions, then is gone for weeks or months at a time. If he attends regularly, you are faced with the real question: HOW CAN I HELP?! Does Gerald have cognitive distortions that need correcting? Does he have an amygdala that needs inhibiting? Does he have conflicts that need interpreting? Does he have avoidance that needs exposing? Does he have eye movements that need desensitizing? Maybe . . . but . . . anything that you do; any distortion that you challenge; any interpretations that you make; any medication that you prescribe; any learning that you condition . . . is undermined as soon as Gerald leaves your office. What do you do?

Gerald travels through the system. He is seen in emergency rooms, residential programs, inpatient units, and outpatient clinics. His care involves mental health, education, social service, and soon the juvenile justice systems. If you are assigned to treat Gerald, then you know that sensible treatment requires a lot of integration with each of these systems. But who has time for that?

He is hospitalized and you see him again. His medications are changed, but you cannot figure out what was done while he was hospitalized. He is failing school. You've gone to a few school meetings and explained about the stress and chaos in Gerald's life. The teachers are tired, and they have to think about the other kids in the class. They don't really know what to do. Gerald is missing school. He is missing appointments. You consider "closing the case" but just can't bear to do it. You've filed a couple of reports with the department of social services, but they are "screened out." What do you do?

There Are No Easy Answers

We wish it were easy. We wish there was that one medication. We wish there was that 12-step, eight-session therapy that would make Gerald's nightmare go away. We know that you wish it too. Sadly, what has created Gerald's nightmare is years of trauma, abuse, and neglect, some of which is ongoing. Real intervention will require rolling up your sleeves and helping to address the reality of Gerald's problems. But how?

This book is about an intervention model that attempts to address Gerald's needs and the tragic needs of children like him. Accordingly, intervention needs to be complex, focused, and intensive. It must be in the home, in the school, and in the neighborhood. It must get to the essence of the problem and stick to it like a dog to a bone, never to let go until the work is done. Intervention must address the numerous barriers that get in the way of families accessing services.

This work is not easy. It requires a lot of energy on the part of clinicians and a lot of support of clinicians from mental health agencies and service systems. Obviously, this type of work exists in a system that is far, far, from perfect. There are enormous public policy concerns related to how services are delivered to traumatized children and how the service system is organized. Nevertheless, there are existing services in place in most states that can be maximized for effective treatment. This book is about using these existing services in a coherent treatment model aimed at maximizing effectiveness.

This book also tries to address the realities of clinical practice. What are these realities?

- The average clinician is busy, probably overworked, and has little extra time or the resources to enhance treatment.
- The average mental health agency is financially stretched and has few funds for the extras such as staff training, supervision, outcome monitoring, or home-based care.
- The average state service system is also stretched and fragmented, with insufficient communication between departments and inadequate cross-system service plans for children with traumatic stress.

We designed our intervention model to address the needs of children with traumatic stress as effectively as possible, given the realities of clinical practice in the United States at this particular time. Accordingly, we designed this intervention using services that are available in most states.

> We designed our intervention model to address the needs of children with traumatic stress as effectively as possible, given the realities of clinical practice in the United States at this particular time.

The answers we propose are not easy; how can they be? We offer a series of solutions that is in no way perfect. Service delivery takes place in a service system that is resource poor and problematic in many ways. Nevertheless, we believe that the solutions we propose will be very helpful for mental health clinicians, agencies, and possibly even service systems as we all try to figure out what to do for children such as Gerald.

Use of Icons

Throughout this manual we use icons to guide you through the elements of our interventions. The icons should be read as symbols that provide "at-a-glance" ideas concerning what a given section is about. The following table describes the six icons that are used in this manual.

ICON KEY		
	Essential Point	An Essential Point indicates a section that contains information that **must** be understood to master the trauma systems therapy treatment approach.
	Academic Point	An Academic Point indicates a section that contains information that is interesting or academically important but is not absolutely necessary for mastering the trauma systems therapy treatment approach.
	Quotation	A Quotation is a piece of writing taken from others that we believe is very important to illuminate the trauma systems therapy treatment approach.
	Case Discussion	Case Discussions are liberally used throughout this manual to illustrate our treatment approach. We believe case discussions are particularly important to understand the concepts described in the manual.
	Useful Tool	A Useful Tool icon is used in our treatment module sections to highlight an intervention technique that is highly useful.
	Danger	A Danger icon indicates a potential pitfall of practice. This icon should serve as a warning to pay attention to the section (or skip at your own peril!).

Who Are We?

We are mental health clinicians, researchers, and educators at the Boston University Medical Center, Boston's inner-city hospital. The children and families we serve contend with considerable social problems, such as poverty, community violence, parental mental illness and substance abuse, homelessness, and racism. Our hospital is a magnet for families that have immigrated to the United States from around the world. Consequently we see many children and families who have experienced war and political violence. We are also a Level 1 trauma center and see most of Boston's children who are injured from assault or otherwise. Many of the families we serve are highly traumatized. Ten percent of children seen in our primary care clinic reported seeing a shooting or stabbing before they were 6 years old (Taylor, Zuckerman, Harik, & Groves, 1994). Sixty-two percent of adolescents seen in our emergency room (for any reason) reported a history of experiencing or witnessing violent physical or sexual assault (Kassner & Karasch, 1999).

We have been trying to help these children and families for many years. Our child psychiatry mental health clinic has been in operation since the early 1960s. We had been trying to do our best for these families with outpatient therapy, including what is considered "empirically validated" treatments and the highest quality psychopharmacology. About 6 or 7 years ago, faced with the frustration of the clinician assigned to Gerald (and a great many other children like him), we began to ask a simple question: Are we helping? We were not able to provide a clear answer to that question. Furthermore, we were getting burned out. Our staff turnover rate was high. People were very frustrated. Frankly, it was feeling as if we were banging our heads against the wall trying to help. We initiated a process of figuring out how we could do better. This book is a result of that process. On the way we investigated many different types of treatments and services for children. We also wanted our work to be helpful to others, so have worked with many people to try to operationalize our ideas into a useable format.

> We began to ask a simple question: Are we helping? We were getting burned out. Our staff turnover rate was high. We initiated a process of figuring out how we could do better. This book is a result of that process.

A huge catalyst for our efforts was the funding we received at the end of 2001 as an intervention development and evaluation center that is part of the new National Child Traumatic Stress Network (NCTSN). We provide details about the NCTSN at the end of this chapter; briefly, this network is the nation's primary response to the problem of treating traumatic stress in children, and it provides the funding and infrastructure to develop new treatments. After we received this funding, our efforts to develop a treatment model to approach the clinical realities of children such as Gerald was conducted as part of our NCTSN center, called the Center for Children At Risk. We call this treatment model trauma systems therapy (TST).

What Is Trauma Systems Therapy?

Traumatic stress occurs when a child is unable to regulate his/her emotional states. This inability occurs when the brain's way of processing emotion is disturbed. We talk a lot more about this in Chapters 2 and 3. For now, it is very important to know that this core problem of dysregulated emotional states is highly reactive to ongoing stresses and threats within the social environment. Because clinic- and office-based practices are removed from the social environment, they frequently are powerless to impact the very factors that drive children's traumatic stress symptoms.

Our treatment is about
interventions in what we call
a *trauma system*.

Our treatment is about interventions in what we call a *trauma system*, a term that refers to the failure to maintain the natural systemic balance between the developing child and his/her social environment. As has been described for decades in the child development literature, healthy development requires a regulatory balance, or a "goodness of fit," between the child and the social environment such that the social environment is properly equipped to help the child. When children enter service systems, this "goodness of fit" then includes the system of care.

 A trauma system is comprised of (1) a traumatized child who has difficulty regulating emotional states and (2) a social environment and/or system of care that is not able to help the child to regulate these emotional states.

TST describes an approach to assessing this "fit" between the child's emotional regulation capacities and the adequacy of the social environment/system of care to help the child and offers a variety of treatment modules based on the outcome of this assessment. We designed our intervention approach to address the severe problems in children's environments and do this work consistent with principles of child development and systems of care. We designed our intervention approach with children such as Gerald in mind. TST is designed to be used by any traumatized child, irrespective of age, who is having difficulty regulating emotional states.

Existing interventions do not offer clear approaches informed by theory about the way the social environment and the developing child interact. As we describe below (and repeat throughout this book), our treatment addresses two core problems of the trauma system: a child with dysregulated emotional states and a social environment/system of care that is unable to help the child regulate these emotional states. Our intervention intensively targets the trauma system. That is why we call our intervention trauma systems therapy.

Four Goals of the Development of TST

In designing our intervention approach, we set four goals for designing this intervention:

1. Treatment must be developmentally informed.
2. Treatment must **directly** address the social ecology.
3. Treatment must be compatible with systems of care.
4. Treatment must be "disseminate-able."

What Does This Mean?

Treatment Must Be Developmentally Informed

 In order to treat Gerald, you need to know certain basic principles about child development. You need to know that the types of interventions effective for a 6-year-old are very different from those for a 16-year-old, and also that a treatment for a child with developmental delays looks different from a treatment for a child without them. You must consider how such areas as attachment, emotional regulation, identity, and cognition, at different ages, can be approached in treatment.

These ideas are very important for a child such as Gerald. What type of attachment relationships might develop for a child who has a depressed mother and a very violent father and brother? What does it do to the sense of identity of a 13-year-old boy to have a father in prison and to have witnessed his father beating up his mother and brother? What does it do to his sense of identity, self-esteem, and feelings of control to have been beaten up by his father? How do these experiences and their influence on attachments and identity formation affect Gerald's ability to regulate emotion? What type of peer groups is he likely to join? How does growing up in terror affect cognitive development and school performance? These types of questions need to be asked and answered in order to sensibly treat Gerald. In Chapters 2, 3, and 4, we describe the developmental principles upon which our intervention approach is based.

> What does it do to the sense of identity of a 13-year-old boy to have a father in prison and to have witnessed his father beating up his mother and brother?

The developmental principles guiding our intervention approach were outlined most specifically in a report in 2000 by the National Research Council/Institute of Medicine called *From Neurons to Neighborhoods: The Science of Early Child Development*. This report describes the science of child development from the earliest years and integrates ideas about attachment, emotional and cognitive development, and identity in interventions for children. In particular, this report describes the influence of adverse environments on these developmental areas and the critically important interacting relationship between the environment and the developing brain.

Intervention Must Directly Address the Social Ecology

 In order to treat Gerald, you must be able to **directly** address the social ecology. If your treatment occurs only in your office, you will be spinning your wheels for a very long time. If you try to approach Gerald's family problems by scheduling the occasional family meeting, you will probably

If your treatment occurs only in your office, you will be spinning your wheels for a very long time.

not help very much. Gerald's problems require treatments on-site that directly address the social-environmental contributors to the problem. Often families of children with traumatic stress experience significant barriers toward receiving appropriate care. Intervention approaches therefore must be flexible enough to surmount these barriers.

Perhaps the most successful intervention model to directly address the social ecology is that of multisystemic therapy (MST) for conduct disorder (Henggeler, Schoenwald, Borduin, Rowland, & Cunningham, 1998). MST uses community-based interventions to specifically target areas of a child's environment that are theoretically related to the development and maintenance of conduct problems. MST has demonstrated effectiveness for aggressive children by successfully targeting for intervention many fields in which they interact: "The child and family, school, work, peer, community, and cultural institutions are viewed as interconnected systems with dynamic and reciprocal influences on the behavior of family members" and are therefore engaged in the treatment process (Henggeler, Schoenwald, & Pickrel, 1995, p. 710). MST targets child and family problems in the multiple systems in which families are embedded, and it delivers treatments in the settings in which they are likely to have the highest impact. Services are delivered in a variety of settings, such as home, school, and the community.

How could you approach Gerald's mental health problems from the distance of a clinic or office?

How could you approach Gerald's mental health problems from the distance of a clinic or office? His severe traumatic stress symptoms are highly reactive to conflicts and threats from his brother. His mother is too depressed to intervene or to reasonably engage in clinic- or office-based treatment. The consequences of these traumatic stress symptoms severely affect Gerald's school performance. Community-based interventions are essential for a child such as Gerald.

- The clinician must go to the home to help Gerald's mother protect him by engaging the police, the social service agencies, relatives, or whoever may help.

- The clinician must actively work with Gerald's mother to ensure that she receives treatment for depression so that she can better protect her son.

- The clinician should go to the school and consult with teachers and other school staff about how to best teach him and help with the construction of an individualized educational plan.

The failure of 2 school years for a child such as Gerald (who has normal intelligence) is a tragedy. Chapters 4, 10, 11, and 12 offer details about the way in which the social environment can be engaged when providing traumatic stress care.

Treatment Must Be Compatible with the System of Care

 In order to treat Gerald, you must be able to clearly link his treatment with the wider system of care. This is not easy, given how fragmented this system has become. Nevertheless, in Chapters 11 and 12 we describe a number of

> In order to treat Gerald, you must be able to clearly link his treatment with the wider system of care.

tools that can help. Gerald, like many children with traumatic stress, is seen in many different service systems. Within the mental health system, children such as Gerald often drift between the inpatient, outpatient, residential, and emergency psychiatry systems. Gerald is currently treated in an outpatient setting. If his suicidal impulses increase, he may be seen in the emergency or inpatient psychiatry systems. If his mother continues to be too incapacitated to protect him, the social services and residential systems may become necessary. There is a clear and reciprocal relationship between his emotional symptoms and his school functioning. His traumatic stress-related anxiety and poor concentration have interfered with his performance at school. This poor school performance, in turn, has contributed to low self-esteem and suicidal impulses. It is hard to imagine a sensible treatment plan that does not fully integrate the educational system.

Clearly, there is a great need for service integration for traumatized children. There is widespread acknowledgment of the need to create integrated systems of care for vulnerable, especially traumatized, children. The surgeon general's report on mental health specifically identifies the need for services integration:

> 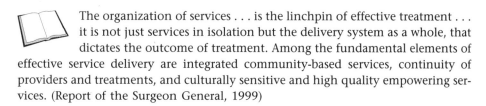 The organization of services . . . is the linchpin of effective treatment . . . it is not just services in isolation but the delivery system as a whole, that dictates the outcome of treatment. Among the fundamental elements of effective service delivery are integrated community-based services, continuity of providers and treatments, and culturally sensitive and high quality empowering services. (Report of the Surgeon General, 1999)

Our overall approach has been strongly influenced by the important national Child and Adolescent Service System Program (CASSP) (Pumariega & Winters, 2003; Stroul & Friedman, 1994). This program was created to guide states and communities in the development of community-based systems of care for vulnerable children, and it outlines a number of important "guiding principles" for effective community-based intervention. These guiding principles concern the need to create individualized, family-oriented services for children that address their physical, emotional, social, and educational needs. These services are "integrated, with linkages between child-care agencies and the programs and mechanisms for planning, developing, and coordinating services" and involve case management to coordinate the broad array of services that children might receive. More details about the CASSP initiative and systems of care are provided in Chapter 4.

What would an integrated and highly coordinated array of community-based services look like for traumatized children? How might the specificity of trauma-related psychopathology guide the development of this array of services? What types of problems would be most likely to change as a result of these services? Our intervention model is designed to provide such an integrated and highly coordinated system of services for individual traumatized children, guided by the specific understandings of the nature of child traumatic stress.

> What would an integrated and highly coordinated array of community-based services look like for traumatized children?

This model views the development of traumatic stress in children as resulting from two main elements:

1. A traumatized child who is unable to regulate emotional states when confronted with a stressor, and
2. A social environment and/or a system of care that is unable to adequately help the child regulate these emotional states.

Our treatment explicitly addresses these two core problems: a dysregulated emotional nervous system and a social environment/system of care that is unable to help the child regulate his/her emotion. Because the social environment (e.g., family, school, peer group, neighborhood) ordinarily plays a central role in helping a child contain his/her emotions or behavior, it is assumed that a child's inability to do so means that there is a diminished capacity of one or more levels of the social environment to help the child. Similarly, the inability to regulate emotional states also implies an inadequacy in the system of care to help the child contain emotions or behaviors. This inadequacy has three possible causes: (1) the child has not yet accessed the system of care, (2) the child is "falling through the cracks," or (3) the services the child is receiving are insufficient in some way to help contain emotions or behavior.

Our intervention approach can be seen as a guide for how services and interventions ought to be put together, given a child's emotional regulation capacities and the ability of the child's social environment and/or system of care to help him/her regulate emotion.

Treatment Must Be Disseminate-able

 In order to treat Gerald, you must be able to work within an agency or service system that supports and pays for this treatment. It is critical that new interventions reflect the financial and human realities of the clinicians, agencies, and service systems that will use them. It is relatively easy to design a "pie-in-the-sky" intervention model that is prohibitively expensive to use. A new intervention must be disseminate-able: That is, it must be described in a clear way and address the clinical realities of practice in this time and place and also incorporate strategies for supporting clinicians in this difficult work. Chapter 9 reviews some of these strategies for supporting clinicians.

> In order to treat Gerald, you must be able to work within an agency or service system that supports and pays for this treatment.

We designed this intervention using services that are available in most states. A multidisciplinary team of clinicians assesses and treats all referred children. This team is typical of most multidisciplinary teams of psychiatrists, psychologists, and social workers, with three exceptions:

1. It has the capacity to deliver home- and community-based interventions in addition to clinic-based treatment.
2. It includes a child advocacy attorney who serves a key consultative role for advocacy for services.
3. It functions from a very specific and operationalized model of assessment and treatment.

The enhancement of treatment with the aforementioned "exceptions" to usual practice was chosen in a way that could be implemented with limited extra resources.

1. *Home- and community-based interventions*: Most states fund short-term home-based intervention. We integrated a home-based team funded by the Commonwealth of Massachusetts Medicaid contract with a conventional multidisciplinary clinical team. This enhancement did not cost extra resources.
2. *Child advocacy attorney*: Many partnerships can be forged between mental health and legal aid clinics, law schools, and pro bono firms. A lawyer from the General Counsel's office, for example, volunteers 2 hours a week on our TST team.
3. *Model of assessment and treatment*: Most of this book is devoted to our description of our model of assessment and treatment. This model is a map that indicates how services and interventions ought to be assembled. Our main aim in this regard is clinical utility.

What's New in TST?

We believe that our main innovation is to create an intervention that allows clinicians to think beyond their office.

There are already a number of good treatments out there for child traumatic stress. We believe that our main innovation is to create an intervention that allows clinicians to think beyond their office. When interventions are conceived that directly address the social environment and system of care and are specifically focused on the child's core problems in regulating emotional states, there is a much higher likelihood of effectiveness. Existing interventions for traumatic stress do not pull the social environment and system of care into treatment sufficiently. Other people have expressed some of these ideas, in other ways, in other formats. We believe one of our main innovations is to pull together these ideas into a useful, focused, and testable framework for treating children with traumatic stress. Many ideas have deeply influenced our thinking; these include:

Ideas about Child Development

As described, we have been particularly influenced by ideas about how the social environment and the child's developing nervous system interact. The National Research Council/Institute of Medicine's *From Neurons to Neighborhoods* report (2000) contains very compelling ideas on this topic. Developmental ideas regarding attachment and self-regulation have also been very important in the development of our approach. Frank Putnam's (1997) concepts about discrete emotional states in traumatized children, based on the infant developmental work of Peter Wolff (1984), are reviewed in Chapter 3. Allan Schore's (1994) work on attachment, self-regulation, and the brain has also strongly influenced our thinking, as well as Robert Pynoos's developmental psychopathology model of traumatic stress (1993; Pynoos, Steinberg, & Wraith, 1995), Bessel van der Kolk's ideas about trauma and self-regulation (1994; van der Kolk & Fisler, 1994; van der Kolk et al., 1996), and Bruce Perry's (Perry & Pollard, 1998; Perry, Pollard, Blakley, Baker, & Vigilante, 1995) and Michael DeBellis's (De Bellis, Baum, & Birmaher, 1999; De Bellis, Keshavan, et al., 1999) ideas about trauma and the developing brain. Barry Zuckerman's (Fitzgerald, Lester, & Zuckerman, 1995) work on translating developmental ideas into public policy has also been very important.

Ideas about the Brain's Processing of Emotion

Joseph LeDoux's books *The Emotional Brain* (1998) and *The Synaptic Self* (2002) have affected our thinking about how trauma influences emotional processing (reviewed in Chapter 2). Other influences include Antonio Damasio (1999), Stephen Porges (1995), Jaak Panksepp (1998), Alan Schore (1994, 2003), and Bruce McEwen (1994).

Ideas about the Social Ecology

Urie Bronfenbrenner's (1979) social–ecological model of mental health, reviewed in Chapters 2 and 4, is fundamental to our treatment approach, as is his extension of this model (with Steven Ceci) (1994) to the interface between the brain and social ecology. These ideas have been extended to traumatic stress by Cicchetti and Lynch (1993), Mary Harvey (Harvey, Milner, & Roberts, 1995), and Anne Kazak (1996).

Ideas about Applying the Social–Ecological Model to Treatment

As described, Scott Henggeler and colleagues (1995, 1998) have been most successful at applying this model to child services with the development of multisystemic therapy. This pioneering model has strongly influenced the way that we operationalize treatment.

Ideas about Child Service Systems

The CASSP initiative (Pumariega & Winters, 2003; Stroul & Freedman, 1994), as reviewed above, has had a great influence on our thinking about the interface between our interventions and child service systems as well as how the system of care ought to be assessed and assembled.

Ideas about Traumatic Stress Treatment

Ideas about developing empirically validated interventions for traumatic stress are fundamental to how we have constructed our treatment approach. This effort most notably includes the work of Terence Keane (Keane, Fairbank, Caddell, & Zimering, 1989), Edna Foa (Foa, Rothbaum, Riggs, & Murdock, 1991), and Patricia Resick and Monica Schnicke (1992). The application of these ideas to children includes the work of William Salztman and Christopher Layne (Saltzman, Steinberg, Layne, Aisenberg, & Pynoos, 2001); Esther Deblinger (Deblinger, McLeer, & Henry, 1990); Judith Cohen and Anthony Mannarino (Cohen & Mannarino, 1996; Cohen, Mannarino, Berliner, & Deblinger, 2000); John March and Lisa Amaya-Jackson (March, Amaya-Jackson, Murray, & Schulte, 1998); and Beverly James (1989). We have been particularly influenced by interventions aimed at enhancing emotional regulation, such as those developed by Marsha Linehan (1993) and Marylene Cloitre (Cloitre, Koenen, Cohen, & Han, 2002).

We are also especially excited to include ideas on treatment initially suggested by Viktor Frankl (1962). Frankl's books, particularly *Man's Search for Meaning*, based on his experiences as a concentration camp survivor, describe psychotherapeutic approaches to trauma. These ideas have been hugely influential in the popular culture but are almost never discussed in academic circles. Our Chapter 16 ("Meaning-Making Skills") is largely about operationalizing these ideas and including them in our treatment approach.

Ideas about the Influence of Intervention on the Brain

The brain is plastic. Just as adverse events can harm the brain, positive events can help the brain. We have been strongly influenced by the recent movement in the mental health field to consider psychosocial interventions as possible psychobiological treatments that enhance brain functioning. This movement was led by Eric Kandel (1998) in his seminal paper "A New Intellectual Framework for Psychiatry."

 Insofar as our words produce changes in our patients' mind, it is likely that these psychotherapeutic interventions produce changes in the patients' brain. From this perspective, the biological and the sociopsychological approaches are joined. (p. 466)

Implementation of TST

Trauma systems therapy has successfully been implemented in Boston and in rural New York State. Our initial outcome study has been published as an open treatment trial and shows very promising effects with the initial 110 families from Boston and New York State over 6 months. This outcome study showed significant decreases in traumatic stress symptoms, emotional and behavioral dysregulation, and an increased stability of the child's social environment. Importantly, 60% of these families started in the intensive home- and community-based treatment phases and 40% started in the less intense office- and clinic-based phases of TST. These percentages were exactly reversed at the end of 6 months when only 40% needed intensive home- and community-based care and 60% needed office- and clinic-based care (Saxe, Ellis, et al., 2005).

At the time of this writing there are eight additional agencies from across the United States that are being trained to implement TST. It is important to note that there is great flexibility about how a given agency may implement TST. Agencies use broad latitude about the type of services that can fit under the TST "umbrella" and use a lot of creativity about forming partnerships and collaborations between agencies to get the right services configuration under this umbrella.

We believe this type of latitude and collaborative creativity is extremely important. TST has been in development for over 8 years as a highly iterative process. Ideas were tried, kept, or discarded based on their clinical usefulness. It is our sincere hope that many different agencies will try TST and adapt it based on their own needs. We would be very glad to learn and try your innovations to TST. We strongly believe that TST sets forth some valuable tools but that utility emerges over time and with diversity of experience. That is a long way of saying that we do not believe that TST is the final answer. We welcome you along our ride.

Outline of the TST Manual

 This book should be read as a manual for implementing the TST intervention approach for working with children who experience traumatic stress. The book has three parts:

I. Foundations
II. Getting Started
III. Doing Trauma Systems Therapy

Part I (Chapters 2–5) describes the theoretical background necessary to implement TST. Part II (Chapters 6–9) describes practical elements of assessment, treatment planning, and teamwork that are necessary to get started in TST. Part III (Chapters 10–16) describes the different treatment modules that offer a hands-on, practical approach to intervention. These chapters are:

PART I. FOUNDATIONS

Chapter 2: Survival Circuits

This chapter describes the interaction between the developing nervous system and the social environment in producing the problems of traumatic stress.

Chapter 3: The Regulation of Emotional States

This chapter identifies how traumatic stress problems are, at their core, a definable inability to regulate emotional states in the face of stressors.

Chapter 4: The Social Environment and the System of Care

This chapter discusses the various interacting levels of the social environment, including the family, school, peer group, neighborhood, and culture. We focus on how these areas of the social environment can serve to promote, or diminish, the self-regulation capacities of the child and how service systems ought to work to promote these capacities.

Chapter 5: Signals of Care

This chapter examines the critical role of the therapeutic relationship for traumatic stress care. We note the importance of building a therapeutic alliance and how to use information derived from the therapeutic relationship to guide treatment.

PART II. GETTING STARTED

Chapter 6: Ten Treatment Principles

This chapter outlines the ten principles that anchor TST treatment. These principles are shown in Table 1.1.

Chapter 7: Assessment

This chapter offers a clear approach to assessing the interface between a child's self-regulation capacities and the social environment/system of care. This assessment approach leads to the approach to treatment planning.

Chapter 8: Treatment Planning

This chapter describes ways of organizing treatment based on our approach to assessment. Briefly, this is a phase-oriented treatment in which each phase corresponds to various degrees of the child's regulation capacities and the stability of the social environment.

Chapter 9: The Treatment Team

This chapter discusses the importance of multidisciplinary teamwork, strategies for creating a supportive team environment, and the role of the team in maintaining treatment fidelity and therapist commitment and energy.

TABLE 1.1. Ten Treatment Principles

1. Fix a broken system.
2. Put safety first.
3. Create clear, focused plans that are based on facts.
4. Don't "go" before you are "ready."
5. Put scarce resources where they'll work.
6. Insist on accountability, particularly your own.
7. Align with reality.
8. Take care of yourself and your team.
9. Build from strength.
10. Leave a better system.

PART III. DOING TRAUMA SYSTEMS THERAPY

Chapters 10–16: Treatment Modules

The remaining chapters of the manual offer hands-on guidelines for providing different types of interventions depending on the assessed degree of self-regulation the child displays and stability that is contained in the child's social environment. Chapter 8 offers guidance on how each module is chosen given this type of assessment.

Chapter 10: Ready–Set–Go

This chapter discusses potential difficulties in engaging families in treatment. It identifies three key areas for successfully engaging families in treatment: building the treatment alliance, providing education and information, and troubleshooting practical problems.

Chapter 11: Stabilization on Site

This chapter describes how a community-based treatment model is interwoven with other service modalities to provide treatment for acutely symptomatic traumatized children. We give clinicians specific skills for providing treatment in the home or community and for coordinating with other providers. This treatment module focuses on diminishing traumatic triggers in the child's social environment. The goals of the approach are described, and the two main treatment areas identified: emotional regulation and environmental stabilization.

Chapter 12: Systems Advocacy

This chapter describes a treatment approach that utilizes legal advocacy in conjunction with traditional treatment modalities to address instabilities in the social environment of traumatized children. We explain how legal advocacy helps clinicians move beyond in-office therapy and psychopharmacology to assist families in changing or overcoming environmental stressors that impede recovery. We also offer guidelines for successful psycholegal collaboration and a discussion of the implications such collaborations have for trauma treatment, specifically, and mental health care, generally.

Chapter 13: Psychopharmacology

Psychopharmacology is an integral part of TST. This chapter shows how the use of psychoactive medications fits within the care of traumatized children and the role of medication in an overall treatment plan to help the child regulate emotion. We focus on the relationship between psychopharmacology and psychotherapy within the TST model and describe the different roles for medication in the various phases of treatment. We also describe the role of the psychiatric consultant on the treatment team and offer practical ideas to enhance the critical communication between psychiatric and nonpsychiatric members of the team.

Chapter 14: Emotion Regulation Skills

The main purpose of this chapter is to teach the clinician specific strategies and exercises that help the family and child improve the child's self-regulation skills. Specifically, the strategies help children and families identify (1) traumatic triggers, (2) internal and external signs that a child's emotional state is changing, and (3) interventions that help the child emotionally regulate him/herself.

Chapter 15: Cognitive Processing Skills

This chapter teaches clinicians how to utilize specific exercises and activities that help traumatized children extinguish maladaptive responses to traumatic reminders and ultimately create meaning out of the traumatic experience. We explain the ways in which the therapist can assist the child in (1) extending his/her repertoire of emotion regulation skills to incorporate cognitive coping skills, (2) increasing his/her tolerance for thoughts/discussions surrounding the traumatic event, and (3) decreasing the intensity of emotion associated with thoughts of the trauma.

Chapter 16: Meaning-Making Skills

This chapter provides clinicians with skills and suggestions for helping clients create meaning out of their traumatic experiences. We explain ways in which the therapist can (1) assist the child in developing new ways of thinking about the traumatic experience, (2) help the child recognize and articulate important lessons learned from the experience, (3) help the child reinvent him/herself and plan for the future, and (4) find ways of turning important lessons learned from the trauma into personal expressions of hope.

Chapter 17: Conclusions

The book ends with a concluding chapter that highlights the possible roles that TST can play in the system of care and the public policy concerns relevant to creating an effective and integrated system of care for traumatized children.

The National Child Traumatic Stress Network

We would like to acknowledge the Substance Abuse and Mental Health Services Administration (SAMHSA) for funding the development of Trauma Systems Therapy and its National Child Traumatic Stress Network (www.nctsnet.org) for being the setting in which many of our ideas have developed. The National Child Traumatic Stress Network (NCTSN) was funded by SAMHSA in October 2001 in order to address the national public health concern of traumatic stress in children. The NCTSN has three components: (1) the National Center for Child Traumatic Stress, a coordinating center based at Duke University, and the University of California at Los Angeles; (2) 15 "intervention development and evaluation centers," which are charged with "identifying, supporting, improving, and developing treatment and service approaches for different types of child and adolescent traumatic events"; and (3) 38 "community treatment and service centers," which are charged with implementing and evaluating effective treatment and services in community settings.

The NCTSN is designed as a highly coordinated network of programs to develop and implement best practices for traumatic stress care in children and to advance their standard of care nationally. Our NCTSN center, the Center for Children At Risk, based at the Child Psychiatry Section at Boston University Medical Center, is one of the intervention development and evaluation centers. Our efforts to develop TST are one of the primary activities of our center.

The mission of the NCTSN is "to raise the standard of care and improve access to services for traumatized children, their families and communities throughout the United States." We hope that you will find our efforts true to this mission and that this manual helps you help all the Geralds in your practice.

PART I
Foundations

Survival Circuits

How Traumatic Stress Is about Survival-in-the-Moment

LEARNING OBJECTIVES

- To understand how traumatic stress responses relate to systems of the brain developed for survival

- To understand how traumatic stress responses relate to "survival-in-the-moment"

- To review neurodevelopmental variables related to traumatic stress responses

- To review the critical relationship between the social environment and the developing brain

---

Traumatic stress is about *survival-in-the-moment*. Survival-in-the-moment is controlled by ancient systems of the brain and body that we call the *survival circuits*. The survival circuits control the way we process traumatic events and the hold that these events may have on us throughout our lives. We begin our discussion of the foundations of TST with a review of these survival circuits and their implications for treating traumatic stress. First, let us briefly think about survival. Any discussion of survival must begin with the amazing work of the 19th-century British naturalist Charles Darwin (1809–1882). As most of us know, Darwin proposed his theory of evolution to explain the natural origins of human beings. Through his observations of animals on the Galapagos Islands, he noted that the animals best equipped to survive were the most likely to live long enough to pass on their survival-enhancing traits to their offspring. Traits that helped promote survival were maintained, and those that did not promote survival died out. Darwin later described this as a process called *adaptation*. New traits can suddenly develop in a given organism out of what is called *chance mutation*. Those new traits that give their owner enough of an advantage to reproduce become integrated into the biology of the species. Over many millions of years, this process creates species with ever-increasing advantages for survival.

> Survival is at the core of traumatic stress. It is enacted at the moment we perceive that our lives are in danger, and the survival circuits control it.

Although Darwin's revolutionary proposal, *The Origin of Species* (1859), was published almost 150 years ago, it anticipated and is supported by groundbreaking work in genetics, molecular biology, and developmental neuroscience that has been published only in the last 10 years. The need to survive has sculpted our biology. This sculpture has occurred over many millions of years and has given us—in our genes, our cells, our brains, and our bodies— powerful mechanisms to survive. Survival is at the core of traumatic stress. It is enacted at the moment we perceive that our lives are in danger, and the survival circuits control it.

Survival Circuits

 We human beings are at the top of the evolutionary ladder. What puts us up there? We have a biology that has been refined over millions of years, giving us amazing systems to master our environments. Our biology gives us the potential to create great works of art, science, mathematics, technology, and culture. Our ability to master our environments, and to achieve enormous advances in diverse areas of pursuit, requires our evolutionarily advanced neurobiological systems to be working properly. The main part of our biology that has allowed us such powerful and flexible adaptive capacities is the brain—particularly the higher-order systems of the brain, located in what is called the *cerebral cortex*.

> One of the primary ways that these advanced, higher-order brain systems become unable to do their great work is if there is a perceived threat to survival in the environment.

Lower-order systems of the brain, such as those that control basic emotionality, physiology, and survival-motivated behavior, are found in the brains of lower animal species and are also powerfully embedded deep within our human brains. These lower neurobiological systems are largely responsible for maintaining our survival, so that our higher-order brain systems can do their great work. However, these advanced, higher-order brain systems become unable to do their great work if there is a perceived threat to survival in the environment. When this occurs, by virtue of millions of years of evolution and adaptation, all neurobiological systems work at only one goal: to foster *survival-in-the-moment*. As described, the survival circuits are responsible for survival-in-the-moment responses. It is the engagement of these survival circuits, in situations where life is not actually in danger, that causes the problem of traumatic stress.

 Once these powerful and ancient systems are triggered, the brain and the body enter a state of processing in order to maintain survival against life-threatening events. The problem, for individuals with traumatic stress, is that most of the time there is no current and immediate life threat. The individual's brain and body are responding to a past life threat in the present. Almost all problems in those with traumatic stress relate to these powerful survival circuits. It is therefore extremely important to understand how seemingly innocuous *stimuli* can create these extreme survival-motivated *responses,* in order to help traumatized children respond in more adaptive ways.

> It is therefore extremely important to understand how seemingly innocuous *stimuli* can create these extreme survival-motivated *responses,* in order to help traumatized children respond in more adaptive ways.

 The importance of these survival circuits will be integrated into the definition of traumatic stress in the next (fifth) edition of the *Diagnostic and Statistical Manual of Mental Disorders* (DSM-V), the important guidebook that defines all mental disorders in the United States and in most areas of the world. The proposed new name for the group of disorders that includes fear, anxiety, and posttraumatic stress disorder (PTSD) will be stress-induced and fear circuitry disorders (First, 2005). These disorders can be understood through the descriptions of the survival circuits provided in this chapter.

Survival-in-the-Moment

 As we will describe, there is a great emphasis within TST on understanding specific moments in a traumatized child's life. In essence, these moments are when the survival circuits get engaged. These are the moments when children feel and do things that become very problematic for themselves and/or others, and lead to the need for mental health intervention. If these moments were somehow magically removed from a child's life, there would be no need for mental health intervention. Traumatic stress, as described, is about survival-in-the-moment. TST is about replacing these survival-in-the-moment responses with responses that allow a child to grow and thrive.

> TST is about preventing survival-in-the-moment responses.

The survival circuits are the means by which the brain processes stimuli that are potentially life-threatening and translates this perception into life-sustaining responses. In traumatic stress, there are fundamental problems with this type of

It is important to know what goes on within the brain and body, between the potentially life-threatening stimulus and the potentially life-preserving response.

processing, and responses become highly maladaptive. In order to understand this more fully, it is important to know what goes on within the brain and body between the potentially life-threatening stimulus and the potentially life-preserving response. We begin the discussion of this fundamental process with a description of an incident of a child with traumatic stress. Consider what happens to Denise, in-the-moment:

Denise is a 16-year-old girl with a history of being sexually abused by her mother's boyfriend. While at a local mall with friends, she saw a man who frightened her. She later reported that this man reminded her of her mother's boyfriend. Denise remembers becoming extremely anxious and being flooded with memories of the sexual abuse. She does not remember walking away. Her friends found her curled up in a bathroom stall, unresponsive.

Denise's case is one of an adolescent with a history of sexual abuse who was functioning well, until she saw a man who reminded her of the man who abused her. When she saw this man, her brain rapidly shifted to *survival-in-the-moment*. It is exactly this moment that must be understood and treated within TST.

Denise generally functions well. Most of the time, her higher-order brain systems are engaged and doing their great work. Denise was at the mall having fun with friends. She was happy, socializing, and very calm. At the moment she saw this man, however, she entered a state of extreme fear and then dissociation. These states of extreme fear and dissociation are entirely motivated by survival. Traumatized children go from the stimulus (a traumatic reminder) to the response (an extreme emotional state) without the ability to think, calm down, and soothe themselves. This response can be immediate, extreme, and outside of conscious control. An essential part of intervention is to help children to calm themselves when they are confronted by a traumatic reminder, so that they do not enter these extreme survival-in-the-moment states. Denise went immediately from the stimulus to this extreme state. If treatment could help her to think before she responded, she might have the potential to calm and soothe herself so that the extreme responses would not occur.

How do children navigate a world full of threats when they have such problems managing their emotions and behavior in response to a threat?

One of the main goals of intervention is to prevent children from going from stimulus to immediate extreme response. A critical problem for traumatized children is that they frequently live in environments riddled with traumatic reminders. The stresses of ongoing family violence, community violence, parental substance abuse, and mental illness, for example, are frequently part of the everyday life of a traumatized child. How do children navigate a world full of threats when they have such problems managing their emotions and behavior in response to a threat? All children must learn to identify, manage, and reasonably respond to signals from their social environment. How does a child with traumatic stress learn to do this when he or she hears any loud voice as angry, or misinterprets a classmate's playful nudge as aggressive? How much more difficult is this task when the child is exposed to ongoing domestic or community violence, endures parental mental illness and substance abuse, or fears impending homelessness? This is the problem that our intervention model is designed to address.

 If Denise did not immediately respond with extreme emotional or behavioral changes and could think about the stimulus of a man who reminded her of her mother's boyfriend, she could perhaps understand that the man was *not* her mother's boyfriend and that more

> How can higher-order brain systems *stay* engaged in situations of threat? TST is designed to help traumatized children's brains do this.

adaptive responses were possible. If Denise could develop the ability to think in this way, a lot of good things could happen for her. The ability to think in this way requires the engagement of the higher-order brain systems that we have described. Again, these higher-order systems are undermined by the lower-order systems in situations of survival-in-the-moment. How can higher-order brain systems *stay* engaged in situations of threat? TST is designed to help traumatized children's brains do this.

TST starts with the understanding that traumatized children frequently live in environments saturated with traumatic reminders (the stimuli) and have limited ability to regulate their emotional and behavioral responses. As Figure 2.1 illustrates, they go from a stimulus to an extreme immediate response (survival-in-the-moment state). Two types of interventions are instituted, as illustrated in Figure 2.2: (1) *social-environmental* interventions and (2) *self-regulatory* inter-

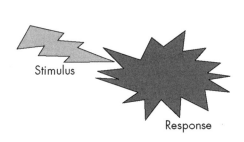

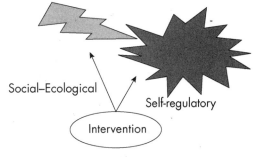

FIGURE 2.1. From stimulus to immediate, extreme response in a child with traumatic stress.

FIGURE 2.2. Two types of interventions for traumatic stress responses.

ventions. Social-environmental interventions are about surveying the social environment for sources of traumatic reminders and trying to diminish these reminders (the stimuli). Self-regulatory interventions are about using both psychotherapeutic and psychopharmacological means to enhance the child's capacity to control the immediate response to the stimuli. As illustrated in Figure 2.3, when the stimuli are diminished and the child has increasing capacity to regulate responses, the potential to think about alternative responses is developed. For reasons that are clear in the illustration, we call this a "wedge" of cognition.

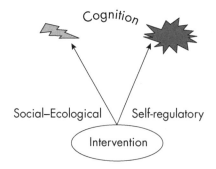

FIGURE 2.3. The wedge of cognition to regulate traumatic responses.

Your Moment in the Zoo

In order to help you understand better how this works, we will take a walk through your brain in a given moment between a stressful stimulus and a response. Please imagine yourself in the following situation:

> You are walking down a path, lost in your own thoughts. It is a nice, sunny day. You feel calm. Suddenly you notice an object coming toward you from the right. You freeze. Your feet are planted in the ground. Your heart is pounding. You are sweating. . . . You then recognize that the object walking toward you is a *lion* . . . you see that it is in a cage . . . and that you are in the zoo. You continue walking and continue to enjoy your pleasant day at the zoo.

The moment described in the scenario above would probably take less than 2 seconds. Within that time, a lot of activity has occurred in your brain that illustrates very important ideas about the emotional nervous system and its integral role in survival. These ideas are very important to understand when we consider the nature of traumatic stress. The moment (illustrated in Figure 2.4 and the following discussion) is adapted from the work of Joseph LeDoux, a neuroscientist at New York University who has conducted some of the pioneering work on emotional processing in the brain, particularly processing related to fear. His books *The Emotional Brain* (1998) and *Synaptic Self* (2002) are very important for understanding how the brain processes threatening stimuli and for understanding survival-in-the-moment. We also rely on Antonio Damasio's *The Feeling of What Happens* (1999) in our discussion of how emotion, memory, and consciousness fit together. In this brief chapter, it is hard to do complete justice to these great areas of research, and parts of the discussion are oversimplified. Nevertheless, there are important components of emotional processing in the brain that help us to understand the nature of traumatic stress and its intervention.

According to LeDoux, there are two emotional processing systems of the brain. These two systems work closely together, such that we are usually unaware that these discrete systems exist. These systems are critical for our survival, and roughly correspond to the aforementioned distinction between the higher-order and lower-order systems of the brain. LeDoux calls these two systems the "low road" and "high road" of emotional processing. We call these systems, considered together, the *survival circuits*.

Figure 2.4 illustrates these two roads of emotional processing. As can be seen, the stimulus of the lion in the zoo passes through the *sensory thalamus* along

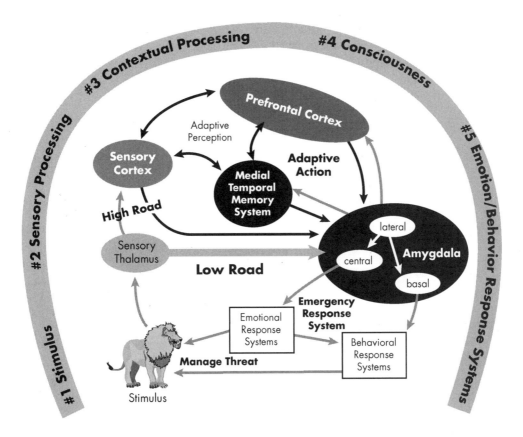

FIGURE 2.4. The survival circuits. Gray arrows, transmissions of danger information; black arrows, transmission of danger *or* safety information.

two separate paths. One path (the low road) goes directly to a structure called the *amygdala* that prepares the body for emergency responses. This pathway is marked by very quick transmission of sensory information to give the organism basic information about danger. This pathway is unconscious and does not contain contextual information. It sacrifices the details in the service of speed so that you can respond before you are eaten! The other path (the high road) travels to cortical areas (the *sensory cortex*, the *prefrontal cortex*, and the *medial temporal lobe memory system*) that process the danger signal, assess its degree of threat, and transmit signals to the amygdala regarding whether the stimulus signals safety or danger. This type of processing can powerfully determine the most adaptive response in-the-moment.

The information processing shared by the sensory cortex, the medial temporal lobe memory system, and the prefrontal cortex is very important for determining an accurate perception of the stimulus and for determining an adaptive response to this perception of the stimulus. The gray arrows in Figure 2.4 indicate transmission of signals indicating danger. The black arrows indicate transmission of signals that may indicate either danger or safety. Safety information traveling from high-road brain systems (the sensory cortex, the prefrontal cortex, and the medial temporal lobe memory system) to the amygdala diminishes amygdala responding and serve to regulate emotion. When danger information is transmitted from these high-road systems, however, it maintains the low-road, survival-in-the-moment response. This type of information could have been transmitted if, for example, the lion you encountered had actually escaped from its cage. The amygdala also communicates directly back to high-road systems. These pathways, indicated by the upward-pointing gray arrows, are very important for understanding the nature of traumatic memory. The remainder of this chapter details the relevance of these concepts for traumatic stress.

Stimulus, Sensation, Context, Consciousness, and Response

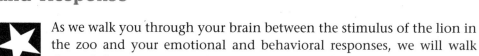 As we walk you through your brain between the stimulus of the lion in the zoo and your emotional and behavioral responses, we will walk through five constructs related to brain processing that are captured by LeDoux's high road and low road of emotional processing. These five constructs, considered together, explain many areas of experience, symptoms, and functioning in individuals with traumatic stress. It is important to note that these five constructs are not necessarily engaged sequentially, but may be involved in parallel at various times in the processing of the stimuli.

1. The Stimulus

People's responses to the external world are based on how they appraise external stimuli. Most stimuli that are processed do not signal a threat to life and limb. Some stimuli, however, indicate such a threat. The way in which people make this distinction is critical for survival and for adaptive responding. At the zoo, you were confronted with a stimulus. How did you eventually decide it was safe? How much did you need to think about the lion walking toward you before you knew that you were (very) unlikely to be attacked? What about Denise in the mall? How did she decide that the stimulus of a man walking toward her indicated that her life could be threatened? How did that appraisal determine a response? As will be detailed next, much of this appraisal is done unconsciously, so that we are completely unaware of the information that bears on survival-laden responses in the moment. It is very fortunate that these responses can be processed outside of conscious awareness. Conscious processing takes time. By the time you needed to think about whether the lion walking toward you was a threat, you might have been eaten (if, for example, the lion had escaped from its cage)!

> At the zoo, you were confronted with a stimulus. How did you eventually decide it was safe? How much did you need to think about the lion walking toward you before you knew that you were (very) unlikely to be attacked?

2. Sensory Processing

All the stimuli that confront us are processed through a structure called the sensory thalamus. This structure has components for processing stimuli from the five senses. The stimuli that you and Denise processed were visual. Once the visual stimulus of the lion in the zoo, or the man in the mall, engages the sensory thalamus, it is transmitted in two possible directions. One direction is to the sensory cortex for higher-order processing, including conscious perception of the stimulus. LeDoux calls this direction the "high road." The other possible direction is straight to the lateral nucleus of the amygdala (the "low road"). We will review amygdala processing in more detail when we discuss emotional and behavioral response systems a little later. What is important to note is that this low road is extremely fast and unconscious. Low-road processing transmits bits of threat-related information very quickly to the amygdala, whose job is then to initiate emergency responses. This type of information does not include the contextual details. It sacrifices these details in the service of speed so that you can respond to maximize your chance of survival, given the threat. The high road—which includes the sensory cortex, the medial temporal lobe memory system (especially a structure called the *hippocampus*), and the prefrontal cortex—is engaged to help get the details of the situation so that the most adaptive response is possible, given the stimulus. These systems working together are what help an individual know just how threatening the stimuli are. In order to do this, the sensory cortex must engage long-term memory stores that contain experience with similar stimuli; the medial temporal lobe memory system must place the stimulus in the proper context of time and place; and the prefrontal cortex must put this information into an individual's direct awareness (working memory) in order for considered action to occur. The low-road amygdala system responds rapidly to incomplete bits of information and facilitates memory storage in such an incomplete way. This is probably why people have flashbacks when they are reminded of a traumatic event. Flashbacks are, in essence, bits or flashes of emotionally laden memory. This type of memory storage is unconscious and is called the *implicit emotional memory system*. This memory system is critical for survival because it stores the memory of survival-threatening stimuli, so that when such stimuli are encountered again, survival-oriented responding can be very quick. Because this storage is so incomplete, however, it leads to misperception of threatening stimuli on future occasions. This helps explain why Denise immediately had a survival-in-the-moment response when she saw the man at the mall.

3. Contextual Processing

As described, the low-road amygdala system does its work in a contextless way. It is *only* concerned with survival. The medial temporal lobe memory system, particularly the hippocampus, provides the contextual details. This is the system that works with the sensory cortex and other areas of the higher-order cerebral cortex to bring accurate, context-laden details provided by the long-term memory systems of the cerebral cortex to help an individual accurately understand the proper time and place of the stimulus.

The low-road amygdala system does its work in a contextless way. It is *only* concerned with survival.

The ability to place a given stimulus accurately in its proper time and place is extremely important. What made you know that the stimulus of the lion was not life-threatening? You could correctly place it in the zoo and connect it with your long-term memory stores of your experiences in zoos. To the degree that none of these memories includes being attacked by a lion in a zoo, but rather pleasant times in the zoo and the safety of lions in zoos, you would feel safe and continue to have your pleasant day at the zoo. In fact, your initial response (heart pounding, sweating, feet planted, etc.) was mediated by the low-road amygdala system, but was terminated so quickly and unconsciously that you could have continued completely unaware that it occurred. What terminated this immediate low-road response? The high-road medial temporal lobe memory system, indicating you were safe by allowing you access to information so that you could correctly recognize the context you were in. This information would include that you have been to the zoo many times before, that you have never been attacked by a lion, that you have never before seen anyone attacked by a lion, and that lions in zoos generally do not leave their cages. Access to this information diminished your body's emergency responses and led to the sense of calmness that you felt only moments after you were alarmed. In Figure 2.4, the black arrow (when it transmits safety information) shows this regulation of response from the medial temporal lobe memory system to the amygdala.

4. Consciousness

Consciousness implies awareness. It is the awareness, *in-the-moment*, of the stimulus, the response, and/or the emotional state of the body. It is also, in-the-moment, the awareness that there is an agent (you) that perceives the stimulus, carries out the response, and/or feels the emotional state of the body. As Antonio Damasio says, consciousness is the bringing together of the self and the object (stimulus) *in-the-moment*. Accordingly, consciousness has a lot to do with our basic sense of identity, or the feeling and thought of who you are. To a great extent, the processing of stimuli and execution of responses occur completely outside of our awareness, as described earlier. Consciousness is when this processing reaches our awareness, or, as Damasio says, when we "step into the light." Consciousness is strongly influenced by the prefrontal cortex, as shown in Figure 2.4. This is related to what is called *working memory*, or the capacity to keep information in awareness, in-the-moment.

Consciousness is very important for traumatic stress. When you were walking in the zoo, you were initially lost in your thoughts and momentarily not really conscious of being in the zoo. Of course, at any moment you could have easily shifted your attention from your thoughts to what you were doing (walking in the zoo), but it is a good thing that you did not need to be completely conscious of

> Consciousness involves the ability to shift attention to the things we want to attend to. When we perceive stimuli suggesting that our life is in danger, however, it is very hard to attend to anything else.

the zoo if you did not need to be. If we do not always need to be conscious of the context we are in, than we can then shift our attention to other things and let our higher-order brain systems do their great work. (Perhaps while you were walking in the zoo you were composing a symphony, solving a scientific problem, or trying to solve an interpersonal conflict.) Conscious thought is experimental action. It allows us to consider our responses carefully before responding. This is the wedge of cognition described in Figure 2.3. Consciousness involves the ability to shift attention to the things we want to attend to. When we perceive stimuli suggesting that our lives are in danger, however, it is very hard to attend to anything else. How might this work for you and for Denise?

You were lost in your thoughts during your walk in the zoo. At some point, the context of the zoo intruded on your consciousness in the form of a lion walking toward you. Prior to your achieving this consciousness, your low-road system was briefly engaged. A moment after your low-road system became engaged, your high-road system processed the sensation of the lion, compared it with previous memories of lions in zoos, accurately brought your current context (the zoo) to your mind, and brought some of that information into your consciousness. Each of the high-road systems—sensory cortex (accurate perception), medial temporal lobe memory system (context), and prefrontal cortex (consciousness)—sent safety signals (see the black arrows in Figure 2.4) to the amygdala, allowing you to enjoy your day. Once Denise was stimulated, she was, sadly, far less able to shift her attention back to her good time at the mall. The stimulus of the man who reminded her of her mother's boyfriend signaled danger; her low-road amygdala system responded rapidly and extremely. Her higher-road systems were not able to perceive the stimulus accurately enough to tell her that the man was not her mother's boyfriend and to keep her in the safer context of the mall. Accordingly, what entered her consciousness was only the context of past abuse. Consciousness involves orientation to time, place, and person. In-the-moment, she was disoriented to when this was, where she was, and who she was. She was a little girl, in her bedroom, being abused.

Another way of describing why your trip to the zoo was calm and peaceful and Denise's trip to the mall was terrifying is that, as LeDoux (2002) puts it, the amygdala leads a "hostile takeover of consciousness by emotion" (p. 226).

 . . . the amygdala leads a hostile takeover of consciousness by emotion. (LeDoux, 2002, p. 226)

In other words, when presented with a stressful stimulus, the emotional nervous system becomes so overwhelmed that what enters an individual's awareness is dominated by low-road amygdala processing (i.e., fast, fragmented, decontextualized, aroused) rather than high-road processing (i.e., slow[er], calm, linear, contextual, and [more] conscious). When Denise saw the man at the mall, the amygdala succeeded in its hostile takeover. When you saw the lion, your higher-order systems fought it back (the amygdala, not the lion).

> When Denise saw the man at the mall, the amygdala succeeded in its hostile takeover. When you saw the lion, your higher-order systems fought it back (the amygdala, not the lion).

5. Emotional and Behavioral Response Systems

The amygdala, via its low-road pathway, is designed to prepare the body quickly and powerfully to react and to survive. Accordingly, it engages the emotional and behavioral response systems of the body. These systems are very important for survival, as they mobilize the body to respond very quickly during situations of danger—so quickly that one is not even aware or conscious of responding. As can be seen in Figure 2.4, the lateral nucleus of the amygdala integrates information from both the sensory thalamus (the low road) and the sensory cortex, medial temporal lobe memory system, and prefrontal cortex (the high road); it then uses this information to guide powerful, evolutionarily driven bodily responses.

Pathways from the amygdala's lateral nucleus go to its central nucleus to engage systems of the body that will *react*. This includes hormonal systems via the hypothalamic–pituitary–adrenal (HPA) axis, which releases energy stores by using the hormone cortisol; the locus coeruleus/norepinephrine system, which activates the heart and focuses attention on the threat; and the polyvagal system, which increases social engagement from the myelinated vagus nerve or immobilization or freezing from the unmyelinated vagus nerve (Porges, 1995). These systems also feed back to the amygdala and to the higher-order cortical systems, and result in our awareness of the feeling state of our bodies. An emotion is the awareness of a feeling state of the body (Damasio, 1999). This process of self-awareness is extremely adaptive. It allows an individual to use emotions as signals for effective action and underlies the critical process of emotional regulation that will be detailed in the next chapter. We use this understanding about consciousness of one's own emotional state to build skills in this area, as described in Chapter 14.

> This process of self-awareness is extremely adaptive. It allows an individual to use emotions as signals for effective action and underlies the critical process of emotional regulation.

The emotional response systems mediated by the central nucleus of the amygdala have strong connections to motivational/behavioral/reward systems mediated by the basal nucleus of the amygdala. The basal nucleus then initiates a pathway that leads to behavioral responses (fighting, running, yelling, etc.) to manage the threatening stimulus. This pathway begins with a structure called the *nucleus accumbens* and directs bodily nerves and muscles to manage the threat. It is also important that the amygdala's central nucleus emotional response system is also connected to these motivational/behavioral/reward systems. This latter pathway leads to the release of dopamine in the nucleus accumbens, which facilitates its response to signals from the basal amygdala (LeDoux, 2002). One important practical implication of this connection is that survival-related emotion can clearly cause survival-related behavior. In children with traumatic stress, this survival-related behavior can be violence, self-mutilation, or suicide. This behavior usually follows extreme emotional states such as panic, rage, dissociation, and depression. As will be detailed in Chapter 7, our assessment approach operationalizes these basic neurobiological processes.

> Survival-related emotion can clearly cause survival-related behavior. In children with traumatic stress, this survival-related behavior can be violence, self-mutilation, or suicide. This behavior usually follows extreme emotional states such as panic, rage, dissociation, and depression.

What about Denise? Denise, as described, does not have a high-road system that will help her correctly identify the stimulus and bring the context of the mall to the moment. Her responses are thus entirely mediated by the very quick pathway from the sensory thalamus to the lateral nucleus of the amygdala. The motivational/behavioral/reward systems activated while in this emotional state included running to the bathroom and freezing (as she lay on the bathroom floor). As described, for Denise this emotional state represented survival-in-the-moment.

The March of the Moments: Traumatic Stress in the Past, Present, and Future

 We began this chapter with a discussion of how traumatic stress responses can be understood via survival-in-the-moment. Our detailing of Denise's response in the mall and your response in the zoo allowed us to describe the neurobiology of these moments through what can be called *survival circuits*. This way of thinking about

Everything is in-the-moment!

traumatic stress is really built on top of how people are put together through the very long process of evolution. This also brings us to an interesting and important idea about human emotion, consciousness, memory, and sense-of-self, which has important implications for treatment: *Everything is in-the-moment!*

As described, consciousness involves the capacity (through working memory) to keep only a small set of things in awareness in any given moment. Human consciousness is *only* a construct for the present. Human consciousness, and therefore the organization of human experience, are moment-by-moment. Memory is the laying down of these present, conscious moments in the brain so that they can be accessible if we need them.

What happens to the moment that has just passed? What makes us know that these moments joined together make up ourselves as entities that travel through time with a continuity of memory and identity?

What happens to the moment that has just passed? What makes us know that these moments joined together make up ourselves as entities that travel through time with a continuity of memory and identity? Our ability to know these critical things requires a process of these moments being laid down, with proper contextual information and relative continuity of emotional experience between moments. In other words, the development of a clear and coherent sense-of-self requires that the high-road systems lay down these moments in memory, rather than the low-road systems. As described, if the pathway from the amygdala to the higher-order systems is very active, then the memory that gets laid down is fragmented, disoriented, and decon-textualized. Individuals construct a sense of themselves through the stringing together of moments. This is what has been called *autobiographical memory*. The ability to access memory consciously in a given moment is greatly facilitated if the memory was laid down in a clear, linear, and context-related way. A person's emotional state in-the-moment facilitates this access. If an individual is in an anxious state, for example, it is much easier to access anxiety-related memories than calmness-related memories. When an individual is in a survival-in-the-moment phase, it is very hard to access memories of calm moments. One of the main functions of psychotherapy is to help an individual have access to these memories, in-the-moment.

Consider the string of boxes in Figure 2.5. Each box indicates a separate moment in time. Each moment in time is marked by a feeling state indicated by a degree of shading. Most people have moment and feeling states that look like Figure 2.5. Moments consist of relatively stable, calm feeling states (the slightly lighter boxes at either side of the present moment in Figure 2.5).

This person occasionally has another, nonextreme feeling state (say, sadness), indicated by the change to a slightly darker shading for the present moment. There is no problem or pathology associated with this feeling state, as it is largely laid down through the higher-order systems. The present moment of sadness is experienced with relative calmness and linear, contextual processing.

To the degree that there is continuity between feeling states in-the-moment, past memory is laid down with relative coherence and is joined with an awareness of the self that is relatively stable over time. In fact, for individuals whose life moments are generally laid down in such calm, contextual, and linear ways,

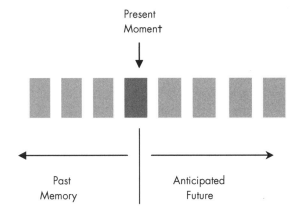

FIGURE 2.5. Moment and feeling states during normal emotional processiong.

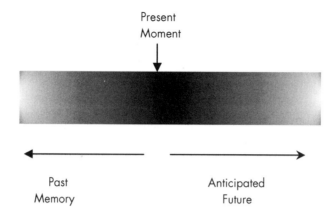

FIGURE 2.6. Continuous experience of the self in normal emotional processing.

their experience of the self looks more like Figure 2.6. Even though conscious-ness works moment-by-moment, the brain has a way of blending moments so that self-experience is continuous.

This fundamental neurological capacity to blend moments is critical for our ability to form a coherent sense of ourselves over time. This capacity is not unlike the way the brain is able to take frame-by-frame images of a movie and construct a complete and continuous story. Consciousness is the "movie-in-the-brain," as Damasio describes it:

> . . . the neurobiology of consciousness faces two problems: the problem of how the movie-in-the-brain is generated, and the problem of how the brain also generates the sense that there is an owner and observer for that movie. (1999, p. 11)

What happens if there is a moment in which survival appears to be threatened?

A moment in which survival is perceived as threatened is indicated in Figure 2.7, where the dark box indicates a survival-in-the-moment state, and the other boxes indicate moments of relative calmness. This experience, like Denise's moment in the mall, is experienced in a highly fragmented, disoriented way. It then gets laid down in memory in such a way that when some of the contextual signals recur on future occasions, there is a higher likelihood of this survival-in-the-moment state recurring. This is why Denise will have such states of survival-related emotion whenever she experiences stimuli of a man reminiscent of her mother's boyfriend. This is also why Denise will have such difficulty blending moments as illustrated in Figure 2.6. Denise's internal world actually looks more like Figure 2.8. Her experience is riddled with episodes of survival-in-the-moment.

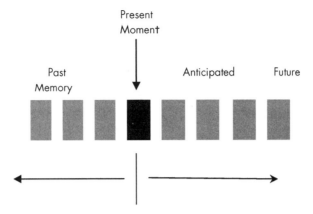

FIGURE 2.7. A survival-in-the-moment state for a person with traumatic stress.

As we have described, in states of survival-in-the-moment, individuals like Denise can become disoriented to time, place, and person. Denise in these moments feels like a little girl out of control and about to be raped. This is very different from how she feels in other moments—that is, calm, happy, and like a competent girl who is in control of her life. In a way, Denise's emotional life looks more like Figure 2.9.

Denise lives parallel lives. Her sense-of-self cannot make the transitions between emotional states, and she grows up with a very fragmented sense of herself. These types of problems occur in certain conditions of psychopathology, such as the dissociative disorders and some of the personality disorders. Such problems—where an individual's sense-of-self can become state-dependent

FIGURE 2.8. Experience of the self in a person with traumatic stress.

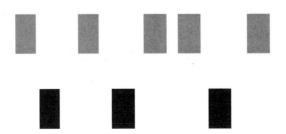

FIGURE 2.9. The emotional life of a person with traumatic stress.

Given the obvious corollary difficulties of forming stable relationships when one's own sense-of-self is unstable, and the emotional fluctuations that are part of this instability, children with traumatic stress often grow up with patterns of painful, unstable relationships.

instead of being state-independent—have also at various times been called *disorders of extreme stress*, *complex PTSD*, and *developmental trauma disorder*. Given the obvious corollary difficulties of forming stable relationships when one's own sense-of-self is unstable, and the emotional fluctuations that are part of this instability, children with traumatic stress often grow up with patterns of painful, unstable relationships. Chapter 3, on emotional regulation, describes some details of this process, including its implications for psychiatric diagnosis of traumatized individuals. Chapter 5, on interpersonal relationships, details how this pattern of unstable emotion and sense-of-self can lead to significant difficulties with relationships. As we will describe, perhaps the only hope of recovery for a child with traumatic stress is the development of stable relationships. It is therefore extremely important that these patterns of survival-in-the-moment are addressed in treatment.

Marching into the Future

One of the most devastating effects of traumatic stress is its effect on children's ability to think into the future.

 One of the most devastating effects of traumatic stress is its effect on children's ability to think into the future. If consciousness is about the present, and memory is about the past, then planning and anticipation are about the future. They involve the use of present consciousness and long-term memory stores to anticipate the risk and reward of future events, and to plan so that one's needs are met into the future.

This ability to see into the future is one of the most powerful functions of the human brain. At a basic level, this ability maximizes survival through the ability to calculate survival-related risk, given the ever-changing environmental variables that are encountered in everyday life. At the zoo, for example, you unconsciously performed a calculation that the lion walking toward you was not likely to pose a risk to your survival, because a series of metal bars mediated your relationship with the lion. This calculation also extended into the future. You (unconsciously) calculated that for the time you would stay in the zoo, you would be safe. This calculation helped preserve your sense of calm safety at the zoo, but was also made with incomplete information. You had no information, for example, about whether the lion's cage was locked or unlocked. You bet your life that it was locked. Our capacity for continual calculation of risk is fundamental for our ability to navigate our world productively. This calculation of risk always involves incomplete information (e.g., your ignorance of whether the cage was actually locked). We must be able to do this well, or we will live our lives completely restricted by survival-related concerns. Our ability to calculate the likely *reward* of specific events in the future is critical for our sense of happiness and pleasure, and to the degree that it motivates behavior to increase the likely reward of future events, it motivates creativity.

The parts of the brain that perform these calculations are located in the area called the *parietal cortex*. The parietal cortex (most specifically, the posterior parietal cortex) performs calculations of the likely risk and reward involved in future events. We need to be able to do this effectively. A calculation of "high risk" of the future event influences the motivational/behavioral/reward circuits to avoid this event. A calculation of "low risk" influences the motivational/ behavioral/reward circuits to engage with this event if there is a sufficient probability of reward related to the event. The posterior parietal cortex calculates probabilities of risk versus reward. The results of these calculations strongly influence emotion and behavior. Neuroscientists have become very interested in understanding these types of calculations as a way to understand how the brain influences motivated behavior. This area of neuroscience has been called *neuroeconomics* (Glimcher, 2003).

In children with traumatic stress, these calculations are extremely important. An overestimate of the likely risk in events leads to the serious problem of avoidance of people, places, and things that might remind a child of the trauma. Traumatized children can therefore lead overly restrictive lives. It is also clinically important that traumatized children can underestimate the risk of danger and put themselves in highly dangerous situations. This can happen when a child is not able to act on interpersonal warning signs and therefore forms relationships with individuals who repeat the trauma. In addition, traumatized children have trouble calculating the likely reward inherent in future events. They underestimate the pleasure that they might experience in relationships and activities. The parietal lobes' calculations of the probability of risk and reward of future events are a part of individuals' ability to visualize themselves in the future. One of the tragic problems of traumatic stress is this lack of ability to see oneself in the future, or, as Lenore Terr (1990) has described it, this sense of a "foreshortened future." Traumatized children will not be able to see their futures if they are fighting for their lives in the present and if they have trouble seeing any likelihood of rewards or pleasure in future events.

> Traumatized children will not be able to see their futures if they are fighting for their lives in the present and if they have trouble seeing any likelihood of rewards or pleasure in future events.

A Picture of the Brain

In order to see how closely many of the areas of the survival circuits work together, it is important to see how close they are to each other in the brain. This is illustrated in Figure 2.10 from the online journal CNSforum.com, where the areas of the brain known to be related to traumatic stress are shown.

As can be seen, the low-road amygdala is situated right beside the high-road hippocampus, a critical part of the medial temporal lobe memory system. Both of these areas are in close proximity to the sensory thalamus, which passes sensory information to the low-road and high-road systems,

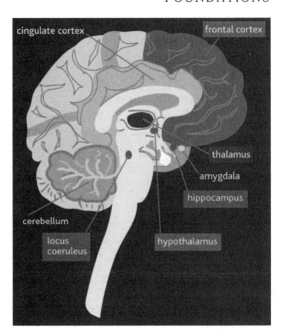

FIGURE 2.10. Areas of the brain known to be related to traumatic stress. Copyright by CNS-forum.com. Reprinted by permission.

respectively. The emotional and behavioral response systems are also closely related anatomically. The hypothalamus is the leader of the HPA axis, which regulates the stress hormones, required for fight-or-flight. Similarly, the locus coeruleus leads the norepinephrine system's response, which causes heightened attention to the threatening stimulus and increases heart rate to help the body respond to the threat. The prefrontal cortex, as described earlier, is critical for holding information in consciousness.

Although this chapter is not intended to provide a full research review of the psychobiology of traumatic stress, it is important to know that many of these systems are affected and even damaged by trauma. Many functional brain imaging studies have reported that the amygdala is active during memory of the trauma (e.g., Rauch et al., 1996, 2000; Shin et al., 2004). Other studies have reported a smaller hippocampal size and diminished hippocampal function in those with traumatic stress (e.g., Bremner et al., 1995, 1997; Stein, Koverola, Hanna, Torchia, & McClarty, 1997). Although this finding has not been replicated in children, Carrion and colleagues (2001) and DeBellis and colleagues (1999) did report a smaller volume of the cerebral cortex in general. There is a large literature on the dysfunction of the HPA axis (e.g.,

Yehuda et al., 1990, 1993) and the locus coeruleus/norepinephrine system in those with PTSD (e.g., Kosten et al., 1987; Southwick et al., 1993). Newer research has focused on the relationship between the high road and low road as described in this chapter. Shin and colleagues (2004) found that during a memory of a traumatic event, the prefrontal cortex was less active in those with traumatic stress, compared to traumatized individuals without traumatic stress. This lower activity of parts of the prefrontal cortex was related to higher activity of the amygdala. Importantly, this lower level of prefrontal activity was also related to the degree of traumatic stress symptoms. In other words, this important functional MRI study reported that the high road has difficulty regulating the low road in those with traumatic stress.

Beyond Survival

TST is about understanding how the child's developing nervous system and the social environment interact. This is reflected in our description of the trauma system. In Chapter 1, we have defined this trauma system as follows:

> TST is about understanding how the child's developing nervous system and its social ecology interact.

1. A traumatized child who has difficulty regulating emotional states.
2. A social environment and/or system of care that cannot sufficiently help contain this dysregulation.

The social ecology (Bronfenbrenner, 1979) of traumatic stress places the child and his or her developing brain in the center of nested levels of a social environment. The parts of the brain described by the survival circuits are at the center of the trauma system. One of the most important implications of the discussion in this chapter on survival circuits is how closely linked these circuits are to social-environmental stimuli. Some of the details of the trauma system are fleshed out in the next few chapters. Chapter 3 details how the critical developmental construct called *emotional regulation* works for the traumatized child. As will be seen, ideas of emotional regulation are highly related to the survival circuits described in this chapter. Chapter 4 details the importance of the social environment and system of care for child development, and describes how exactly these systems can go wrong for traumatized children. Chapter 5 details the importance of interpersonal relationships for helping or hindering the healthy development of traumatized children. These interpersonal relationships are considered to be the cusp of the trauma system and strongly mediate the relationship between emotional regulation and the social environment/system of care.

The quality of earliest interpersonal relationships sculpts the brain's survival circuits to make the child more or less able to regulate emotion when faced with a stress.

The quality of earliest interpersonal relationships sculpts the brain's survival circuits to make the child more or less able to regulate emotion when faced with a stress. These "working models" of relationships described in the attachment literature help or hinder the regulation of emotion in future relationships. We call strong attachment relationships *signals of care,* because they work exactly to counteract survival-in-the-moment when a child is confronted with signals of danger. As will be described, if children live in social environments and systems of care that contain sufficient signals of care, this will go a long way toward minimizing the risk of a survival-in-the-moment response. TST has a strong focus on building these signals of care in the lives of traumatized children.

We end this chapter with some evidence that the survival circuits can be changed through the right types of experiences. Peter Kirsch and colleagues (2005) at the National Institute of Mental Health recently reported that the amygdala, the leader of the low-road system, can be regulated by a chemical called *oxytocin*. Oxytocin is critical in human life for a lot of reasons. It strongly influences a woman's labor and delivery of her baby. It also strongly mediates breast-feeding and is a chemical known from animal and human research to be critical for bonding and healthy attachment. Oxytocin is naturally released during social bonding from the earliest phases of development and is one of the critical mediators of social attachments. The release of oxytocin during safe social contact causes a sense of calmness. Figure 2.11 shows the results of the Kirsch and colleagues experiment.

Individuals were shown pictures of frightening faces and of frightening scenes. In the placebo condition, the areas of the brain that were most active, indicated by the light patches near the bottom of the two top images, was the amygdala on both sides of the brain. When these same individuals were given a dose of oxytocin and shown the very same frightening pictures, the amygdala was no longer active.

The profound implications of this experiment go far beyond the possible therapeutic value of giving

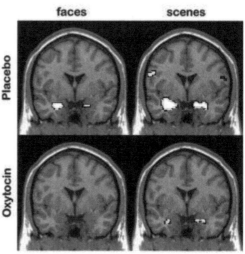

FIGURE 2.11. Oxytocin diminishes amygdala response to frightening faces and scenes.

frightened people injections of oxytocin. We all release oxytocin naturally in the context of safe and caring relationships, and the release of this chemical leads to our feelings of calm contentment in these relationships. If the leader of the survival circuit is the low-road amygdala, and the amygdala is regulated by oxytocin, then strong, safe, caring relationships will help to regulate the amygdala and therefore the survival circuit.

The silver lining in the cloud of trauma is that just as bad events can change the brain in deleterious ways, good events can change the brain in beneficial ways. We designed TST to help the brain, and the child who owns it, to have experiences that will move them toward the future they deserve.

The silver lining in this cloud of trauma is that just as bad events can change the brain in deleterious ways, good events can change the brain in beneficial ways.

The Regulation of Emotional States

How Child Traumatic Stress Is a Disorder of the Regulation of Emotional States

---

LEARNING OBJECTIVES

- To understand how traumatized children enter extreme emotional states
- To understand how intervention approaches depend on the emotional state of the child
- To learn principles of assessing emotional states in traumatized children

---

The dysregulation of emotional states is a defining feature of child traumatic stress. What are emotional states? How are they defined? How are they assessed? We introduced the importance of emotional states and how they relate to the survival circuits in Chapter 2. We discussed how traumatized children go from stimulus to immediate, extreme response when exposed to a stressor. In particular, we discussed how the amygdala leads a "hostile takeover of consciousness by emotion" (LeDoux, 1998, p. 226) when a traumatized child is triggered by a traumatic reminder. In this chapter we describe these extreme, immediate emotional responses in more detail and how to assess them. In Chapter 7 we discuss how the assessment of emotional states fits in the overall assessment of traumatized children. Chapter 14 discusses how to help children with these emotional states.

Recall that problems with the regulation of emotional states are half of our formula for what produces traumatic stress in children. Therefore, it is very important to clearly understand emotional states. Unfortunately, it is not easy to understand exactly what is meant by the term *emotional states*. Emotional states are most clearly understood via an example:

Consider Robert . . .

 Robert is a 10-year-old boy with a history of severe physical abuse from his stepfather. He has a long history of extreme and impulsive aggressive behavior. While at recess, another child made a demeaning comment about Robert. Without thinking, Robert lunged at him and continued to pound him in the face with his fists until the school monitors pulled him off.

Robert and Denise (from Chapter 2) each enter extreme emotional states when reminded of prior traumatic events. As described in Chapter 2, the reactions of both children can be understood through a review of neurobiological systems that are responsible for defensive behavior in the face of threat and are experienced as survival-in-the-moment states. Think about what is going on inside of Denise as she is curled up on the bathroom floor. Think about what is going on inside Robert as he lunges after the boy on the playground. Think about both these children in the instant before they behaved in these extreme ways. Now think about what changed after both these children were reminded of a traumatic event. If you have a good sense of what changes, then you know what an emotional state is. The rest of this chapter is devoted to describing these changes.

What Are Emotional States?

 Frank Putnam, at the Cincinnati Children's Hospital Medical Center, was the first to describe the importance of discrete emotional states for traumatized children. Putnam (1997) reviewed one type of emotional state, dissociation, but his ideas are also useful for many other clinical problems encountered by children with traumatic stress. The term *discrete emotional states* refers to special patterns of thinking, feeling, and acting that go together and change dramatically when a person is presented with a stressor. Lichtenberg, Lachman, and Fosshage (1992) offered a good definition of an emotional state as

... a constellation of relatively stable repeated patterns of motivational variables and patterns of self experience characterized by specific forms of activity, cognition, affect, and relatedness. (p. 157)

It is important to understand that this "constellation" of special patterns of behavior, thinking, and feeling is relatively stable and highly related to an individual's sense of him/herself and to the way he/she relates to other people. In traumatic stress conditions this pattern can be so separate (or discrete) that when people finally calm down, they do not remember what they said or did when they were in this changed emotional state. Even a person's sense of who he/she is can be different in different emotional states.

The psychopathology of child
traumatic stress is a definable
deviation from normal child
development.

The psychopathology of child traumatic stress is a definable deviation from normal child development. The regulation of emotional states is a key task that infants and young children must acquire. Peter Wolff (1987), at Children's Hospital in Boston, developed important theories, based on infant research, for the regulation of emotional states in all infants. According to Wolff, infants are born with unique, distinct, and regularly fluctuating emotional states that are defined by such variables as respiratory rate, motor tone, activity level, vocalization, and facial expression. He describes basic emotional states that can be defined by the unique configuration of these variables. Infants regularly fluctuate through these emotional states, which are the basic building blocks of emotion and consciousness. Changes between states are regular, predictable, and in response to stimuli in the infant's external or internal environment. As infants grow, states become more elaborate and complicated and involve more thinking. New states develop in order to respond to the increasing environmental demands placed on the developing child. As Putnam (1997) says:

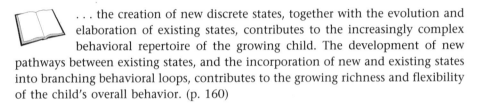

... the creation of new discrete states, together with the evolution and elaboration of existing states, contributes to the increasingly complex behavioral repertoire of the growing child. The development of new pathways between existing states, and the incorporation of new and existing states into branching behavioral loops, contributes to the growing richness and flexibility of the child's overall behavior. (p. 160)

A key job of the infant is to attain control over the switches between emotional states so that a more desired state is maintained for longer periods of time and across different situations. The parent's role is to help the infant transition from less desired states to more desired states. An infant's cry means that he/she is in a distressed state. Parents hear the cry and respond by distracting or soothing the infant and leading him/her back to a calm state. When parents do this hundreds or thousands of times, the young child learns how to calm and self-soothe. In Putnam's or Wolff's language, this means they are able to transition from an emotional state of distress (with clear behavioral and physiological signs) to a state of calmness. Learning to make this transition is one of the key ways that children learn to manage emotion and behavior. In situations of family trauma, abuse, and neglect, the parent on whom the infant depends for calming and soothing is either causing the distress or ignoring it. This pattern can create lifelong difficulties with emotional state regulation.

As described in the previous chapter, the focus of attention, orientation to surroundings, emotions, and behaviors all change together, affecting another key task of infancy: learning to transfer information acquired in one state to other states. Young children have great difficulty doing this. The capacity to transfer or generalize knowledge across contexts and emotional states is important for the development of a sense of self. As Putnam (1997) describes:

> In normal individuals, mood state has a lesser but still noticeable impact on how an individual perceives and represents himself or herself . . . specific state-dependent senses-of-self are sufficiently integrated with one another that the individual maintains a sense of continuity of self across state and context. (p. 164)

We talk a lot more about this sense of self later. For now it is important to know that the sense of self develops over time and is one of the most important things that is injured by traumas. Next we review the process by which emotional states change in traumatized children.

The Three A's and the Four R's (or How the Elements of Emotional States Change across Phases)

Emotional states are very important for assessment and intervention in TST. When emotional states are a part of traumatic stress, we call them "survival-in-the-moment" states. In order to make this concept clear and relatively easy for assessment, we have tried to operationalize it as best we can. The rest of this chapter describes a clinically useful approach to understanding emotional states. An emotional state is a unique pattern of experience in response to a stressor. What are the elements of this unique pattern? We call the elements of emotional states the three A's:

- Awareness (or consciousness)
- Affect (or emotion)
- Action (or behavior)

What happens when an emotional state changes? We call these changes the phases of emotional states. There are four phases—the four R's:

- Regulating
- Revving
- Reexperiencing
- Reconstituting

Now let's take this one step (or letter) at a time.

What are the three A's and the four R's and why is it important to know about them?

Elements of Emotional States

As described in Chapter 2, children with traumatic stress go from stimulus to immediate, extreme responses when confronted by a traumatic reminder or stressor. An extreme, immediate response in a traumatized child is a discrete emotional state and involves dramatic changes in a number of areas of experience. Discrete emotional states are more than just emotions; they involve complex patterns of feelings, thoughts, and behaviors that change *together* after a child is stressed. Consider Denise and Robert in the moment just before and just after they were reminded of their past traumas. Please pay attention to the three areas of experience that we call the three A's. While you are paying attention to these three A's, think about what we described in Chapter 2 about survival-in-the-moment. It is this survival-related emotion that determines the dramatic shift in each of the three A's.

> Discrete emotional states . . . involve complex patterns of feelings, thoughts, and behaviors that change *together* after a child is stressed.

 It is also important to be aware of how important the three A's are to the survival of a person. Awareness, affect, and action have evolved to help us survive in the face of threat and are mediated by the brain's *survival circuits* (described in Chapter 2). Accordingly, it makes sense that an event or events that challenge a person's survival (a trauma) would cause changes to these three elements.

Awareness (or Consciousness)

In the moment just before and after a traumatized child is reminded of the trauma, there are huge shifts in the child's awareness of what is going on. Before a traumatized child experiences a stressor, he/she is most likely aware of, and engaged in, the external world and the relevant tasks at hand. After the traumatized child is stimulated, he/she is usually aware of only very specific features in the environment that are important for survival. The child also may be more focused on his/her internal state than the external environment as old traumatic memories begin to dominate consciousness. In other words, there are dramatic shifts in the focus of attention.

Awareness, or consciousness, also implies a sense of self: there is a subject (person) who is aware or is conscious. Antonio Damasio (1999), in his great book *The Feeling of What Happens: Body and Emotion in the Making of Consciousness,* defines consciousness as "the unified mental pattern that brings together the object and the self" (p. 11). According to Damasio, consciousness is a critical evolutionary advance that allows an individual to be aware of the environment and his/her internal states in order to decide on the most adaptive response for a given stimulus (or object).

 At its simplest and most basic level, consciousness lets us recognize an irresistible urge to stay alive and develop a concern for self. At its most complex and elaborate level, consciousness helps us develop a concern for other selves and improve the art of life. (Damasio, 1999, p. 5)

There are three main components of awareness (or consciousness) that must be assessed:

- *Attention*: The degree to which the child's shifts in focus of *attention* changes his/her awareness of what is going on around him/her after being stressed.
- *Orientation*: How the child's experience of place and time changes after experiencing a stressor.
- *Sense of self*: How a child's experience of who he/she is changes after experiencing a stressor.

Affect (or Emotion)

The child's emotions dramatically shift after experiencing a stressor. Affect, or emotion, has two key biological functions: (1) to produce a specific reaction to a stimulus (e.g., fight–flight–freeze) and (2) to help regulate the internal state of the individual so he/she can be prepared to react to that stimulus. Emotions have evolved to be highly adaptive. Unfortunately, these emotions can be highly maladaptive in traumatic stress conditions. In reexperiencing emotional states children can have intense feelings of anger, fear, dysphoria, guilt, or shame. These feelings are profound and disorienting. Robert entered a state of intense anger when he punched his classmate. Denise experienced a state of intense anxiety when she saw a man at the mall who reminded her of her mother's boyfriend. These affects, or emotions, are experienced because they may have facilitated survival in the context of trauma. The problem is that the child is unable to see that the context has changed.

Action (or Behavior)

A child's behavior may change dramatically after perceiving a stressor. Some-times these dramatic changes are motivated by efforts to diminish the intense and painful emotions that were elicited. Behaviors such as running away, self-mutilation, suicide, aggression, substance abuse, binge eating and purging, fire setting and compulsive sexual behavior can be behavioral means of managing posttraumatic emotion. Robert, for example, discharges rageful emotions through aggressive behaviors. Again, as in the case of awareness and affect, the behavior has developed to facilitate survival. **The action or behavior of a traumatized child in a posttraumatic state is motivated by survival. From the child's point of view, this behavior is a matter of life or death.** The behavior of a traumatized child in this type of state, no matter how extreme, dangerous, or destructive, is his/her way of surviving. As we discuss in other sections, if we expect children to stop doing what they do in order to survive, we had better have something *effective* with which to replace it.

> . . . if we expect children to stop doing what they do in order to survive, we had better have something to replace it with.

Let's consider Denise and Robert (and their three A's) in the moment just before and the moment just after they were reminded of a traumatic event (Denise was reminded of the man who raped her; Robert was reminded of his stepfather, who abused him). As soon as Denise and Robert are presented with the stimulus (the reminder of a trauma), they go into an extreme, immediate response with clear changes in *awareness*, *affect*, and *action*. These changes are summarized in Table 3.1.

TABLE 3.1. Changes in Awareness, Affect, and Action after Denise and Robert Experienced a Stressor

Three A's	Denise before	Denise after	Robert before	Robert after
Awareness	Fully aware and engaged in surroundings of shopping mall. Experiencing herself as "a good friend" and "in control."	Disoriented, feeling as if she is back "in her bedroom" in her old house; believes she is about to be raped.	Fully aware and engaged in surroundings of basketball game with friends in schoolyard.	Awareness narrowed; he is thinking only of this peer and the demeaning comment; forgets to take into consideration school rules, that the peer can't hurt him, and that he doesn't want to get in trouble.
Affect	Feeling good, enjoying herself with friends.	Feeling terrified, then numb.	Feeling good, happy, enjoying basketball game.	Feeling rage.
Action	Shopping, laughing.	Running away, then curling up in ball in bathroom.	Shooting baskets, talking with friends.	Punching other child in face.

Phases of Emotional States

Children with traumatic stress can go from calm, engaged states to states of extreme emotion very quickly. If these children are assessed very carefully, four phases can be identified. These four phases are important because they give unique opportunities for intervention. For example, Robert was having a good time in the schoolyard and was calm and engaged in the basketball game. When another boy made a demeaning comment about him, Robert lunged at him, pounding his face. A moment-by-moment analysis of Robert's emotional states suggests four phases of regulation. The phases are illustrated in Figure 3.1 and described below.

The Regulating Emotional State

Traumatized children spend most of their time in regulating states of emotion. These states are characterized by calmness, continuity of experience, control over emotions and behavior, and engagement in the environment. During *regulating states* children are learning, playing, working, talking, and otherwise fully engaged in, and responsive to, their social environment. Robert was in a regulating emotional state prior to hearing the demeaning comment. Similarly, Denise was in this emotional state while at the mall before seeing a man who reminded her of her mother's abusive boyfriend. When a child is in a regulating emotional state, higher-order brain systems

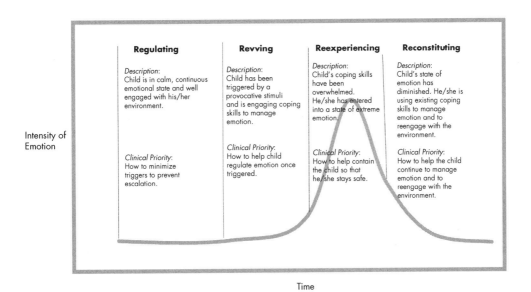

FIGURE 3.1. Phases of emotional state regulation.

are working. The amygdala has not yet begun its "hostile takeover of consciousness."

The Revving Emotional State

During a *revving state,* a child with traumatic stress has encountered a stimulus that consciously or unconsciously reminds him/her of a traumatic event. During this phase, children's coping skills are challenged as they attempt to utilize existing coping skills to calm and self-soothe. They may seek others whom they expect will help them to manage emotion. The three A's are beginning to change in a *revving* state. The child may begin to get disoriented as his/her focus of attention shifts (awareness), affects change, and actions escalate into defensive behaviors. When Denise was becoming anxious after seeing a man who reminded her of her mother's boyfriend, and as she began to experience memories of the assault, she was in a *revving* emotional state. This emotional state is a critical focus of intervention. Children send out signals of distress in this phase. If intervention does not happen, it is very easy for them to enter the *reexperiencing* emotional state. In a *revving* emotional state the hostile takeover is only beginning. Now it becomes a question of whether the child has the emotional "assets" to thwart this hostile takeover.

The Reexperiencing Emotional State

During *reexperiencing* emotional states, children are often flooded with feelings that remind them of their trauma, including flashbacks where the child actually perceives elements of the trauma in the present. The three A's have shifted dramatically. The child's awareness of, and engagement in, the environment change markedly. This state is survival-in-the-moment. As the child reexperiences the trauma, he/she becomes disoriented to time and place. The child may feel as if he/she is "back then" and "back there." The way the child feels about him/herself is very different in a *reexperiencing* phase, and at the extreme, he/she may become disoriented to his/her own identity (dissociative identity disorder). Similarly, the emotions and behaviors that emerge to manage these emotions also change dramatically. We saw how each of these changed for Denise and Robert in Table 3.1.

The amygdala's emergency response system is highly relevant here. The "hostile takeover of consciousness by emotion" is in full swing. Amygdala-mediated information processing prepares the body to fight, flee, or freeze in order to maximize the chance of survival. The speed of information processing necessary for survival sacrifices the details of the context. As contextual processing diminishes, the child becomes disoriented. When a child is in a *reexperiencing* emotional state, he/she experiences flashes and bits and pieces of highly threatening information.

The Reconstituting Emotional State

As described, *reexperiencing* states are marked by extreme emotion and behavior with changes in awareness or consciousness (attention, orientation, sense of self). Once these states are terminated via therapeutic means or otherwise, the child transitions back to the regulating emotional state. This transition requires a period of time wherein the child reorients to his/her surroundings and tries to calm and soothe him/herself. This reconstitution period is very important because the child is particularly vulnerable at this time to trauma triggers and at risk of reentering the *reexperiencing*, survival-in-the-moment state.

Why Phases Matter

Why does it matter whether we know which phase of state regulation a child is in? Because how you intervene is very different depending on the phase. Figure 3.1 summarizes our state-dependent intervention approach. Many of these ideas are detailed in Chapter 14.

- **During the regulating phase,** children are calm. They are fully aware (focus of attention and orientation) of the external world. It is in this regulating state, therefore, that they can be best engaged in treatment. Efforts are then devoted to improving their emotion regulation skills in case they get stressed (described in Chapter 14). As children practice these skills, their ability to cope with a traumatic reminder or stressor is maximized. Efforts are also devoted to surveying the environment (e.g., home, school) to look for sources of stress that can lead to dysregulation.

- **During the revving phase** (which can be very brief), children's coping skills are challenged. Interventions are acute, devoted to removing the immediate stimulus and working with their existing coping skills to help them manage their emotion and return to the baseline regulated state. Without immediate intervention, children may escalate to more difficult or even dangerous feelings and behaviors—as they enter a reexperiencing emotional state. During the course of a traumatized child's day, there may be many revving episodes. These episodes terminate due to the implementation of sufficient coping skills to regulate emotion and therefore to transition back to the regulating state, or they escalate into the reexperiencing state.

- **During the reexperiencing phase,** it is assumed that children are both disoriented and experiencing the environment as highly threatening. All efforts are devoted to ensuring that the environment is safe, that the children are reassured that it is safe, and that they are properly oriented to their surroundings. If they are engaging in physically dangerous behaviors, all efforts must be devoted to ensuring that others in their vicinity are safe and to immediately summon authorities who can ensure their safety.

- **During the reconstituting phase,** efforts are devoted to reorienting children and working with them to calm themselves, to self-soothe, to get back to the regulated emotional state. During this phase, children are still at risk of being easily triggered back to the reexperiencing emotional state.

The Moment-by-Moment Assessment

The proper assessment of emotional states requires the moment-by-moment understanding of how the elements of state regulation change across its phases.

The proper assessment of emotional states requires the moment-by-moment understanding of how the elements of state regulation change across its phases. Phase changes are defined by shifts in awareness (attention, orientation, sense of self), affect, and actions.

Children may not be aware of how they have experienced these changes or why. The clinician must note all occasions of emotional states and interview the child and observers, such as parents or teachers, to fully assess this area. A child's entry into a discrete emotional state during a clinical session is a particularly valuable opportunity for assessment, because the clinician can see what has precipitated the episode and how the child appears during it. Clinicians should note and assess each time a child enters such a state in order to construct a reasonable understanding of how a child's emotional life is put together.

We offer examples of questions to help assess the three A's in Table 3.2. These questions are just meant as examples. They should not all be asked. They should be woven into a clinical interview with the child that focuses on a particular episode of emotional state dysregulation and how awareness, affect, and action change when the child is stressed. The questions are intended to help the clinician understand the types of questions to ask but how the questions are asked and which questions to ask depend on the clinical situation. In order to illustrate how this questioning can be used in practice, we give an example of a clinical interview with Robert about the episode of dysregulation described in the vignette at the beginning of this chapter. The interview (and our commentary) is shown in Table 3.3.

Robert's Assessment

 The case of Robert provides a useful example of this type of assessment. In Table 3.3 the interview appears in the left column and our commentary on the right.

TABLE 3.2. Examples of Questions to Ask to Assess Awareness, Affect, and Action (the Three A's)

Awareness (consciousness)	Affect (emotion)	Action (behavior)
What were you noticing?	What were you feeling?	What did you do?
Did what you notice seem different? (*attention*)	Did your feelings change?	Did your behavior change?
Was it harder to pay attention to what was going on around you? (*attention*)	How strong were the feelings? Were they more intense, less intense, or about the same as before? Did you feel angrier?	Sometimes kids do things that aren't very safe when they feel the way you described, such as throwing things or hitting or running away. I'm wondering if you felt like doing any of these things. What did you do?
What do you remember about what happened?	Did you feel sadder? Did you feel more scared?	
Do you have trouble remembering what happened? (*attention*)	Did you have less of any of these feelings?	Did you yell or cry or feel like doing those things?
Did it feel like something that happened before was happening again? (*orientation*)	Sometimes feelings seem really big and strong or really far away and hardly there. Sometimes they're in the middle of those two extremes. What were your feelings like?	What did people around you do about what you were doing? Did people notice that you seemed different?
How long was this going on? Was it harder to keep track of time? (*orientation*) Where did this take place? Did you forget where you were? (*orientation*)	Was it harder to control any of these feelings? Did you have trouble feeling anything at all?	Did you feel like hurting yourself? Did you try? What did you do that made you feel better? What did other people do to make you feel better? What do you think would have helped?
Did it seem like you were back at the time or place of the bad thing that happened to you? (*orientation*) What did your body feel like? Did your body feel different? (*sense of self*)	Often people have more than one feeling at the same time. Did you have any other feelings? Tell me about those feelings.	Did you use drugs or alcohol? Sometimes kids do things sexually when they feel really upset, such as touching other kids in private places or saying sexual things. Do you ever feel like doing those things? Did you do anything like that?
Did it seem like you were younger (or older)? (*sense of self*) Did you feel like you were a different person? (*sense of self*)		What about eating? Tell me what your eating was like during that time. Did you eat something or get rid of what you ate?

TABLE 3.3. Robert's Assessment and Our Commentary

Interview	Commentary
CLINICIAN: So I understand you had some difficulty in school today.	Clinician asks open ended, nonthreatening question.
ROBERT: Yeah. John bothers me.	Clinician must first understand the context of the episode: "what happened," "what caused it," "how the child experienced it."
CLINICIAN: Is John the kid you hit?	
ROBERT: Yeah.	
CLINICIAN: Well, what happened?	
ROBERT: I hit him.	
CLINICIAN: What do you remember about hitting him?	It is important to assess memory during an episode.
ROBERT: He bugged me and I jumped him.	
CLINICIAN: Do you know why you jumped him?	Clinician assesses Robert's understanding and insight into his behavior (higher-order cognitive processing).
ROBERT: No.	
CLINICIAN: OK. Let's talk about exactly what happened. What were you doing before you jumped John?	It is very important to determine a moment-by-moment understanding of the episode. This involves trying to assess how the three A's change when the child was triggered.
ROBERT: I was playing basketball.	
CLINICIAN: How were you feeling while playing basketball?	Clinician assesses affect and action in regulated state.
ROBERT: Good. I love to play.	
CLINICIAN: Were you having a good game?	Clinician assesses awareness in regulated state.
ROBERT: Yeah. I scored a couple of baskets. Me and my friends were gonna win.	
CLINICIAN: Were you feeling upset about anything while you were playing?	Clinician assesses the triggering stimulus and its specific meaning for Robert.
ROBERT: No. It was going great. I was just thinking about scoring baskets and winning.	
CLINICIAN: Then what happened with John?	Clinician assesses the emotional meaning of the stimulus.
ROBERT: He was on the other team. He's bugged me before, saying he's going to beat me up. I wasn't thinking about that during the game. Under the basket, he elbowed me and I fell. I got up and looked at him. He called me a fairy and a loser. I just jumped him.	
CLINICIAN: What did you do when you jumped him?	Clinician assesses awareness, affect, and action in revving and then reexperiencing states.
ROBERT: I don't know, it happened so fast. I'm not sure I really remember.	Client describes level of awareness.
CLINICIAN: What was the next thing you remember after John called you a fairy and a loser.	
ROBERT: I don't really know. I guess I was on the ground on top of him, punching, and the monitors were pulling me off him.	Client describes awareness.
CLINICIAN: Do you remember jumping at him?	
ROBERT: Not really.	

(continued)

TABLE 3.3. *(continued)*

Interview	Commentary
CLINICIAN: OK, let's talk about just before you jumped him. John called you a fairy and a loser. What did you feel when he said that?	Clinician assesses awareness.
ROBERT: I dunno.	
CLINICIAN: Please think back with me to that time in the schoolyard. You were playing basketball and having a good game until John elbowed you under the net. You fall and then when you get up he calls you a fairy and a loser. Do you remember anything you felt then?	Clinician continues to try to assess awareness and affect in the revving or reexperiencing state. Robert's confusion is apparent.
ROBERT: Scared.	Robert begins to describe affect in the revving phase.
CLINICIAN: What scared you?	
ROBERT: The way he said it.	
CLINICIAN: What was it about the way he said it that scared you?	Clinician tries to get details of Robert's experience during the revving phase.
ROBERT: I felt small. Really small.	Robert begins to describe awareness in the revving phase—initial evidence that he is becoming disoriented.
CLINICIAN: Can you tell me more about feeling small?	
ROBERT: A little like I felt when my stepdad would say things to me, calling me a girl and that type of stuff.	
CLINICIAN: So when John said that to you, it reminded you of some things your stepfather had said to you?	
ROBERT: Yeah. Before he gave me a beating.	
CLINICIAN: Can you tell me more about how you felt after John said those things to you?	Clinician tries to get more detail about Robert's experience after he was triggered.
ROBERT: I guess I felt like I was going to explode, and the next thing I remember, they were pulling me off of him.	
CLINICIAN: Do you mean, you felt angry?	
ROBERT: Yeah. I could'a killed him.	Robert describes affect (anger) during reexperiencing phase.
CLINICIAN: What happened after they pulled you off him?	
ROBERT: I dunno. I remember trying to fight. Then I let them pull me off and I sat down on the grass with a monitor. I felt kinda limp and confused. I had a headache.	Client describes awareness during reexperiencing phase.
CLINICIAN: Confused?	Clinician assesses awareness, affect, and action during the reconstituting phase.
ROBERT: Yeah. For a minute it was like I forgot where I was. I felt spaced out. Then I felt calmer.	
CLINICIAN: What happened next?	
ROBERT: I went to see the principal and they put me in an ambulance to see you.	

Discussion of Robert's Assessment

There are a number of principles to consider in Robert's assessment. Robert is initially very vague and confused. It is important to be very specific about how he is thinking, feeling, and behaving before, during, and after the episode of dysregulation. The clinician conducts this questioning in a moment-by-moment way; first trying to understand Robert at baseline—whether he was in a regulating state prior to the episode—then to find out exactly what triggered him and to assess each of the elements of emotional state regulation change after he is triggered. Finally, the clinician tries to ascertain how the episode ended and Robert's experience during the reconstituting phase. The clinician should always be aware of the phases of emotional state regulation (the four R's) and its elements (the three A's) and to gather and organize information accordingly.

States and Traits

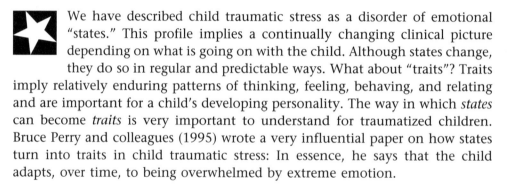 We have described child traumatic stress as a disorder of emotional "states." This profile implies a continually changing clinical picture depending on what is going on with the child. Although states change, they do so in regular and predictable ways. What about "traits"? Traits imply relatively enduring patterns of thinking, feeling, behaving, and relating and are important for a child's developing personality. The way in which *states* can become *traits* is very important to understand for traumatized children. Bruce Perry and colleagues (1995) wrote a very influential paper on how states turn into traits in child traumatic stress: In essence, he says that the child adapts, over time, to being overwhelmed by extreme emotion.

- What does it do to a child's sense of self-esteem and self-control to grow up continually having difficulty controlling affect, awareness, and actions? How much worse is the impact of this state regulation problem if the child has difficulty remembering what he or she said or did in a given emotional state?

- What does it do to a child's sense of identity to grow up having dramatically different feelings about him/herself in different emotional states? What does it do to a child's sense of identity, over time, when the sense of self is dependent on the state the child happens to be in?

- What does it do to a child's capacity to learn when he/she is regularly overwhelmed with emotion and consequential changes in attention and information processing?

- How does the experience of the trauma and the child's continuing state regulation problems affect the way he/she thinks about him/herself in relation to other people, to the world, and to the future?
- How do these changes in affect, awareness, and actions influence the child's relationships over time?

We do not have clear answers to all these questions. Nevertheless, traumatic stress in children is more than a disorder of extreme emotional states. It is also a disorder that includes a child's chronic adaptations to these states. Some of these chronic adaptations can be thought of as changes in the child's cognitions. Aaron Beck (Beck, Rush, Shaw, & Emery, 1979) introduced the cognitive triad of depression, which identifies changes in thinking about

- The self
- The world
- The future

Many of the chronic adaptations of traumatized children concern enduring changes in cognition about each of these three domains of the cognitive triad. Our intervention modules on cognitive processing (Chapter 15) and meaning making (Chapter 16) address these chronic adaptations to traumatic events.

What about PTSD?

 Why have we hardly mentioned posttraumatic stress disorder (PTSD) in this manual of trauma treatment? Although the diagnostic category of PTSD has its utility, we have two main concerns about it:

1. The DSM-IV definition of PTSD does not include a sufficient account of how symptoms and the social environment fit together.
2. The DSM-IV definition of PTSD does not include a sufficient account of the primary developmental psychopathology of trauma—the dysregulation of emotional states.

PTSD and the Social Environment

What social environment? We have described repeatedly that the core problem of traumatized children involves the "fit" between the social environment or system of care and the child's capacity to regulate emotional states. There is no mention of the social environment within the definition of PTSD. The DSM includes an Axis-IV dimension titled "Psychosocial and Environmental Prob-

The core problem of traumatized children involves the "fit" between the social environment or system of care and the child's capacity to regulate emotional states. There is no mention of the social environment within the definition of PTSD.

lems." Axis IV is helpful but very limited. Although it lists a variety of environmental problems (e.g., educational, occupational, housing), the list items are not integrated with psychopathological items. This list could only become clinically meaningful if there were a clear way to relate the identification of any of these problems with psychopathology and translate both into treatment planning. We have aimed our assessment approach at exactly this type of specificity.

PTSD and the Regulation of Emotional States

Our primary concern about the diagnosis of PTSD is that it obscures the main developmental pathology of traumatized children: the dysregulation of emotional states when confronted by a stressor.

Our primary concern about the diagnosis of PTSD is that it obscures the main developmental pathology of traumatized children: the dysregulation of emotional states when confronted by a stressor. The understanding of this critical developmental psychopathological process—and particularly how awareness, affect, and action can dramatically change when the child is confronted with a stressor—gives the clinician a very rich way of comprehending psychopathology in traumatized children. The way in which children chronically adapt to this state regulation problem is also helpful, as described in the previous section on how states become traits.

The utility of the diagnosis of PTSD is that it casts a "fishnet" that captures many children (and adults) who have this basic developmental problem related to the dysregulation of emotional states. In other words, using the symptom groupings of PTSD will identify many children who have problems regulating emotional states, as described in this chapter. The symptom groupings of PTSD are, however, a poor way of describing and organizing the symptoms and experiences that are most relevant for the psychopathology of trauma. The most important psychopathological process that must be identified is how awareness, affect, and action fluctuate when a child is confronted by a stressor and how a child adapts to these fluctuations. The symptom groups of PTSD may be a proxy for this process, but not a very good one.

Consider these symptom groupings of PTSD:

A. Trauma exposure
B. Reexperiencing (e.g., flashbacks, nightmares, intense distress at reminders)

C. Numbing or avoidance (reduced emotional responses, restricted activities related to fear)

D. Increased arousal (e.g., poor sleep, poor concentration, startle, hypervigilance)

These symptom groups are, to be sure, an important part of the trauma response and describe certain types of emotional states (e.g., anxious states, numb states, perhaps dissociative states). The problem is that this profile captures little about the variety of posttraumatic responses, particularly the key developmental psychopathological process described above.

Other symptom clusters have been proposed as alternate ways of classifying traumatic stress responses. These have been called, at various times, disorders of extreme stress, complex PTSD, or complex trauma. The DSM-IV includes these additional symptoms under the heading of the associated features of PTSD:

• Impaired affect modulation
• Self-destructive and impulsive behavior
• Dissociative symptoms
• Somatic complaints
• Feelings of ineffectiveness, shame, despair, or hopelessness
• Feeling permanently damaged
• Loss of previously sustained beliefs
• Hostility
• Social withdrawal
• Feeling constantly threatened
• Impaired relationships with others
• Change from the individual's previous personality characteristics.

Although these symptoms can be relevant to traumatized children, many of them can also be understood through the lens of development and particularly through understanding the dysregulation and adaptation of emotional states. Table 3.4 shows how the listing of symptoms in PTSD (and its associated features) can be classified according to the changes in the three A's (or chronic adaptations to these changes). The advantage of using an emotional state regulation model is that it captures the process by which symptoms fit together for a given individual.

Consider the case of Denise. We could say that she has PTSD (and its associated features). She has:

TABLE 3.4. PTSD Symptom Groupings and State Regulation

Dimension of state regulation	PTSD symptom or associated feature
Awareness (consciousness) • Sense of self • Attention • Orientation	Reexperiencing; dissociation; poor concentration; hypervigilance; feeling of detachment or estrangement
Affect (emotion)	Intense distress at reminders; reduced emotional responses; irritability or impaired affect modulation; somatic complaints; hostility; feeling constantly threatened
Action (behavior)	Aggression; self-destructive and impulsive behavior; restricted activities
Adaptation (chronic adaptation to state regulation problems)	Feelings of ineffectiveness, shame, despair, or hopelessness; feeling permanently damaged; a loss of previously sustained beliefs; sense of a foreshortened future

- Intense distress at traumatic reminders
- Flashbacks
- Reexperiencing of the trauma
- Restricted activities related to fear about the trauma
- Hypervigilance
- Irritability or impaired affect modulation
- Feelings of ineffectiveness, shame, despair, or hopelessness

We could also say that Denise transitions from regulating states, when confronted by reminders of sexual abuse from her mother's boyfriend, to reexperiencing states marked by changes in *awareness* (fragmented memory, disorientation in place and time, depersonalization), *affect* (terror, possibly numbness), and *action* (running away, curling up in a ball). One of her chronic adaptations to this response is feeling continually ashamed. These states are repeatedly provoked by stressors in her social environment, including exposure to domestic violence and lack of privacy.

Similarly for Robert, we could say that he has PTSD (and its associated features). He has:

- Intense distress at traumatic reminders
- Flashbacks
- Reexperiencing of the trauma
- Restricted activities related to fear about the trauma

- Hypervigilance
- Irritability or impaired affect modulation
- Aggression
- Self-destructive and impulsive behavior

We could also say that Robert transitions from regulating states, when confronted by reminders of physical abuse, to reexperiencing states marked by changes in *awareness* (fragmented memory, disorientation in place and time, loss of awareness of surroundings and context, hypervigilance), *affect* (rage), and *action* (aggression).

We believe that this latter way of describing Denise and Robert is truer to their experience and has much greater clinical utility.

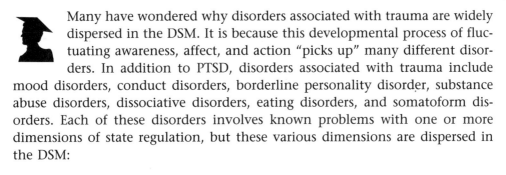

Many have wondered why disorders associated with trauma are widely dispersed in the DSM. It is because this developmental process of fluctuating awareness, affect, and action "picks up" many different disorders. In addition to PTSD, disorders associated with trauma include mood disorders, conduct disorders, borderline personality disorder, substance abuse disorders, dissociative disorders, eating disorders, and somatoform disorders. Each of these disorders involves known problems with one or more dimensions of state regulation, but these various dimensions are dispersed in the DSM:

- **Awareness (elements of attention, sense of self, orientation)**—attention deficit disorder, dissociative disorders, somatoform disorders, personality disorders
- **Affect**—mood disorders, personality disorders
- **Action**—conduct disorders, personality disorders, mood disorders, eating disorders, substance abuse disorders

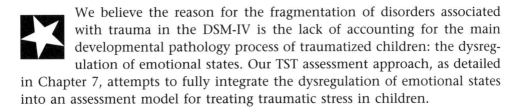

We believe the reason for the fragmentation of disorders associated with trauma in the DSM-IV is the lack of accounting for the main developmental pathology process of traumatized children: the dysregulation of emotional states. Our TST assessment approach, as detailed in Chapter 7, attempts to fully integrate the dysregulation of emotional states into an assessment model for treating traumatic stress in children.

In Chapter 2 we noted how in DSM-V posttraumatic stress disorder may be included as part of the new "stress-induced and fear circuitry disorders." This new conceptualization offers great hope for capturing the process of traumatic stress described in this chapter and in the previous chapter.

CHAPTER 4

The Social Environment and the System of Care

Traumatic Stress Responses Are Embedded in a Social Context

LEARNING OBJECTIVES

- To understand how the social environment influences the emergence of the child's affective and behavioral regulation capacities
- To understand how the social environment is affected by traumatic stress
- To understand how different levels of the social environment can be enlisted to support the child in the wake of traumatic events
- To appreciate cultural influences in the expression and treatment of trauma

---

As described in the earlier chapters of this book, our approach focuses on a "trauma system." To restate a central point, the trauma system consists of:

1. The traumatized child's difficulty in regulating emotional states.
2. The inability of the social environment and/or system of care to help the child effectively manage these emotional states.

Chapter 3 reviewed what it means to regulate emotional states; this chapter considers how these signals may be expressed across the social environment and system of care. In order to best address this topic, we briefly digress to discuss an experiment with young rats.

(What does an experiment with young rats have to do with the social context? Keep reading . . .)

We would like to acknowledge the invaluable contribution of Wanda Grant-Knight, PhD, in the development and writing of this chapter.

What Rats' Play Tells Us about Traumatized Children

Almost all young mammals play. As professionals concerned about the mental health of children, we know the importance of play and, in particular, when play stops or goes wrong. Some of the first treatments in the field of child mental health involved play. Why do human and nonhuman children play?

Jaak Panksepp, a neuroscientist at Eastern Michigan University, believes that play is a substrate of the emotion of joy and has important evolutionary value. Panksepp studies young rats at play and is able to quantify their play in their cages. In that environment, as in their natural habitats, these rat pups, like all other young mammals, *play.*

Panksepp (1998), in his influential book *Affective Neuroscience,* reports on his study of young rats at play. He observes these animals playing for several days and keeps track of the number of play initiations and episodes of rough-and-tumble play they display under normal conditions.

He then introduces a minimally threatening stimulus into this environment— a hair from a cat. He leaves the hair in the cage for only 24 hours and then removes it. What happens to play after the cat hair is introduced and then is removed?

It's important to realize that these experiments are conducted with lab rats (see Figure 4.1): They have never actually seen a cat. Figure 4.2 shows what happens. The vertical axis shows the amount of play. The horizontal axis shows "successive test days." As you can see, in both the figures the young rats are happily playing for 4 days. On the day the cat hair is introduced, play completely stops. Even after the cat hair is removed, play never returns to the level where it was before the time the hair was introduced.

What is at stake here? Why is the play behavior of rat pups relevant for our chapter on the social environment? What, exactly, does a lab rat experiment have to do with traumatized kids?

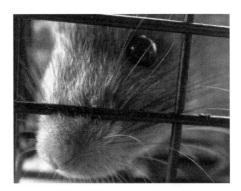

FIGURE 4.1. A young rat.

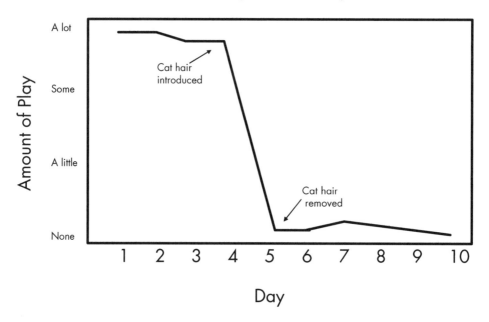

FIGURE 4.2. The introduction of cat hair stops play in lab rats. Adapted from Panksepp (1998).

We, of course, understand that our human social environments are immeasurably more complex and sophisticated than that of a young lab rat. It is worthwhile to consider, however, whether our need for safety and security is any more complex or sophisticated. What happens when a signal of danger is introduced, even briefly, into our social environment? It changes everything. Life is never the same again. This signal of danger for those unfortunate lab rats is a single hair from a cat. Think about the traumatized children with whom you work. Think about Denise or Robert and their survival circuits.

How does this information contribute to our treatment of traumatized children?

What if we told you that Denise's story continues like this?

Denise's friends repeated her name and asked if she was OK. Denise became aware of their presence but did not fully calm down until about an hour later. Denise reports frequent nightmares. She "always" feels ashamed. Denise lives with her mother and her mother's boyfriend (not the one who abused her) and three siblings in a two-bedroom apartment. The apartment would be considered substandard (if it were inspected). Of note, Denise does not have a bedroom door. Her older brother stares at her, in her doorway, while she is changing. She hears (and sometimes sees) violent fights between her mother and her mother's boyfriend. She has not slept for days because she is sure that something "awful" will happen to her or her mother if she goes to sleep. She cannot concentrate at school and will "fail" again this year.

What if we told you that Robert's story continues like this?

 Robert was sent by ambulance, in restraints, to an emergency room. He did not finally calm down until about an hour after his arrival, when he fell asleep. He was awakened by a loud argument in his room between his stepfather and a nurse. His stepfather was insisting to take Robert home because "this is a family matter. I know how to discipline my boy!" Hospital security was called when Robert's stepfather became agitated and threatening. They escorted him into another room. The psychiatrist then evaluated Robert, who reluctantly disclosed that he is beaten with a belt by his stepfather almost every night (and sometimes his fists). His mother tries to help, but she is "given a beating if she gets in his way." Robert reports that he is sure that he will either "be killed, kill someone, or kill himself" in the near future. He is in a regular, overcrowded class at school. He has been suspended 10 times over the past 6 months for "fighting" and is "about to be kicked out."

As Panksepp's experiment illustrates, if there is a single cat hair in the environment nothing else is important. Similarly, if there is a real threat in a child's social environment, it makes no sense to address anything else. The child cannot possibly attend to anything else if a signal in the environment represents threat. Denise and Robert cannot possibly recover if the "cat hair" in their environment is not clearly and effectively addressed in treatment.

In Denise's case the cat hair is:

1. Seeing her brother in the doorless doorway.
2. Seeing and hearing violent fights between her mother and her mother's boyfriend.
3. Seeing men at the mall.
4. Failing at school.

In Robert's case the cat hair is:

1. Undergoing beatings by his stepfather.
2. Seeing his stepfather beat his mother.
3. Hearing noise and threatening voices.

What is simply and tragically true for Denise and Robert, and more traumatized children than any caring adult would like to admit, is that they are living in cages full of cat hair—and sometimes they are living with the cat!

caring adult would like to admit, is that they are living in cages full of cat hair—and sometimes they are living with the cat!

In Chapter 2 we quoted Joseph LeDoux (1998) who said that "the amygdala leads a hostile takeover of consciousness by emotion." That statement is not entirely true: *Cat hair* (so to speak) leads the amygdala to lead this hostile takeover of consciousness by emotion. If we want to help traumatized kids, we must know where the cat hair is and help to remove it.

What Do We Mean by *Environment*?

Looking at Urie Bronfenbrenner's (1979) social–ecological model of human behavior is a helpful start to understand how the social environment can be addressed via interventions. As illustrated in Figure 4.3, this model describes

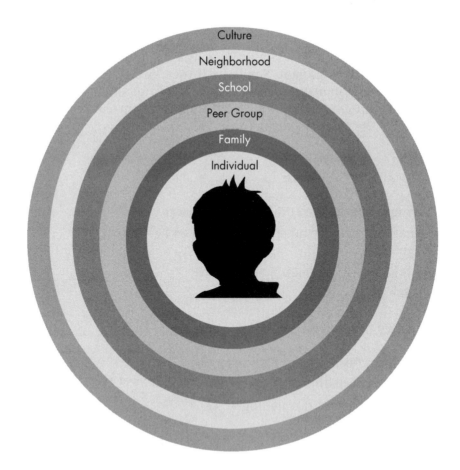

FIGURE 4.3. The social–ecological model.

nested levels representing the multiple layers of a child's social ecology. By including different levels of the social ecology, Bronfenbrenner points to important roles played by larger institutions and cultural contexts in shaping a child's development. Each level of the social ecology plays a key role in some aspect of healthy child development, and as such, may serve an important recovery function when the child is exposed to traumatic stress.

There are ongoing transactions between the levels of this social environment/social ecology that shape all aspects of development. To further understand the ways in which levels impact child development, a brief description of each is provided.

The individual level encompasses what the individual brings into any situation, including biology as well as the lessons and skills a child has learned up to a given point in time. Children's experiences determine the emotional, cognitive, and behavioral resources (i.e., strengths and weaknesses) they have available to them as they interact with the world around them and are critical in determining their responses to traumatic events. If children have developed good, adaptive resources, they will be fairly resilient in the face of trauma, but if they do not have good resources, they may experience poor adaptation to traumatic events and possibly even develop psychopathology as an outcome. This individual level of the social ecology "houses" the child's emotional regulation capacities.

According to Bronfenbrenner, the next level of the social ecology is the **microsystem** that includes the family environment and encompasses such factors as parenting styles, family dynamics, developmental histories, psychological resources of all family members (e.g., their strengths and weaknesses), financial stresses, and members' own experiences with, and reactions to, traumatic events. These factors not only influence the family's functioning but also the way in which parents help children learn to regulate their emotions and behavior. The way in which a family responds to a child's traumatic experiences will significantly impact the child's adaptation to them. Similarly, the child's distress level will affect how the family copes as well.

The next several rings of the diagram represent the **exosystem** that includes formal and informal social structures that influence children's immediate environment, such as school, peers, social networks, church, availability of organized support systems and services, and employment opportunities. The risk and resilience features of these elements of the environment have important implications for development. An exosystem that provides children with an appropriate educational placement, a safe community with opportunities for prosocial peer and support network interactions, and sustaining employment opportunities for caregivers will affect children's development very differently from one in which children are not being appropriately educated or supported in school, where neighborhood conditions are violent and residents feel unsafe, where peer and social support networks are engaged in unproductive or criminal activity, and where poverty, hopelessness, and despair abound. As one might imagine, these environments too will have very different implications for how children recover from traumatic events.

The outer level of the diagram, the **macrosystem**, encompasses the cultural beliefs and values that permeate societal functioning in general and family functioning in particular. In essence, this outer ring of culture surrounds and infuses every other level of children's worlds with meaning and influences the way the individual and family interact with the other levels of the social ecology. These cultural forces also shape how members understand what trauma is, what are appropriate and inappropriate reactions to it, and what interventions are needed to address it.

Bronfenbrenner's model provides us with a way to understand how children are influenced by, and influence, their world throughout development. These mutual influences, or transactions, highlight ways in which healthy development is either promoted or inhibited.

Bronfenbrenner's microsystem, exosystem, and macrosystem relate to the second part of the TST framework: the ability of children's social environment and/or system of care to help them regulate emotion.

In a way, these ecological levels outside the individual child represent his/her "rat cage." Signals of threat or danger at any of these levels will produce an important challenge to development, especially regarding emotional regulation. What purpose do these social–ecological levels serve? Ultimately, they insulate the individual from the inevitable bumps of life. The profiles of children with traumatic stress often show clear breakdowns in many of these levels. Think about Denise and Robert and count the number of breakdowns in their environments. WE ARE NOT SAYING THAT HUMANS LIVE IN RAT CAGES! We are saying that humans' behavior dramatically changes (like that of a lab rat) when a signal in the environment indicates danger.

> WE ARE NOT SAYING THAT HUMANS LIVE IN RAT CAGES! We are saying that humans' behavior dramatically changes (like that of a lab rat) when a signal in the environment indicates danger.

 As we described, a traumatic event does not just impact the individual; it impacts every aspect of the individual's social ecology. To truly understand the impact of trauma, you must appreciate its effect on each environmental system as well as how it impacts the transactions between systems. To effectively intervene, you must enlist those systems to collaboratively support the child. First, however, you must know where the cat hair *is*.

As we describe in Chapters 7 and 8, it is extremely important to identify the signals of danger for a traumatized child at each and every level of the social ecology and to construct intervention plans to get rid of them.

However, as we all know, there is no way to completely remove all evidence of the "cat hair" from the environment. We cannot remove all the dogs that bite, all pools where children might drown, all wars, all natural disasters, all abusers, or all those who might remind children of their abusers from the world. In Denise's case, for example, it is unlikely that a plan to remove all men from a shopping mall who might appear threatening to Denise would work. It would deviate from one of our main principles of TST, detailed in Chapter 6: "Align with reality." For this type of problem (i.e., one that cannot be changed) a much better solution would be to help Denise acquire the emotion regulation skills to cope with seeing a man who might appear threatening to her. On the other hand, such "cat hair removal strategies" as installing a bedroom door and effectively addressing domestic violence in the home can be extremely helpful.

As is examined in Chapters 7 and 8, our job is to do everything we can to work with any member of the social ecology who is willing to work with us to remove as much cat hair (danger) as possible, and to create plans to address the cat hair that we cannot remove. Sometimes this goal requires removing the child from the environment.

Trauma and the Social Environment

Following a trauma, the role of the social environment is to support the child's regulatory capacities so that he/she can effectively manage the ensuing emotions. Members of the child's social environment need to recreate a sense of stability, control, and order in this new, posttraumatic world.

> Following a trauma, the role of the social environment is to support the child's regulatory capacities so that he/she can effectively manage the ensuing emotions.

Trauma, however, has the potential to disrupt the very environmental systems on which the child has depended to manage and cope over the course of his/her development. Events such as traumatic injuries or physical and sexual abuse of the child, house fires, and murders in families primarily impact the individual and microsystem levels of the ecology and send ripples through the other levels. The impact of such events on the microsystem might include making caregivers or loved ones physically unavailable to children through separation or loss, or by rendering them emotionally unavailable because of their own reactions to traumatic events. Robert's mother, for example, was simply unable to help him due to fear for her own life.

Larger-scale traumas, such as terrorist activities and natural disasters, more directly impact multiple levels of children's social ecology. In these instances, extended families, religious and neighborhood organizations, and schools—all of which serve as potential protective factors for children coping with trauma— may be disrupted by trauma and therefore be less able to perform their important functions in the survival and healthy development of children. Similarly, cultural rituals and beliefs may be broken down by traumatic events in ways that alienate people from their histories. These disruptions then may exacerbate and complicate a child's experience of traumatic events and complicate his/her ability to cope.

Complex Problems Need Comprehensive Solutions

What do we know so far? Traumatic events can disrupt the functioning of children and families as well as different levels of the social ecology. The aftermath of trauma can overwhelm children's coping skills, decrease their ability to enact adaptive behaviors, and increase their display of maladaptive behaviors. Trauma also can impair the ability of environmental support systems to help children cope.

Clearly, interventions on the individual level are not sufficient to address all these issues. Comprehensive interventions are required to support children and improve the ability of the different levels of their social ecology to support them in the process of recovery from traumatic events. The TST model prescribes a way to identify which services need to be part of the intervention, how to apply them, and how to coordinate them in order to ensure maximal success in the child's, as well as the family's, recovery from trauma. As we have noted, many different systems are involved in the growth and development of children. That means that there are many different systems that can help children when traumatic events occur. That's the good news. The bad news is that unless these different systems work together in a coordinated fashion, they may be useless or—worse still— get in each other's way. TST recognizes the many different players (systems) in a child's life and works to weave them together so that everyone is working toward a common goal: fixing a broken system (more on what this means in Chapter 6).

> There are many different systems that can help children when traumatic events occur. That's the good news. The bad news is that unless these different systems work together in a coordinated fashion, they may be useless or—worse still— get in each other's way.

TST addresses children's multiple needs partly by coordinating different systems of care. This focus is consistent with the Child and Adolescent Service System

Program (CASSP) and System of Care (SOC) approaches, which recognize that many children with severe emotional disturbances do not receive appropriate services and that the services they do receive often have limited effectiveness because they are poorly coordinated. In short, they noticed that teachers aren't talking with doctors, who aren't talking with lawyers, who aren't talking with social service workers, who aren't talking with. . . . Everyone might mean well, but unless the different systems work *together*, services are unlikely to do much good. The interventions provided under CAASP and SOC follow core SOC principles that include the following:

1. Tailoring interventions to reflect the unique needs of children and to build upon their existing strengths.
2. Empowering family members to be full partners in the process of decision making and treatment planning for the child.
3. Delivering services in the child's home community to promote successful participation in the community.
4. Involving multiple relevant systems in the child's care and facilitating collaborative treatment planning and service coordination between them.
5. Appreciating and incorporating the cultural values of the family in a sensitive manner.
6. Providing services in the least restrictive manner possible.

TST builds on these principles, as you will see in Chapter 6.

What Systems of Care Are Part of TST?

Roughly speaking, we can divide a child's social ecology into two sections: what is already there, and what (sometimes) needs to be there. The first section ("Levels of the Social Ecology") describes naturally occurring connections that the child has in the world around him/her. Family, peers, school, and neighborhood are all part of "what is already there"—for better or for worse. Because these parts of a child's social ecology are, and always will be, important parts of his/her environment, they are considered essential parts of the treatment. Depending on the child's needs and the circumstances of the social ecology, interventions may not take place directly with, or in, those parts of the social ecology—but they are always considered when we think about the child's social environment. The next section ("Outside Agencies") describes "what (sometimes) needs to be there"—for example, agencies that might be enlisted to support a child after a traumatic event. These agencies, though not typically part of a child's social environment, often need to be included in the child's treatment to either support the child or to enhance the ability of those other levels of the child's social ecology—such as family—to help the child more effectively. As these agencies become involved in the child's care, they become other levels of the social ecology. One important note: Just because an outside agency is already involved in a child's life doesn't necessarily mean that it's helping! As we mentioned earlier, unless these agencies and the rest of the social ecology are working together toward a common goal, there could be a lot of "noise but no music." Under TST we figure out (1) who is involved, (2) who else needs to be involved, and (3) how we can get all those players working together toward the common goal. First, let's talk about who is involved.

Levels of the Social Ecology (or What Is Already There)

Family

The family is the child's first significant environment. It is through contact with caregivers in the family environment that children develop their first attachments, learns about the world around them, appreciate the impact of their behavior on the world around them, begin to regulate emotions, engage in social exchanges, and incorporate cultural values and beliefs. If all goes well, the family environment supports children's development in these areas and serves as the base from which they branch out into other levels of the social ecology, carrying these lessons with them.

Sometimes families have trouble supporting their children's development. Sometimes their own reactions to their child's trauma, their own problems (e.g., substance abuse), or even their own capacity to hurt their child gets in the way of supporting their child. No matter what a family system looks like, it's an important part of a child's social environment. Under TST, the goal of working with the family is to help family members function at their best so that they can help support the child's recovery. This goal can look pretty different depending on the family resources. At one sad end of the continuum, the goal is to keep the family from hurting the child. At the other end of the continuum, families become active helpers, healers, and essential treatment team members. No matter where a family falls on the continuum, however, TST assesses the impact of the family on the child and helps to build the family's strengths.

> No matter where a family falls on the continuum, however, TST assesses the impact of the family on the child and helps to build the family's strengths.

But first a reality check: Although families are almost always an essential part of a child's social environment, mental health clinicians and TST treatment teams are not. What? TST teams aren't essential?

Let's phrase that a different way. Families are a basic part of a child's life, but families have a choice about whether or not to make mental health clinicians or TST teams a part of that life. We're part of that outer layer of the social ecology—the "needs to be there" group of agencies. Fundamentally, a family needs to *want* TST to be a part of the child's social environment. So the first step in successfully working with a family is *building a treatment alliance*. We talk at length about this later in the manual but raise it here as a reminder: Without the treatment alliance, there is no treatment.

> Without the treatment alliance, there is no treatment.

Peers

Next to family members, peers are the primary socializing influences in children's lives. They can influence all aspects of children's belief systems. Peer influences can affect children's understandings of the way the world works (information that is as likely to be accurate as inaccurate), the importance they place on education, how they negotiate and problem-solve in social situations, how they initiate sexual contacts, what they identify as appropriate goals (e.g., from striving to attend an Ivy League school to joining a gang), and how they cope with difficult circumstances (e.g., experimenting with substance use, cutting, running away, attempting suicide).

As with family, peers can be positive supportive influences or part of the "cat hair" in the child's social environment. Think back to Denise, who was curled up in the bathroom stall. Her friends, who found her there and stayed with her until she was calm and oriented, were very positive, helpful members of her social environment. Depending on how Denise feels about it, they may be important players to bring into the TST team. Or, if not that, they may at least be important people for Denise to talk about and learn to call on when she's having trouble at school.

Now think back to Robert. Robert recently got into a fight after a peer made a demeaning comment. We don't know a lot about his other peers or his friends, but from what we *do* know right now some aspects of his peer environment are making it harder for him to manage at school. Depending on whether the TST team sees this as a priority problem (more on how to define priority problems later), they may decide that this level of the social ecology is an important place for intervention. Exactly how you intervene in the peer ecology will vary depending on multiple factors—maybe the school needs to be more involved in monitoring the playground, maybe Robert needs to be transferred to a more structured school—but the key is to identify this part of the social environment as an arena for change.

Schools

The school environment rivals the home environment as the setting in which children spend most of their time. Schools do a lot more than teach the three

R's: They provide opportunities for children to engage in social exchanges, vocational training, athletic activities, and, in some schools, religious instruction. Schools are also mandatory for children to attend! Put these factors together and it's easy to see that schools are (1) a really important part of every child's social ecology and (2) an essential element of intervention in the lives of traumatized children.

Unfortunately, the same factors that make schools so important in a child's life—being responsible for so many facets of children's development and for so many children—can make it difficult for teachers or school personnel to attend to specific trauma-related needs of individual children. Many teachers or administrators simply haven't had the opportunity to learn about how trauma affects kids and how they, as school personnel, can help. As mental health clinicians, we know that traumatic stress affects not only children's feelings and behavior but also their attention, processing of information, memory, and learning. What looks like dissociation to us might look like daydreaming or laziness to a teacher. Unless we help make these connections for teachers and school administrators, we're contributing to that age-old problem of the mental health clinician not talking to the teacher, and so on.

> What looks like dissociation to us might look like daydreaming or laziness to a teacher.

One aspect of working with the school as a part of the child's social environment is to help teachers understand the core and associated features of traumatic reactions, such as appreciating differences between inattention and dissociation, and between hyperactivity and the increased arousal and watchfulness (hypervigilance) that might characterize reactions to trauma. Teachers could also benefit from support that recognizes the difficulties that they face in handling the challenges presented by working with traumatized children in the context of their other professional responsibilities. Think about the times that a certain child in one-on-one therapy is just about all you can handle—now imagine doing that in a classroom of 30! Depending on the situation, teachers may need some additional support to become equipped to work with a traumatized child in a classroom, or the classroom itself may need to be changed. Specific ways this information might benefit children is by having their Individualized Education Program (IEP) address problems of traumatic stress, such as via behavioral modification plans, curriculum adaptations, coordinated counseling services, transportation, social skills training, help with activities of daily living (ADLs), attendance at summer school, use of in-school respite workers, supportive tutoring, and tracking and investigating the causes of school absences (such as trauma-related avoidance). Don't worry about how

> The important point to remember is that schools are a key part of a child's social environment, and if the school is a priority problem . . . then there are lots of ways to help it become a more supportive presence for the child.

to do all of this just now. The important point to remember is that schools are a key part of a child's social environment, and if the school is a priority problem (more on this later), then there are lots of ways to help it become a more supportive presence for the child.

One other important "plus" of working closely with school personnel: They see the kids all day long and in many different contexts. Teachers can be very important partners in identifying what leads to a child's experience of dysregulation and what helps him/her stay regulated.

Neighborhood

As discussed previously in reference to Panksepp's work, the environment in which a child lives can contain traumatic reminders that inhibit adaptive behavior and increase maladaptive behavior. On the neighborhood level, such traumatic reminders would include local violence and crime. Other associated features in the environment, such as vacant buildings, gang and drug activity, and limited advancement opportunities for community members, although not directly reminders of traumatic events, create the kind of environment in which traumatic events can continue to occur. Similarly, factors such as racism, disenfranchisement, and limited opportunities also imbue the environment with a sense of bleakness that can interact with traumatic reactions in a way that slows down recovery. Given that children spend considerable amounts of time in their neighborhoods (whether or not they have the luxury of being able to play outside or walk to school or stores without fear), their perceived level of safety in the environment is key to their ongoing adaptation to traumatic events.

> The environment in which a child lives can contain traumatic reminders that inhibit adaptive behavior and increase maladaptive behavior.

It might not be realistic to include, as part of a TST treatment plan, the directive "Replace all broken windows in eight-block area." But for starters, we can try to understand how the child feels about the neighborhood and what kinds of frank threats do exist there. This focus on neighborhoods is all part of the assessment of the social environment and, depending on the priority problems, may be important enough to really rally around. Chapter 12 on systems advocacy provides tools for chiseling away at big systemic problems that are fundamental contributors to a child's dysregulation.

Sometimes problems with neighborhoods need to be handled by helping other layers of the social ecology—the family, the individual child—think creatively about how best to protect the child from neighborhood threats. For some families, making a difference in their neighborhood may be something they choose to do when they reach the meaning-making section of treatment (see Chapter

16). Activities that demonstrate a sense of commitment to, and pride in, neighborhoods might emerge, such as establishing neighborhood watches or making links with local police agencies to advocate for better surveillance and protection for community residents.

It's also important to keep in mind that many neighborhoods, even if they have some problems, have some really great strengths—and in TST one of the fundamental principles is to "build from strength." Just as important as your assessment of the traumatic stressors in the neighborhood is an assessment of the strengths. Are there neighborhood recreational centers, churches, "watch blocks," or even crossing guards whom the child knows and trusts? Are their neighbors whom the child knows and can trust? Factor these into discussions of who, in the social environment, can help create a sense of safety in the child's daily environment.

Outside Agencies (or What Sometimes Needs to Be There)

Child Protective Services and Foster Care

Social service agencies are often involved in the lives of traumatized children. If a child's trauma results from abuse or neglect, these agencies may already be involved when we TST clinicians come on the scene. If a child discloses some form of ongoing abuse to us for the first time, we may be required to bring an agency onto the scene. Either way, if child protective services is involved with a child, then we need to be involved with the child protective services.

The overarching goal of child protective services and TST is, in theory, the same: protect the child. But underneath that shared goal can be a lot of different opinions about how best to provide that protection and different assessments of what is urgent or important to do for any given child. Again, if the systems aren't working toward a common goal, there can be a lot of wasted energy—and a lot of wasted time in a child's life.

As with just about every other system we've discussed, child protective services fall along a continuum. Sometimes, at the sad and ugly end of things, we need to do battle with child protective services to get them on board with taking the necessary steps to protect and help a child. This is not to suggest that anyone goes into a child protection job with the intention to do harm to a child—but in the midst of dwindling resources, overburdened caseloads, and seemingly unfixable problems, people sometimes turn their faces away. If this is the case, TST clinicians need to use advocacy skills (see Chapter 12) to bring those faces back to the problem at hand and create a safer environment for the child. Happily, on the other end of the continuum are child protection workers who are willing to go the extra mile to get a child what he/she needs. In these cases TST clinicians have a receptive audience eager to learn more about the effects of trauma and trauma-related symptoms (or the caseworker may already know), and are willing to develop treatment plans in lockstep with the agency and worker.

Ongoing contact with caseworkers and supervisors after a case has been supported is important because service plans can be developed that are based on a comprehensive understanding of the elements needed to provide adequate support for the child, facilitate recovery, and ensure appropriate delivery and coordination of these services.

Legal/Court Systems

Occasionally children's traumatic experiences lead to involvement with legal or court systems; for instance, as a result of (1) a child's behavioral dysregulation, which lands him/her in juvenile court; (2) an investigation of a child's abuse for the purpose of the offender's prosecution; or (3) a refugee family's petition for political asylum claim. The legal process can often be drawn out and difficult for families. Under TST, the role of the court and legal system may be important to consider if (1) the problem being addressed is a traumatic trigger for the child (e.g., the threat of deportation to a country where the child witnessed war); (2) the legal process itself is a traumatic reminder (e.g., the child must testify about abuse); or (3) the child is being prosecuted for something he/she did in a traumatized state (e.g., he/she was dissociated at the time of a crime). Each of these scenarios presents a different reason for TST clinicians to get involved, and the involvement for each would take a different form. At the heart of any decision to become more closely involved with the legal system, however, is a fundamental question: Is the child's priority problem in some way related to the legal proceeding? If it is, then involvement as an advocate for the child or trauma educator for the courts may be essential. As with any layer of the social ecology, the legal service system may need bolstering and insight from a trauma-trained clinician to make it the most helpful, and least hurtful, for a child.

> As with any layer of the social ecology, the legal service system may need bolstering and insight from a trauma-trained clinician to make it the most helpful, and least hurtful, for a child.

Medical Care

In instances where children have experienced medical illness or injuries that require the involvement of medical professionals, connecting with health care providers and agencies is a very important aspect of their care. Issues of how a physical illness (e.g., an asthma attack) or a physical injury (e.g., a surgical scar or amputated limb) can serve as a traumatic reminder, and the implications of this reality in relation to the child's and family's adjustment to the condition and their compliance with medical interventions needs to be sensitively navigated in order to best help. Similarly, helping medical professionals understand the interactions between traumatic reactions and grief (as might be experienced in response to a considerable change in a child's level of function as a result of trauma) could impact the way they convey information about a child's condition to the child and family.

Cultural and Religious Agencies

Many children and families have spiritual and cultural connections that help to define how they see themselves. Given the important role that these systems can play in a child's and family's recovery from traumatic events, it is important to attend to ways that these levels of the social ecology can be included in the child's treatment.

What comfort do family members derive from their religion or culture? How does that religion or culture view the healing process? In investigating this area, you may find common points of view in the approaches to supporting people in the wake of trauma. These common views can be drawn upon to provide consistency in care provided to families.

Mental Health Centers/Community Agencies

And, yes, mental health agencies can be a part of a child's social environment. We're not around as early or as much as parents, we don't see kids as much as schools do, and we don't hold the power that child protective services agencies do. But don't underestimate the role we can play in a child's life! For the TST team, the goal is not to *become* the child's social environment but to set in motion a cascade of changes through those other layers of the social environment—all the way down to the child him/herself and his/her regulatory skills—so that we can step out of the scene entirely. We want to stick around long enough to be a catalyst for really positive change and then leave once we're confident that change is around to stay.

> For the TST team, the goal is not to *become* the child's social environment but to set in motion a cascade of changes through those other layers of the social environment—so that we can step out of the scene entirely.

You may not be the first mental health agency worker to be involved in a child's life. Before assuming you are walking into a social ecology that just can't *wait* for your involvement, remember to assess past mental health agency involvement—and present!—in the same way that you would any other level of the social ecology. Has the family been involved with other mental health systems? What was their experience? Did family members feel heard? Are they feeling heard by the TST team? One of the very important principles to be discussed in Chapter 6 is to insist on accountability—particularly your own. Examining your role in the child's social environment is a first step toward achieving this accountability.

What Is the TST Approach to Coordinating Services?

We have identified the levels of the social ecology and outside agencies that may be involved in a child's care and talked about why they are each so important in helping a child recover from traumatic experiences. Now that you know all this information, how do you put it together in a way that will really meet the child's and family's needs? As you might imagine, the process of coordinating services becomes increasingly complex as the number of services, and agencies providing them, increases. Once you start inviting the neighborhood basketball team into your office, things really get busy.

Just because we listed a lot of different agencies and groups doesn't mean that they all need to be, or should be, intimately involved in treatment—more is not always better. Certainly we want to *assess* each of those layers of the ecology and think about the strengths or weaknesses and dangers of each layer. But in terms of who is actually involved in the treatment, a careful decision needs to be made in coordination with the family. Essentially, we want to involve the players or agencies most likely to influence the priority problems that have been identified for treatment. Other people or agencies may come into play later—but we can't do it all at once, so we put scarce resources where they'll work (yes, that's another treatment principle) and pick the team that makes the most sense for the problem at hand.

Once these steps have been taken, the TST provider plays several key roles in ensuring that all goes off without a hitch. First, the TST provider serves as the "single point of contact" for the family. That means that the TST provider is the person with the primary responsibility for working with the family to ensure that the child and family are active participants in the treatment planning and development process. Second, the TST therapist sets the tone of the collaboration between the other levels of the social ecology and how they interact with the family and with each other. Thus the tasks of the TST provider are many. Through successful balancing of these many tasks, the TST therapist helps to guarantee that the services provided to children and families are integrated, rather than fragmented, and that all effort is focused on a common goal.

The services administered as part of TST care build upon a foundation of strengths in the child, family, and service systems. TST provides a framework for bringing together the layers of the social ecology in a way that makes available the best help and protection possible for a traumatized child.

CHAPTER 5

Signals of Care

*The Importance of Caring Relationships
for Traumatized Children*

LEARNING OBJECTIVES

- To help clinicians understand the importance of the therapeutic relationship in TST

- To help clinicians gather critical information based on the therapeutic relationship

---

- To identify and avoid potential barriers that may prohibit a therapeutic relationship
  from forming

Relationships are the matrix upon which everything happens in TST. It is easy to get lost in our special lingo and procedures, but the bottom line is that everything stands or falls on the quality of relationships. It is usually some type of relationship problem that initially brings the traumatized child to the professional for care, and it is the quality of the relationship that the professional forms with the child (and family) that offers the only hope for bringing them back (to recovery). The therapeutic relationship exerts its effect in very specific ways; psychotherapy, from whichever theoretical perspective, works only if very specific things are put in place regarding the specific role of relationships in helping the child recover. **The therapeutic relationship is the necessary condition for all effective treatment**. A mental health professional will therefore either conduct their work knowledgeable or ignorant of this simple fact.

Why are relationships especially important for effective treatment of traumatized children? Where do relationships fit within the TST framework?

The Primacy of Relationships

 We always go back to first principles. We think of the trauma system: emotional regulation in its social context. Relationships stand on the cusp of the trauma system. They are the mediator between the child's emotional regulation capacities and the capacities of the social environment to help the child regulate emotion. How does this work?

As we described in Chapter 3, the regulation of emotional states grows out of the quality of interpersonal relationships. In very early development regulatory tasks are not seen as capacities of the individual infant but as transactions between infant and caregiver. The caregiver's response to the infant's distress is all about regulating that distress. Over time, as the infant increasingly develops the capacity to regulate his/her own distress, these developments are constantly refined by ongoing transactions with caregivers.

The infant's job, as previously noted, is to attain control over the switches between emotional states so that a more desired state is maintained for longer periods of time and across different situations. The parent's role is to help the infant transition from less desired states to more desired states. If these ongoing transactions between the child and parent are distressed or neglectful, there may be critical effects on the brain systems involved in the development of emotional and behavioral control. Because these are the systems that must be prepared to help the child cope with threat throughout life, damage to them creates a developmental cascade of dysregulation.

Signals of Care within Systems of Care

 These ideas, based largely on attachment theory, show why the quality of relationships sits right on the cusp of the two components of our trauma system: emotional regulation and the social environment. In essence, the quality of these relationships can be described as signals of care within systems of care.

> The quality of relationships sits right on the cusp of the two components of our trauma system: emotional regulation and the social environment.

The quality of the child's earliest relationships sets the stage for the child's ability to regulate emotion in the face of threat throughout his or her life. In addition, the quality of these earliest relationships creates memories of relationships that are only available implicitly (through the "low road" of emotional processing described in Chapter 2) instead of through conscious declarative memory processes (the "high road" of emotional processing described in Chapter 2). In this way, the child (or adult) responds to interpersonal signals without knowing why (because he/she does not consciously have access to these memories). Accordingly, subtle interpersonal signals (e.g., a harsh look, a detached tone of voice) can lead to dysregulation in a given moment without the child knowing to what he/she is responding or why.

These signals, both subtle and not so subtle, are often the "cat hair" (described in Chapter 4) and can be ubiquitous in the social environment. Other types of interpersonal signals, also both subtle and not so subtle, can remedy the emotional dysregulation precipitated by the provocative interpersonal signals. These "signals of care" usually communicate warmth, empathy, and positive regard. If these signals of care form a "critical mass" within a level of the child's social environment, the child will feel "cared for" and will be much less likely to have an episode of dysregulation in a given moment, regardless of the nature of a given signal on a given occasion.

The systems of care (described in Chapter 4) must be built on top of this critical mass of signals of care from people within the systems. If there is no such critical mass of signals of care, the child (or any human being) will feel apprehensive, uncomfortable, and unsafe, and he/she will be much more likely to have an episode of dysregulation when provoked. Interpersonal relationships both create the child's emotion regulation capacities and the environments in which the child is more or less likely to respond with emotional dysregulation when provoked. In this way, relationships are the cusp of the trauma system.

The therapeutic relationship is critical in this regard; it must create a social environment filled with signals of care. The therapeutic relationship can also offer a very important opportunity to understand how subtle interpersonal signals can lead to emotional dysregulation and reregulation when the reaction occurs in clinical session. Even if a child's primary trauma is not defined as interpersonal, these ideas are still relevant. In some of our research (Saxe et al., 2005), for example, we found that the single greatest predictor of the eventual development of traumatic stress in a child who is hospitalized for a burn is separation anxiety. In other words, a burned child in the hospital is much more likely to get traumatic stress if he/she feels anxious that there is no one there to help him/her. Any traumatized person will ask him/herself the same question, consciously or unconsciously: Who is here to help me through this? In this sense, *all* trauma is interpersonal.

The Therapeutic Relationship

How do we create therapeutic relationships saturated with signals of care with our child clients? The therapeutic relationship may be the first "healthy relationship" some traumatized children have ever had. For this reason, in forming a relationship with you, they may be embarking on an entirely new journey. They may expect that you will abandon them, hurt them, or abuse them in some way. And when you don't, it can be an extremely powerful and transformative experience. The signals of care you give go exactly counter to all the interpersonal signals of danger in the child's environment, present and past.

Traumatized children often have memories of relationships as riddled with conflict, strife, betrayal, violence, loss, and abandonment. There are a great many consequences to these memories. Perhaps at a most basic level these memories indicate to children that they are unloved and unlovable, uncared for

> Traumatized children often have memories of relationships as riddled with conflict, strife, betrayal, violence, loss, and abandonment.

and unworthy of care. These memories and expectations lead to lifelong difficulties with relationships and a poor sense of self. These difficulties, described in Chapter 3 as *chronic adaptations* to trauma, can be described as the avoidance of all relationships, the failure of self-protection within relationships, or patterns of strife, conflict, and violence within relationships.

 There are four reasons why the therapeutic relationship is critical in TST:

1. **The experience of feeling "cared for" is a necessary precondition of the child's and family's engagement in treatment.** If the child and family do not feel sufficiently cared for in treatment, nothing you do will really matter. Traumatized children and families vigilantly appraise whether the relationship that has been set up is safe enough. They vigilantly scan your words, face, and body for signals that suggest danger. They test you to see if you are safe enough. Setting up the therapeutic relationship to be safe and creating an environment filled with signals of care often work against the child's and family's entire history of interacting with people in authority. When we say "I will help you," the child and family members are often thinking, whether expressed verbally or not, "Sure, just like the 30 other therapists I have worked with who said the same thing."

It is important to understand that this type of reluctance to form a therapeutic relationship is self-protective and should be encouraged. When a traumatized person opens up to a new relationship, it leads to intense vulnerability. It is far healthier for a child or family member to enter a relationship with wariness and self-protection than to jump right in and get overwhelmed. Clinicians should support the self-protection by saying things such as, "I don't blame you for not wanting to do this, given what I understand you have been through. I don't expect you to trust me right away, nor do I think that would be a good thing. Hopefully, over time, I will earn your trust." In the next chapter on treatment principles we say the clinician should "insist on accountability, particularly your own." We will only be able to earn the family's trust and thereby facilitate a therapeutic relationship if we are vigilant about our own accountability. If we are able to do this, we will have earned the possibility of forming a therapeutic relationship. The first treatment module, Chapter 10, concerns engaging with the family in treatment and forming the treatment alliance. We call this process "ready–set–go" because we cannot really start treatment until there is a treatment alliance, and we cannot form a treatment alliance unless the family feels sufficiently cared for.

> The invitation to a safe and healthy relationship that the initiation of treatment signals is bound to suggest some danger. Therefore, it will be tested in many different ways. Clinicians should expect this testing and manage it by, again, understanding that this behavior is a form of self-protection (a good thing).

The invitation to a safe and healthy relationship that the initiation of treatment signals is bound to suggest some danger. Therefore, it will be tested in many different ways. Clinicians should expect this testing and manage it by, again, understanding that this behavior is a form of self-protection (a good thing).

2. **Information exchanged within the interpersonal relationship may offer a critical window into the child's emotion regulation problems within interpersonal relationships.** Interpersonal signals, no matter how subtle, can frequently be a stimulus that leads to emotional dysregulation in a child who has experienced interpersonal trauma (e.g., abuse, assault). It is sometimes hard to know exactly what leads to dysregulation in the life of an abused child. Directly observing how these signals can work within the therapeutic relationship opens the possibility of knowing how they work in all relationships and then doing something about them. This process is illustrated in the following case.

 Serena is a 7-year-old girl who was referred to treatment due to oppositional behavior both at home and at school. She was recently brought to the emergency room because she threatened to stab one of her teachers with a knife. Serena is currently in her fifth foster care placement. During the initial intake evaluation with Serena's foster mother, the therapist discovers that Serena had been severely beaten by her biological mother until the age of 4, at which point she was removed from the home. She had been transferred from foster home to foster home due to the fact that she was "difficult to handle" and would often initiate physical fights with other children in the home. During the first therapy session, the clinician introduces Serena to the toys in her office and tells her that they need to be cleaned up before the end of the session. Serena throws several toys onto the floor and yells at the therapist, "You clean up this mess!" When the therapist offers to help Serena clean up the mess that she made, Serena says, "If you don't clean this up right now, I'm going to smack you." The therapist calmly explains that the therapy room is a safe place where no one gets hurt and no one is allowed to hit anyone. She then says to Serena, "Even if you make a mess, I'm not going to hit you. Lots of kids worry that if they do something bad, they might get hurt, but that doesn't happen here." Serena pauses to look at the therapist and slowly starts to clean up the toys.

The therapist needs to be a keen observer of the subtle interpersonal transaction between him/herself and the child. This observation nets critically important information about how subtle interpersonal signals can lead to dysregulation outside the session. Serena threw the toys and yelled at the therapist after being given a subtle warning about cleaning up the toys. We do not know much about Serena's history, but it is not a great leap to imagine that she was given threats around cleanup or other chores. Serena may be thinking, consciously or unconsciously, "or else . . . what??" What will the therapist do if Serena does not clean up? This line of thinking may then lead to linkages with other episodes in which she was found to be "difficult to handle." In Chapter 3 reviewed the moment-by-moment assessment used to understand how a signal can lead to dysregulation on a given occasion. When we see this dysregulation occurring directly in front of us, caused by an interpersonal signal we just gave, we have a golden opportunity to understand the child.

Serena also illustrates other ideas on the therapeutic relationship described above. In this first session of treatment Serena was appraising whether the therapist was sufficiently safe or trustworthy. Serena needs to know that she will be cared for even if she is "difficult." The therapist's response to this difficulty can be judged according to whether she "passed the test" in the moment.

3. **The experience of feeling cared for can be transformative.** As noted, a strong therapeutic relationship can often counter the negative impact that previous neglectful or abusive relationships may have had on the child. Signals of care diminish a life history of signals of danger. The experience of feeling cared for is often so novel that it directly addresses such critical human needs as self-worth and value.

> Signals of care diminish a life history of signals of danger. The experience of feeling cared for is often so novel that it directly addresses such critical human needs as self-worth and value.

One of the most important lessons that a traumatized child can learn in therapy is that he or she is worthy of attention—the good kind of attention. In fact, many of the children we see have never had an adult pay more than a few minutes of attention to them, unless it was due to their misbehavior. Consequently, with the establishment of a strong therapeutic relationship, children eventually learn that they can get their needs met without having to "act out." We also see many children who have internalized their neglect and abuse experiences so that they come to believe that they deserve to be treated this way.

The therapeutic relationship can be reparative for these children, who now experience a relationship filled with positive interactions and mutual trust—life-enhancing moments they can take with them beyond the therapeutic experience. The therapeutic relationship can help them to form an internal model of what a "healthy" relationship looks like and feels like so that they can replicate it in the future. In this way the simple experience of being cared for can be transformative for a traumatized child.

4. **The emotions experienced by the clinician can have powerful benefits and costs.** The therapist's experience of contributing to the transformation of a traumatized child can be particularly sustaining, despite the difficulties of the work. On the other hand, working with children who have experienced sexual and physical assault and abuse can elicit very uncomfortable feelings in the therapist. Feelings such as hopelessness, withdrawal, anger, aggression, or sexual arousal are part of the human mix of working with traumatized children. It is very important to be aware of these feelings, to think about them, and to consider how they might impact the treatment. The psychodynamic literature refers to this process as *countertransference*. Whichever term is used, it is extremely important to be aware of these feelings so that they do not get enacted with the child. Enactment often occurs when our feelings make us withdraw or retaliate in even subtle ways. These behaviors then become perceived as signals of danger, and a very difficult trauma-related transaction ensues. (In Chapter 9 we discuss the importance of the treatment team for helping with this common problem, and in Chapter 6 we discuss one of our principles, "Take care of yourself and your team," as a means of minimizing the likelihood of enactment.)

> Feelings such as hopelessness, withdrawal, anger, aggression, or sexual arousal are part of the human mix of working with traumatized children.

It is always a good idea to think about how you are reacting to a particular child. Most likely, others are reacting to that child in a similar way. For example, is this a child who makes you feel irritable as soon as they enter the office? Is there a specific behavior that seems to be eliciting your reaction? This may be something that you can address with the child directly in therapy. Or is this a child who makes you feel extremely sad because he or she appears to be so lonely and withdrawn? The child may not be able to tell you verbally how he or she is feeling, but your own reactions can often tell you even more about the child's internal experience.

Final Thoughts on Signals of Care

Signals of care is the TST way of describing the importance and meaning of interpersonal relationships for the traumatized child. Many of the stimuli that will lead to emotional dysregulation in the traumatized child concern subtle interpersonal cues that signal danger for the child as only the child would know given his or her trauma history. It is therefore extremely important for the TST clinician to be keenly aware of how these signals may lead to dysregulation in the child's social environment and, particularly, within the therapeutic relationship. Although dysregulation within the therapeutic relationship can be very painful for all concerned, it may reveal aspects of the child's problems that were previously not apparent and therefore offers golden opportunities of intervention. As described, if the trauma system is riddled with signals of danger, the child's only hope is for enough signals of care to be developed. If this transformation can occur, it offers the child a dramatically increased chance at a future of health and happiness.

We now turn our attention to Part II of this book, Getting Started, to begin to understand how this trauma system can be so transformed.

PART II
Getting Started

CHAPTER 6

Ten Treatment Principles
The Principles That Guide TST

LEARNING OBJECTIVES

- To introduce the 10 treatment principles of TST

- To describe how these principles guide treatment

TST is guided by 10 treatment principles. These principles are based on some of the foundations described in the previous chapters, and their implementation is described in the chapters that follow. Table 6.1 shows the 10 principles. The rest of this chapter discusses them. Our treatment fidelity approach is anchored by these 10 principles (see the Appendix).

TABLE 6.1. Ten Treatment Principles

---

1. Fix a broken system.
2. Put safety first.
3. Create clear, focused plans that are based on facts.
4. Don't "go" before you are "ready."
5. Put scarce resources where they'll work.
6. Insist on accountability, particularly your own.
7. Align with reality.
8. Take care of yourself and your team.
9. Build from strength.
10. Leave a better system.

Principle One: Fix a Broken System

As we noted in Chapter 1, the trauma system is defined by

- A traumatized child who is not able to regulate emotional states.
- A social environment/system of care that is not sufficiently able to help the child regulate these emotional states.

What is different about TST is its relentless focus on fixing the trauma system. TST assembles interventions in a clear, integrated, and organized way in relation to this focus.

The trauma system is a broken system. TST is devoted to fixing this broken system. Many people have asked us how TST is different from other models of treatment. We always say: TST uses a lot of elements from other types of treatment. What is different about TST is its relentless focus on fixing the trauma system. TST assembles interventions in a clear, integrated, and organized way in relation to this focus. A corollary to Principle One is:

If it is not about the trauma system, it is not TST.

Treatment within TST always boils down to fixing a broken system. If a clinician or team cannot clearly see how a particular intervention helps a child regulate emotional states, helps the social environment and/or system of care to help the child regulate these states and, ultimately, improves the interaction between these two, then the intervention is not part of TST.

The nine other principles are all about what it takes to fix a broken system.

Principle Two: Put Safety First

All kinds of risks are involved when clinicians enter the trauma system. The child can be at risk to hurt him/herself or other people. The child can be at risk to be hurt by family members or others in the social environment. Sometimes even the clinician can be at risk for harm, particularly during the surviving and stabilizing phases of treatment (introduced in Chapter 8), but risk can occur during any of the phases. The surviving phase is, in fact, defined by this risk. The important part of Principle Two is that clinicians and teams must be vigilant about assessing risk and proactive about reorganizing treatment based on the results of this assessment. A clinician, prepared to focus a session on emotional regulation skills, for example, gets information from the child about suicidal ideation or about child abuse. Accordingly, all plans stop in order to address the child's safety. This principle is, of course, simply good clinical care, but in the messiness of treatment it can sometimes be missed. In other words, when a safety concern is raised, all treatment resources are devoted to addressing the safety concern. The treatment plan is not resumed until the safety concern is over.

Principle Three: Create Clear, Focused Plans That Are Based on Facts

TST is about focus. It requires the specific gathering of clinical evidence to decide about the child's level of emotional dysregulation and the level of instability in the child's environment and system of care. Chapters 7 and 8 describe the framework that must be used to assess and develop a treatment plan for a child and family within TST. This framework can only be used if facts are gathered methodically and clearly. A disorganized assessment will lead to an unfocused treatment plan, which will lead to ineffective treatment.

Once the team develops a clear notion about the treatment plan, it must be communicated to the family as part of the ready–set–go module (described in Chapter 10). This plan forms the foundation for building a treatment alliance and troubleshooting practical barriers to care. It also contributes to what we call *transparency*—an openness and honesty with ourselves and the families about the treatment. The construct of transparency is very important within TST. Unless everything is clear to all stakeholders (not the least of whom is the clinician and TST team members), treatment will not work.

> A disorganized assessment will lead to an unfocussed treatment plan, which will lead to ineffective treatment.

 Once the plan is set up, it is very important for the team to marshal a high degree of focus on the specific treatment goals. A TST clinician needs to be tenacious. The TST clinician must stick to the plan like a dog to a bone! But whereas the clinician's focus on the plan must not waver, the plan itself needs to be flexible in response to new information or new circumstances. TST requires the continual gathering of clinical evidence and changing of the plan based on new evidence. This point is part of Principle Two regarding changing the plan when there is new evidence of safety concerns, but it is relevant to any type of new evidence. The TST clinician and team are always proactive about gathering clinical evidence and redoing the plan based on new evidence. What remains constant is a dedication to focusing the plan on the most critical elements for fixing the trauma system.

The need to be proactive about redoing the plan is especially important when treatment is not working. When things are not going as planned, the team members must always be asking themselves: "What am I missing? What are we missing?"

If team members are not asking "What are we missing?" at least twice per meeting, then they are surely missing something!

If team members are not asking "What are we missing?" at least twice per meeting, then they are surely missing something!

Principle Four: Don't "Go" before You Are "Ready"!

As we explore in Chapter 10, before treatment can really begin, three components must be in place:

- There must be the beginnings of an alliance with the family about a specific treatment plan.
- There must be troubleshooting of practical barriers to treatment (e.g., transportation, child care, appointment times).
- There must be some psychoeducation regarding traumatic stress responses and what involvement with TST will entail.

It is a common mistake in almost every type of psychotherapy to dive into treatment without a clear treatment alliance with the family. In our consultations with many clinicians who are doing TST, the most common reason for treatment failure is that the ready–set–go format is not properly completed. Often when clinicians think they have a good alliance with a family, it is based on their idea that the family likes them and they like the family. Under TST, liking each other is not enough!

The treatment alliance is very specific. **It specifies that the family and the clinician agree to work on a problem that addresses something that the family is motivated to change, and that the family and the clinician agree that the TST treatment plan can help to change that problem.** In Chapter 10 we outline the ways in which the ready–set–go module can be completed and the parameters by which the team should know that the child and family are, indeed, ready. Of course, building a solid alliance takes time (particularly with families that do not easily trust strangers [you!]). Accordingly, we do not believe that a treatment alliance must be absolutely and completely in place before anything else is done. It is a question of how much alliance is enough to *go*.

We ask a lot of families in TST. For a family to be motivated to do what we ask them to do in TST, they must have clarity on two points:

- That the treatment plan addresses an important source of their pain.
- That the treatment plan can, to some degree, alleviate their pain.

If the family does not have clarity on these two points, why in the world would they want to work with us?

Principle Five: Put Scarce Resources Where They'll Work

TST addresses difficult and complex problems within the child, the social environment, and the system of care. Frequently these problems have existed for years before the TST team is put in place.

> Treatment will only work if the team is strategic about its resources.

Accordingly, it is presumptuous to even suggest that a treatment can change everything. Even if a treatment team were given endless resources, they still wouldn't be able to change *everything*. And nobody has endless resources. In reality, mental health resources are very limited. So how can we begin to help?

We have suggested a series of intervention modalities that we believe can help (e.g., home-based care, emotional regulation skills training, psychopharmacology, advocacy) and put them into a framework where they can fit together and strengthen each other. We believe that this is a great advance from previous interventions for child traumatic stress—**but this framework is still not sufficient**. We can't, and shouldn't, give every service to every person. We need to be strategic about the way we use our resources.

Mental health interventions are expensive. Mental health clinics and agencies struggle to make ends meet. Given the limited (scarce) resources contained within a clinic or agency and placed on a TST team, these resources must be allocated with a high degree of strategy. Milton Erickson, the founder of strategic therapy, said that psychotherapy is like helping with a logjam. The question is finding the right log to kick. The TST clinician, like the good strategic therapist, is always searching for the right log to kick that will get the logs flowing down river. The TST clinician is also a good economist and knows that there are not unlimited resources that can be used to find and kick the right log. Therefore the TST clinician and team are always asking, "How can we get the best solution at the least cost (or the best flow for our kick)?"

As we describe in Chapter 9 regarding the treatment team, the team is the holder of these scarce resources and is entrusted to use them strategically and effectively. This principle is true in the context of a given child and family, for whom the team must make decisions about the use of its home-based, psychotherapy, psychopharmacology, and advocacy resources. It is also true at a macro level, where a team must decide, given its limited resources, how many children will be able to get the various service elements at a given time. These types of decisions are not easy but will set the stage for effective (and efficient) interventions.

Principle Six: Insist on Accountability, Particularly Your Own

Why should family members trust you? Family members may have been violated by those in authority and may have long histories of adversarial relationships with authorities such as teachers, social service workers, court officers, police, or previous mental health clinicians. Why should they trust you? You are usually of a different race, class, or ethnic group. If they do trust you on your first meeting, that may even signal a "red flag."

We discussed the issue of trust in detail in Chapter 5 on the therapeutic relationship. What is most important regarding the building of trust is accountability; doing what you say you will do. This point is very important. We all know that *action speaks louder than words*. When a clinician enters the therapeutic relationship with an individual who has been traumatized, frequently there is the unspoken scanning of the clinician for evidence that he/she will be "just like everyone else." A clinician's failure to keep his/her word, no matter how unavoidable the circumstances, is a sure sign, from the family members' perspective, that their fears are real.

The root of the word *accountability* is "count." Accountability is about the indispensable question that clinicians and families ask (to themselves) of each other: "Can I count on you?"

As clinicians, we must understand that accountability is extremely important and that our communication, via our behavior more than our words, is critical. When we fail, addressing our failure up front and with authenticity will help a great deal. We are building trust in people who have no implicit reason to trust us, and we are modeling something very important for the building of other positive relationships and for good parenting. Some of the ideas mentioned earlier about transparency and alliance building are very important for communicating to families the value of accountability. The root of the word *accountability* is "count." Accountability is about the indispensable question that clinicians and families ask (to themselves) of each other: "Can I count on you?"

The other part of insisting on accountability is insisting on the child's and family members' accountability, as well as others in the child's social environment and system of care (including professionals). An important reason for our development of the TST Treatment Planning Form (introduced in Chapter 8) is to elicit accountability from everyone who is involved in implementing the treatment plan, including family members. The Treatment Planning Form outlines the treatment plan and specifies who is responsible for what: it includes a space for signatures. The only way that TST clinicians can be in a position to insist on families' accountability is by being meticulous about our own.

This principle is extremely important because family members may never have had an experience in which expectations were communicated in such a clear way. What are these expectations? Family members are expected to fulfill their specified part in the treatment plan. This part may include activities that are very difficult to complete. However, if the ready–set–go part of treatment is properly instituted, family members will know what they have to do, why they have to do it, and how it can benefit them and their child. Additionally, they will have agreed to do the specified activity beforehand. These agreements can include such challenges as the following:

- Stopping the use of drugs and starting drug abuse treatment.
- Asking a partner to leave and completing a restraining order.
- Calling the police to help with a violent child or partner.
- Taking psychiatric medications regularly.
- Participating in a Department of Social Services investigation.
- Allowing a home-based team into the home.

Every session of TST includes a check-in period to ascertain what was agreed to during the previous session. When agreements are kept, family members are given a lot of credit. When agreements are not kept, the inaction is discussed explicitly, including going back to the original treatment agreement and evaluating whether family members will be able to keep that agreement. This discussion may include renegotiating the treatment plan, troubleshooting practical barriers again, reexamining the treatment plan in light of new information, or providing further psychoeducation. The important point is that agreements are attended to and accountability is expected. TST clinicians must be vigilant about this principle if their hard work creating a treatment plan and building an alliance is to pay off.

Principle Seven: Align with Reality

 Align with reality? What does this mean? Whose reality? Clinicians and families must work within the bounds of reality no matter how strong the pull is to enter a fiction of a simpler, happier world.

Without getting too far into philosophy, it is important to note that TST makes certain assumptions about reality in relation to TST. We discuss Principle Seven in more detail than the others because we believe it is extremely important and often missed.

- Decisions that reflect the practical realities (i.e., that align with reality) are more likely to succeed. A decision to place a child in a supportive classroom with 2:1 supervision and an emphasis on teaching Latin may be just what the child needs, but if that classroom doesn't exist—if it isn't real—then the plan will fail. Similarly, although it might be easier to believe the parent when she says "Oh, Jinny is lying about my hitting her!" we can't believe her just because it's easier. If we don't make our decisions based on what's real, we won't succeed.
- The high level of emotion contained within a trauma system can interfere with making decisions that conform to the practical realities. These mistakes can be made by everyone inside this system (including the TST clinician).
- The TST clinician has an important role to play in helping children and families take into account the practical realities of their situation and to build skills toward making reality-based decisions.
- The TST treatment plan is built within the bounds of practical realities and is a map of the best decisions possible—given reality.

In order to illustrate what we mean by "staying within the bounds of practical realities," we offer the following case illustration.

 Nicole, a 14-year-old girl, recently was discharged from a hospital after a serious suicide attempt. You see her for a first visit after the discharge. Just prior to the hospitalization she had disclosed to her mother that her mother's boyfriend had sexually abused her. The Department of Social Services investigation is ongoing, but her mother has said that this abuse is "impossible." The night before this visit Nicole and her mother had a big fight about the allegation. Nicole's mother called her a "liar"; Nicole called her mother a "bitch." Nicole then went to her bedroom and cut her arms. At this visit, Nicole and her mother are both agitated and angry. You raise the possibility of Nicole's going back to the hospital. Nicole becomes more upset, saying that she hated the hospital and could never stand to be "locked up again." She says that she learned her lesson and will never hurt herself again. She begs you not to send her to the hospital and says she will call you if she has new thoughts of hurting herself. Nicole's mother, in frustration and anger, states, "I don't care what you do with her." There are no other friends or relatives that can be identified to help.

Commentary

This case brings up a number of reality-based concerns. What decisions best reflect the practical realities of this clinical situation? Nicole's understanding of reality is that she has "learned her lesson" and does not need to go to the hospital. Furthermore, she "contracts for safety" by promising to call you. What is the practical reality?

This is an adolescent who was recently hospitalized following a serious suicide attempt in the wake of disclosure of sexual abuse. She impulsively cut her arms after a fight with her mother over the reality of the abuse. She is currently quite agitated, and her mother is not displaying evidence of being able to help minimize risk. There are no other members of the social environment who can be engaged to help. The clinician's appraisal of the reality of risk, based on this clinical data and knowledge of the literature on suicide risk, is that it is very high. Thus, aligning with reality, the clinician initiates another hospitalization—it is a prudent decision but what does it mean for the treatment alliance? It all depends on how this alliance was initially constructed. Presumably, with Nicole, this alliance would include working together to minimize the risk that she would hurt herself. According to Nicole's understanding of her current reality, she is not at risk. On the contrary, your understanding of the practical realities suggests very high risk. An important corollary of Principle Seven is:

> The alliance with the child and family is always constrained
> by the alliance with reality.

The TST clinician must always be asking him/herself about the practical realities of the clinical situation, despite huge pressures to ignore them (as illustrated in this case). The TST clinician must never deviate from this understanding. In this way, TST is a treatment model that is strongly grounded in reality.

 After Nicole is hospitalized, you have a session with her mother in which you review Nicole's suicide attempts and her allegation of abuse by the mother's boyfriend. Nicole's mother becomes angry at you for bringing this up. She says, "You're not going to believe *her*, are you?" You ask why she believes the abuse is "impossible." She says that she knows how to "read people" and she can tell that her boyfriend is not an abuser. She also says that Nicole "lies about everything." She has complied with the Department of Social Services (DSS) request that her boyfriend not come to her apartment, but she admits that she has met him elsewhere two or three times since this request was made. When asked about their relationship, she says he is "the perfect gentleman." When asked, she admits that he hit her "once or twice when he was using . . . but he's clean now." You raise the concern about what it means for Nicole that her mother believes the abuse is "impossible" even before the DSS investigation is completed. Her immediate response is, "I can't believe a word that kid says."

Commentary

 One of the main factors that interferes with good decision making within the trauma system (and elsewhere) is the difficulty in distinguishing a wish from reality. From the details presented, Nicole's mother so strongly wishes that her boyfriend has not abused her child that she is not even willing to consider the possibility that it might be true. This wish can be motivated by, among other factors, guilt for letting a dangerous man into her home or for her own urgency for companionship. Her decision to not consider the possibility that her daughter might be telling the truth is not prudent, because it raises the real risk that she will not protect her child from a man who might be dangerous, and it does not include the reality of what her blanket denial can mean for her daughter's mental health and for her future relationship with her daughter. The TST clinician aligns with reality by keeping these facts on the table. The function of aligning with reality is not unlike the psychoanalytic notions of the ego's main function as one of helping individuals understand reality in the face of their wishes, emotions, and impulses.

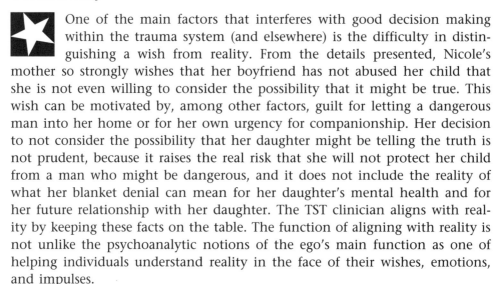 After meeting with Nicole's mother, you call the DSS worker to get information on the investigation. The DSS worker appears stressed and rushed and says that the case is being "screened out." She says that she tried to interview Nicole during her first hospitalization, but Nicole would not speak to her. Furthermore, staff at the unit confirmed that she does "lie" and that they had difficulty trusting her. The DSS worker also interviewed the mother, who, consistent with what she had told you, reported that her boyfriend could not possibly have abused Nicole and that Nicole was never alone with her boyfriend. The DSS worker also reported that the mother's boyfriend completely denied the abuse. When you bring up issues such as the boyfriend's past domestic violence and drug abuse, Mother's possible motivations for believing the abuse is "impossible," Nicole's possible reasons for not wanting to be interviewed on one occasion, and the need to integrate a full psychological evaluation in this decision, the DSS worker replies, "It's too late, the decision has already been made."

Commentary

None of us is immune to factors that can interfere with our ability to align with reality. The DSS worker likely has a large caseload and is managing a lot of pressure in discharging her cases. She may not have had the time to conduct a reasonable evaluation. Nevertheless, the decision making of this worker does not reflect the practical realities of the current situation. Accordingly, you protest this decision and, using advocacy skills (see Chapter 12), write a letter to the director of the DSS area office, outlining the realities.

Obviously, TST clinicians are only human and do not have the market cornered on access to reality. Furthermore, when the TST clinician enters the trauma system and is confronted with the many reality-bending emotions contained within this system, it can be difficult to "see" the practical reality of a given situation and to make good decisions. Accordingly, we have built certain "safeguards" into TST. These include team discussions and decision making (reviewed in Chapter 9), supervision, and the clarity of a structured treatment model. Further, the next principle addresses ways to manage emotion so that prudent decision making is enhanced.

> When the TST clinician enters the trauma system and is confronted with the many reality-bending emotions contained within this system, it can be difficult to "see" the practical reality of a given situation and to make prudent decisions.

Team decision-making processes that adhere to Principle Seven are peppered with such questions as "Is it practical?," "What is the reality?," and "Can it work?" Given the difficulty of discerning practical realities across language or culture, it is, of course, important to get consultation when indicated or, even better, to have diverse cultural groups represented on the team.

Principle Eight: Take Care of Yourself and Your Team

 When oxygen levels drop on an aircraft, there is always an announcement to parents to put on their *own* oxygen mask before their child's. Why? Isn't a parent's main concern during an emergency the safety of his/her child? The airlines have wisely discerned that for parents to most effectively attend to their child's safety, they must be strong enough to do it by ensuring that *they* have enough oxygen.

The trauma system is like an oxygen-poor environment in which it is easy to get weakened, sick, disoriented, and hurt. In order for clinicians to manage what they must do to *fix a broken system* (Principle One), they must take care of themselves and be sufficiently cared for by their team, agency, and organization (we review some of these ideas in Chapter 9). Trauma clinicians face some of the following challenges on a daily basis:

> The trauma system is like an oxygen-poor environment in which it is easy to get weakened, sick, disoriented, and hurt.

- Facing the cruelty of life by hearing stories of children assaulted, tortured, and murdered.
- Facing the randomness of life by hearing stories of children unexpectedly injured or ill.

- Trying to help children and families in great need, without a lot of resources to help.
- Experiencing the extreme emotions that trauma elicits and which are sometimes directed at the clinician.
- Making decisions that contribute to a parent losing custody of his/her child.
- Making decisions that contribute to the child staying in the home, when the clinician is unsure whether the home is really safe.
- Making decisions related to whether a child will hurt him/herself or someone else.

Such ubiquitous challenges can corrode the humanity in us if we are not careful. In particular, repeatedly bearing witness to the harm that one person can cause to another, particularly to a child, can lead to withdrawal, burnout, and personal life stress. Clinicians with their own histories of trauma can be especially vulnerable.

The emotional toll that this work takes can affect clinical decisions. It is hard to make good decisions when one is burned out or fed up. Similarly, emotions related to this work can lead to the clinician's withdrawing from the child or family or being overly punitive. Chapter 5 described ways in which this challenge can adversely affect clinicians and influence clinical decision making. Chapter 9 describes ways in which the team can be organized to take care of its members. All teams must be on top of how its members are responding emotionally and contribute to the effort of making this important work rewarding and fulfilling.

Principle Nine: Build from Strength

People are resilient. Our families are resilient. People have, over time, developed ways of coping with their situations that are adaptive, notwithstanding other ways of coping that may be highly maladaptive.

Given the degree of emotion and need expressed by some children and families, it is easy to see them as driven by pathology. However, the strengths and ways of coping that children and families have developed over time comprise powerful means of managing emotion and should be explicitly integrated into care. This notion of strength-based care is often given only lip service in mental health systems but is, truly, an effective approach to treatment. Traumatized children often have many social, intellectual, artistic, or athletic skills that can help them a great deal to manage their emotion.

It is not only individual strengths but community and cultural strengths that can be used. Cultures have developed rituals over the centuries to help their members manage adversity; these resources should never be ignored. This point is consistent with Principle Three, to *put scarce resources where they will work*. Given that mental health treatment resources are scarce and expensive, it is highly strategic to integrate individual, family, and cultural coping mechanisms into the treatment plan. Before these can be integrated, the clinician must, of course, know what they are. In Chapters 7 and 8 we discuss ways of assessing strengths and integrating them into the treatment plan.

> Cultures have developed rituals over the centuries to help its members manage adversity. These should never be ignored.

Building from strength is also a principle that is important for alliance building. Why would anyone want to ally with us about anything if they believe we only see their weaknesses? When children and families see that *we* see their strengths as well as their vulnerabilities, they are more apt to feel that we view them as people worthy of care and want to work with us toward maximizing this care.

Principle Ten: Leave a Better System

The operative word here is *leave*. Notwithstanding the considerably complex problems that TST is meant to address, it is not meant to be a long-term support for a child and family. There are significant downsides to long-term treatment, not the least of which is the development of dependence on the treatment team. A piece of wisdom transmitted across the ages is:

> If you give a man a fish, you feed him for a day.
>
> If you teach a man to fish, you feed him for a lifetime.

TST is about teaching people to fish. *Never do for a family what you believe they can do for themselves*. This does not mean that the TST clinician and team do not do things for children and families. Families are in great need, particularly early in treatment, and TST clinicians are correspondingly active. The guiding principle is that over time, children and families should be doing more and more for themselves. Our job is to (1) enter the trauma system, (2) assess the problem with focus, (3) construct a treatment plan that strategically allocates intervention resources, (4) conduct the plan mindful of the changes that need to be made for treatment to end, and (5) to leave children and families with the skills necessary to do enough of this work on their

> Never do for a family what you believe they can do for themselves.

own, and with services in place that maximize the chance of their sustaining lasting change.

Principle One, *fix a broken system*, is about intervening in the trauma system when:

- A traumatized child who is not able to regulate emotional states;
- A social environment/system of care that is not sufficiently able to help the child regulate these emotional states.

Principle Ten, *leave a better system*, involves imagining, from the start, what needs to be in place in the child's emotional regulation capacities and the capacities of the social environment/system of care in order for treatment to end.

 Will we leave a perfect system? None exists on earth. Our goal is to leave a system that is *good enough* to help the child manage emotion when he/she is faced with a reasonable range of stressors and reminders.

- *Leaving a better system* means giving the child the right emotion regulation skills (Chapter 14), cognitive processing skills (Chapter 15), and some semblance of meaning and perspective toward the traumatic event(s) (Chapter 16).
- *Leaving a better system* means giving parents the right skills to help their child manage emotion and to protect themselves from threat.
- *Leaving a better system* means giving parents the right skills to advocate for themselves and their children within the system of care.
- *Leaving a better system* means instituting processes within the system of care to help and protect the child after treatment ends. Such processes might include a more appropriate Individualized Education Program (IEP) or social service plan.

 Leaving a better system can have important public policy implications. Although TST is not explicitly about changing public policy, the TST clinical team comes face-to-face with public policy issues every day. The specific focus on advocacy, systems of care, and the mental health needs of traumatized children gives the TST team unprecedented information that can be useful for improving public policy. Similarly, it is our hope that using an intervention model that is comprehensive, focused, integrated, and testable will influence other treatment providers and public policymakers to build a better system for addressing the needs of traumatized children.

Assessment

How to Assess Child Traumatic Stress

LEARNING OBJECTIVES

- To learn the TST Assessment Grid
- To develop skills in assessing emotional regulation
- To develop skills in assessing the social environment

How do we assess traumatized children? As we have noted, our aim in assessing traumatized children is to ascertain their ability to regulate emotional states and the ability of their social environment and/or system of care to help them with this regulation. How do we do this? In order to best describe our ideas about assessment, we expand the discussion of Denise that began in Chapters 2 and 3 and also introduce the case of Lena. First, we restate the basic facts of Denise's case.

 Denise is a 16-year-old African American girl with a history of sexual abuse from her mother's boyfriend. While at a local mall with friends, she saw a man who frightened her. She later reported that this man reminded her of her mother's boyfriend. Denise remembers becoming extremely anxious and flooded with memories of sexual abuse. She does not remember walking away. Her friends found her 30 minutes later, curled up in a bathroom stall, unresponsive. Her friends repeated her name and asked if she was OK. Denise became aware of them but did not fully calm down until about an hour later. Denise reports frequent nightmares and "always" feels ashamed. She lives with her mother and her mother's boyfriend (not the one who abused her) and three siblings in a two-bedroom apartment. The apartment would be considered substandard (if it were inspected). Of note, Denise does not have a bedroom door. She hears (and sometimes sees) violent fights between her mother and her mother's boyfriend.

Lena is a 10-year-old girl of Albanian ethnicity from Kosovo. She lives in the United States with her uncle. Her uncle brought her to treatment because of a recent episode in which she was almost hit by a car after running into traffic. She was a passenger in the car with her uncle when she suddenly opened the door and ran into traffic. Her uncle immediately followed her and brought her back into the car. She reported no memory of this episode. Upon careful questioning, her uncle reported that he heard her scream just before she fled the car. He remembered that he had mentioned her father's name to his girlfriend in conversation just before this episode occurred. He mentioned that this type of episode (suddenly fleeing and then being confused) happens a few times a year and that she frequently gets very upset for no apparent reason. In Kosovo she witnessed extreme violence. She saw her father murdered and her mother and adolescent sister raped and murdered by members of the Serbian militia. She was rescued by her uncle when she was 6 years old, and they fled to the United States with the help of relief agencies. Lena gets very poor sleep and has frequent nightmares. She awakes screaming 3–5 nights per week. Lena is often worried that people will break into her apartment and kill her uncle. Lena's uncle appeared very supportive and helpful during the interview. He was very worried about Lena. Lena reported feeling loved and supported by her uncle. Although Lena's uncle reported his own traumatic stress symptoms, there was no evidence that these reduced his caregiving abilities.

Overview of Assessment and Intervention

How do we assess Denise and Lena? What type of information will help the most for planning and organizing treatment? TST Principle Three tells us to create *clear, focused plans that are based on facts*. Which facts? The facts that will help most are those that give information related to *fixing a broken system* (Principle One). What is a broken system? A broken system (or a trauma system) is comprised of:

1. A traumatized child with difficulty regulating emotional states, and
2. A social environment and/or system of care that is not able to help the child contain this dysregulation.

Assessment must proceed from this understanding about how traumatic stress works. Our assessment approach determines how emotion regulation and the social environment/system of care *fit together*. The notion of *goodness of fit* (Chess & Thomas, 1973) has a long and successful history in helping us understand mental health problems, and it informs the TST assessment approach. What is the fit between Denise and her social environment (e.g., family, peers, school)? How equipped is her social environment to help with her difficulty in regulating her emotional states? What is the fit between Lena's emotion regulation capacities and her uncle's capacity to help her?

The TST Assessment Grid

In order to graph this fit between the child and his/her social environment (in particular, the fit between the child's self-regulation capacities and the social environment/ system of care's readiness to assist with these capacities), we have constructed the TST Assessment Grid. This grid is shown in Figure 7.1. The clinician rates the child's emotion regulation and social–environmental stability on this grid. Based on this bidimensional assessment, the child is placed in one of five phases of treatment. Intervention is then constructed around the particular phase in which the child is assessed to fit. Each phase of treatment involves a different theme of TST. These five phases of treatment are described in detail in Chapter 8, where we review treatment planning. What is important to understand here is that the phase of treatment in which the child is placed depends on his/her capacity to regulate emotional states and the capacity of the social environment/system of care to help him/her with that regulation.

> The clinician rates the child's degree of emotion regulation and social–environmental stability. Based on this bidimensional assessment, the child is placed in one of five phases of treatment.

Treatment is considerably different for a child in Phase 1 (dysregulation of behavior/threatening social environment) than for a child in Phase 4 (dysregulation of emotion/stable social environment). Chapter 8 provides details on how these various phases differ. This chapter discusses how to use the TST Assessment Grid to determine treatment phase.

What is a *distressed social environment*? How is this descriptor defined? How does the clinician make such a determination? Similarly, what exactly is *emotional dysregulation*? How is it distinguished from behavioral dysregulation? Why are these distinctions important? Is Lena behaviorally dysregulated?

> What is a *distressed social environment*? How is this descriptor defined? How does the clinician make such a determination?

Is her social environment stable or distressed? How should we classify Denise's social environment? The rest of this chapter describes how to acquire the skills

		Social–Environmental Stability		
		Stable	Distressed	Threatening
Regulation of Emotion	Regulated	**Phase 5**	**Phase 4**	**Phase 3**
	Dysregulation of Emotion	**Phase 4**	**Phase 3**	**Phase 2**
	Dysregulation of Behavior	**Phase 3**	**Phase 2**	**Phase 1**

FIGURE 7.1. TST Assessment Grid.

to make these clinical determinations. We start with definitions of terms used to discuss the regulation of emotional states.

The Regulation of Emotional States

 In Chapter 3 we discussed the regulation of emotional states and its assessment. Many of the ideas about regulation described in this chapter are defined in Chapter 3. Recall that children with traumatic stress transition from a regulating emotional state to a revving, then a reexperiencing, and finally a reconstituting emotional state (the four R's). During these transitions, there are changes in awareness (or consciousness), in affect (or emotion), and in action (or behavior) (the three A's). Our TST Assessment Grid collapses the details of this moment-by-moment assessment process to essential features that must be used for treatment planning. These essential features are viewed along a continuum from *emotional regulation* to *emotional dysregulation* to *behavioral dysregulation*.

There are four key points to consider when assessing whether a child is experiencing emotion dysregulation, behavioral dysregulation, or neither. They are:

1. **Changes during the episode of dysregulation**. How is dysregulation distinguished from the experience of an emotion? As detailed in Chapter 3, dysregulation is identified by how the three A's change when the child is presented with a stressor. We define an episode of dysregulation as *changes in awareness, affect, and action when the child is presented with a stressor*. If these three changes do not occur, we do not consider a child to be dysregulated.

2. **Frequency of dysregulation**. How frequently does the dysregulation occur?

3. **Impact of dysregulation**. Does the dysregulation cause a problem? An episode of dysregulation affects some part of the child's functioning. There must be some evidence that the dysregulation episode caused a problem for the child at school, with family, in peer relationships, or internally (self). This problem can either be related to the dysregulation episode itself or to feelings or behaviors related to the anticipation of a dysregulation episode. For example, a child who does not go to school because he/she is afraid of having an episode of dysregulation would be considered to have a dysregulation problem.

4. **Safety during dysregulation**. Does the dysregulation jeopardize someone's safety? The answer to this question is how we differentiate emotion dysregulaton from behavioral dysregulation. When some children become dysregulated, they engage in potentially dangerous behaviors

such as aggressive, suicidal, self-mutilatory, or otherwise impulsive behaviors. When children engage in potentially dangerous behaviors during an episode, we say they are behaviorally dysregulated.

The application of these four constructs allows the clinician to determine whether a child is regulated, emotionally dysregulated, or behaviorally dysregulated and helps him/her complete the TST Assessment Grid.

The Emotionally Regulated Child

The child who is emotionally regulated has pretty good control over his/her emotional states and spends most of his/her time in a regulated emotional state. This child may become upset and express negative emotions such as anger, sadness, fear, shame, or guilt, but he/she also has a good ability to self-soothe and return to a state of calmness and engagement with the environment.

> The child who is emotionally regulated has pretty good control over his/her emotional states and spends most of his/her time in a regulated emotional state.

- The regulated child does not have changes in *all* three systems of awareness, affect, and actions when faced with a stressful provocation (he or she may, however, have changes in two of these elements when stressed).
- On almost no occasion will the regulated child act dangerously when stressed (e.g., engage in self-destructive, aggressive, substance-abusing, extreme eating, or sexual behavior).

The Emotionally Dysregulated Child

The child who is emotionally dysregulated has difficulty controlling his/her emotional states. Although this child may spend most of his/her time in a regulated emotional state, he/she expresses negative emotions such as anger, sadness, fear, shame, or guilt relatively often and has limited ability to self-soothe and reinstate calmness and engagement with the environment. The transitions from a regulated state occur with typical changes in awareness (or consciousness), affect (or emotion), and action (or behavior). The changes in behavior, however, do not involve risk (e.g., self-destructive, aggressive, substance abusing, extreme eating, or sexual behavior). Dyregulation takes place at least once a month, and the episodes cause problems at school, home, personal relationships, or for the child him/herself.

> The child who is emotionally dysregulated has difficulty controlling his/her emotional states . . . and has limited ability to self-soothe and reinstate calmness and engagement with the environment.

- The emotionally dysregulated child has changes in awareness, affect, and action when faced with a stressful provocation.

- The emotionally dysregulated child has an episode of dysregulation at least once monthly that interferes with functioning.

- On almost no occasion will the emotionally dysregulated child behave dangerously when stressed (e.g., engages in self-destructive, aggressive, substance-abusing, extreme eating, or sexual behavior).

- The emotionally dysregulated child has problems in functioning. There must be some evidence that the dysregulation episode caused a problem at school, with family or peer relationships, or for the child him/herself. This problem can either be related to the dysregulation episode itself or to feelings or behaviors related to the anticipation of a dysregulation episode.

 In essence, the dividing line between the emotionally regulated child and the emotionally dysregulated child concerns the experience of the three A's, the frequency of episodes and the impact of the dysregulation. If the child does not have each of the four features outlined above, he/she is considered regulated.

The Behaviorally Dysregulated Child

The child who is behaviorally dysregulated has difficulty controlling his/her emotional states, and this difficulty is expressed in potentially dangerous behaviors.

The child who is behaviorally dysregulated has difficulty controlling his/her emotional states, and this difficulty is expressed in potentially dangerous behaviors (e.g., self-destructive, aggressive, substance abusing, extreme eating, or sexual behavior). Although this child may spend most of his/her time in a regulated emotional state, he/she expresses negative emotions such as anger, sadness, fear, shame, or guilt often and has limited ability to self-soothe and return to a state of calmness and engagement with the environment. The transitions from a regulated state occur with typical changes in awareness, affect, and action. In contrast to the emotionally dysregulated child, the changes in action (behavior) are frequently extreme and involve risky behaviors, as noted.

- The behaviorally dysregulated child has changes in awareness, affect, and action when faced with a stressful provocation.

- The behaviorally dysregulated child has an episode of dysregulation at least once monthly that interferes with functioning.

- The behaviorally dysregulated child behaves dangerously when stressed (e.g., engages in self-destructive, aggressive, substance-abusing, extreme eating, or sexual behavior), and this dangerous behavior has occurred at least once within the last 3 months.

- The behaviorally dysregulated child has problems in functioning. There must be some evidence that the dysregulation episode caused a problem at school, with family or peer relationships, or for the child him/herself. This problem can either be related to the dysregulation episode itself or to feelings or behaviors related to the anticipation of a dysregulation episode.

 In essence, the dividing line between the emotionally dysregulated child and the behaviorally dysregulated child concerns whether the child engages in potentially dangerous behavior during a dysregulated emotional state.

Gray Zones

 Because the real world is hard to define and assess, there are multiple "gray zones"—types of problems that fall on the border. For example, there are a number of gray zones in the assessment of emotion regulation. We organize this discussion by the frequently asked questions that we have encountered during trainings.

1. **Is behavioral dysregulation always more extreme than emotion dysregulation?** We make no claims that behavioral dysregulation is more extreme from every possible frame of reference. We approach this problem, however, from the frame of reference of treatment planning. At least from this perspective, we consider behavioral dysregulation more extreme than emotion dysregulation. The distinction between emotional and behavioral dysregulation is defined by the tendency to discharge emotion into potentially dangerous behaviors. From our point of view the treatment approach is different when the clinician is working with a child who is engaging in potentially dangerous behaviors. We believe this position is well reflected in our TST Assessment Grid where the phase of intervention also depends on the degree of social–environmental stability. That is to say, the type and intensity of an intervention for a child who is engaging in risky behaviors differs in relation to how well the social environment/system of care is equipped to help manage the emotion or behavior. When risk of harm is involved, a level of containment must be built into the treatment that is not necessary when this risk is not present. There are other frames of reference in

> We make no claims that behavioral dysregulation is more extreme from every possible frame of reference. We approach this problem, however, from the frame of reference of treatment planning. At least from this perspective, we consider behavior dysregulation more extreme than emotion dysregulation.

which a given episode of emotion dysregulation may be regarded as more "extreme" than a given episode of behavioral dysregulation. A given episode, for example, may have a higher score on some defined psychophysiological parameter such as heart rate.

2. **Are all occasions of behavior change following a stressor considered behavioral dysregulation?** No. Many (all?) children express emotions through behavior. Play therapy, for example, is based on this construct. This is particularly the case for younger children, who have a limited ability to verbalize emotion and instead enact it. We define behavioral dysregulation as occurring when the child, confronted by a stressor, has changes in awareness, affect, and action, and the action (behavior) is potentially dangerous. These behaviors may include aggression, suicidality, self-mutilation, running away, substance abuse, or risky eating or sexual behaviors. There must be some risk associated with the behavior for it to be considered behavioral dysregulation.

3. **Are all occasions of risky behavior considered behavioral dysregulation?** No. Many children engage in risky behavior for reasons that have nothing to do with traumatic stress. Some risky behavior, however, is very much a part of traumatic stress. We consider risky behavior to be a part of traumatic stress when it occurs in the midst of an episode of dysregulation. There must be evidence that the behavior was precipitated by a stressor or traumatic reminder, and there must be evidence of changes in awareness, affect, *and* action. These two areas can be assessed in the moment-by-moment fashion described in Chapter 3.

What about Denise and Lena?

We have just reviewed operational definitions of different levels of dysregulation. What can these tell us about Denise and Lena?

Denise was confronted by a traumatic reminder (a man who looked like her mother's boyfriend), became extremely anxious and disoriented as she reexperienced the trauma, fled, and was found in a dissociated state in the bathroom. There is thus evidence of changes in awareness, affect, and action. There is also no evidence that she engaged in risky behavior during this event, although this is, of course, possible. If evidence emerges that these types of episodes occur at least monthly, we would say that she is emotionally dysregulated. If evidence emerges that on this or other occasions she engaged in potentially dangerous behavior, we would say that she is behaviorally dysregulated. We include Denise's TST Assessment Grid in Figure 7.2. As can be seen, Denise will receive treatment Phase 2, 3, or 4 (shaded), depending on the stability of her social environment/system of care. The assessment of this domain is described in the next section.

		Social–Environmental Stability		
		Stable	Distressed	Threatening
Regulation of Emotion	Regulated	**5**	**4**	**3**
	Dysregulation of Emotion	**4**	**3**	**2**
	Dysregulation of Behavior	**3**	**2**	**1**

FIGURE 7.2. Denise's TST Assessment Grid.

Lena runs out of her uncle's car while in traffic (not the first time) when reminded of her father's murder. During this episode there is also evidence of changes in the three A's:

1. Awareness: She does not remember the episode and was also confused
2. Affect: Her scream suggests a sudden change in emotion
3. Action: She runs out of the car.

Lena is *behaviorally* dysregulated because running into traffic is clearly dangerous. We include Lena's TST Assessment Grid in Figure 7.3. As can be seen, Lena will receive treatment Phase 1, 2, or 3 (shaded), depending on the stability of her social environment/ system of care.

The Stability of the Social Environment/ System of Care

In Chapter 4 we described what constitutes stability in the child's social environment and/or system of care. Recall that children with traumatic stress may live in environments riddled with stressors, and they may have family members or areas of the service system that are ill equipped to help them regulate emotion. Because the social environment (e.g., family, school, peer group, neighborhood) ordinarily has a core function of helping a child to contain emotions or behavior, it is assumed that a child's lack of ability to do so indicates diminished capacity of one or more levels of the

		Social–Environmental Stability		
		Stable	Distressed	Threatening
Regulation of Emotion	Regulated	5	4	3
	Dysregulation of Emotion	4	3	2
	Dysregulation of Behavior	3	2	1

FIGURE 7.3. Lena's TST Assessment Grid.

social environment to help the child. Similarly, this problem also implies an insufficiency in the system of care in helping the child contain emotions or behaviors. This insufficiency is a result of (1) the child' lack of access to the system of care, (2) the child's "falling through the cracks," or (3) an ineffectiveness in the services the child is currently receiving.

This problem also implies an insufficiency in the system of care in helping the child contain emotions or behaviors. This insufficiency is a result of (1) the child's lack of access to the system of care, (2) the child's "falling through the cracks," or (3) an ineffectiveness in the services the child is currently receiving.

The TST Assessment Grid evaluates the social environment/system of care along a continuum that ranges from a *stable* social environment/system of care to a *distressed* social environment/system of care, to a *threatening* social environment/system of care.

The constructs of *help* and *protect* are critical in defining the distinction between these three levels of stability.

- **Help:** Implies the capacity of the social environment or system of care to help the child manage emotion. This capacity is defined by the caregivers' (including professional caregivers) ability to be:
  - *Attuned* to the child's emotional needs.
  - *Able* to assist the child with these emotional needs; in the case of children with traumatic stress, assistance usually means helping them self-soothe when they are distressed and enhancing their developmental capacities to manage emotion.

- **Protect:** Implies the capacity of the social environment or system of care to protect the child from stressors that may lead to dysregulated emotional states. This capacity is defined by the caregivers' (including professional caregivers) ability to be
  - *Attuned* to the child's history of trauma and reactions to it, such that stimuli that remind the child of the trauma are identified.
  - *Able* to change the environment to diminish the stimuli.

The Stable Social Environment/System of Care

The child's social environment/system of care is considered stable when the child's family has the capacity to **help** him/her manage emotion and to **protect** him/her from stressors.

The child's social environment/system of care is considered stable when the child's family has the capacity to **help** him/her manage emotion and to **protect** him/her from stressors. Often, if the child's family is not able to help and protect, others in the social environment, such as extended family, friends, and neighbors, might serve this function for the child. Systems of care such as school, social services, or mental health systems are designed to support the child, his/her family, and extended social network in service of the child's optimal functioning (in the case of a child with traumatic stress, optimal functioning usually means the regulation of emotion, as defined above).

A stable social environment is defined by the following factors:

- The child's immediate caregivers are able to **help** him/her regulate emotion and to **protect** him/her from stressors.
- The child's extended family, peer group, or neighbors are able to support the child, such that any limitations of the immediate family in their ability to **help** the child regulate emotion or to **protect** him/her from traumatic reminders are mitigated.
- The child's system of care has been accessed and, if the child's immediate family or extended social network is unable to **help** the child regulate emotion or to **protect** him/her from traumatic reminders, services are in place that effectively provide these functions.

The Distressed Social Environment/System of Care

The child's social environment/system of care is considered distressed when the child's family has difficulty **helping** him/her manage emotion or **protecting** him/her from stressors. In addition, others in the social environment, such as extended family, friends, and neighbors, cannot adequately help and protect the child, and the system of care has not been accessed or services are not in place to adequately help the child regulate emotion or to protect him/her from stressors and traumatic reminders.

Examples of a distressed social environment include the following:

- Caregivers are incapacitated with mental illness or substance use and are limited in their ability to understand or help their child with emotion regulation or to protect him/her from stressors.
- Caregivers are incapacitated with physical illness and are physically limited in their ability to help their child with emotion regulation or to protect him/her from stressors.
- Caregivers are frequently absent, at work or otherwise, and are not sufficiently present to help their child with emotion regulation or to protect him/her from stressors.
- Caregivers have limited financial resources and are not able to care adequately for the child's physical needs (excluding homelessness and hunger).

Examples of a distressed system of care include the following:

- A school that does not provide a child with an adequate Individualized Educational Program (IEP), thus exposing the child to the possibility of school failure and ongoing frustration and assaults on self-esteem.
- A social service agency that is not able to adequately investigate or provide appropriate child protective services to the child.
- A mental health system that does not address the social context of the child's problems or provide sufficient services to adequately address these problems.
- A mental health system in which various levels of care (outpatient, inpatient, emergency, residential) are not easily accessible and are fragmented.
- A community that does not offer adequate social, developmental, or recreational services for children.

A distressed social environment/system of care displays all of the following:

1. The child's caregivers (usually legal guardians) are not able to adequately help him/her regulate emotion or to protect him/her from stressors, *and*
2. The child's extended family, peer group, or neighbors are unable to support the child, such that any limitations of the immediate caregivers in their ability to help the child regulate emotion or to protect him or her from stressors are mitigated, *and*
3. #1 and #2 are met and the child's system of care has not been accessed or services are not in place that effectively help the child regulate emotion or that protect him/her from stressors.

The Threatening Social Environment/System of Care

The child's social environment/system of care is considered threatening when the child's immediate caregivers have difficulty helping him/her manage emotion and protecting him/her from stressors and traumatic reminders and when there is a threat of harm to the child. Others in the social environment, such as extended family, friends, and neighbors, either cannot adequately help and protect the child from this threat or are causing this threat. The system of care either has not been accessed to protect the child, or (tragically) the system of care itself is threatening to the child.

Examples of threat from the social environment include the following:

- Ongoing physical or sexual abuse
- Ongoing threats of violence

- Ongoing domestic violence
- Ongoing community violence
- Ongoing child neglect
- Ongoing severe deprivation, including hunger and homelessness

Examples of threat from the system of care include the following:

- Violence or threats of violence at school for which the school does not intervene
- Boundary violation (including sexual) by a professional
- Lack of intervention from a social services agency following an investigation for child abuse when child abuse is, in fact, occurring (think of what this means for an abused child)
- Use of mechanical restraint in a mental health program with a child who has been physically or sexually abused

A threatening social environment/system of care displays all of the following:

1. The child's caregivers pose a threat of harm to the child, *and*
2. The child's extended family, peer group, or neighbors cannot adequately protect the child from this threat, *and*
3. The child's system of care either has not been accessed or has not adequately protected the child from this threat, *or*
4. There is a threat of harm to the child from a source outside the immediate caregivers (e.g., extended family, peer group, neighbors, professionals) that is not sufficiently mitigated by the involvement of others in the social environment or system of care.

Gray Zones

 As we discussed in the section on emotion regulation, our definitions of the three levels of stability in the social environment/system of care are meant to be as clear and discrete as possible. Nevertheless, clinical practice is rarely clear and discrete. Therefore there are a number of "gray zones" in the assessment that must be addressed. We organize this discussion by the frequently asked questions that we have encountered during trainings.

1. **If a threatening social environment involves risk of harm, doesn't this risk require referral to the state social services agency?** We work closely with our state social services agency and not infrequently engage their services in our roles as mandated reporters. However, in usual practice there is frequently some level of ongoing risk. Many of the cases we treat with a

"threatening" designation have already had a social services investigation, and a social services worker may consequentially be involved along with our services. We also frequently work with the "new" environment if an out-of-home placement is mandated. Sometimes our interventions offer the stability needed to preserve in-home placement.

2. **What if there are no traumatic reminders in the social environment but the family has problems helping the child regulate emotion. Is this situation considered unstable?** The distinction between a stable social environment and a distressed social environment concerns whether the social environment/system of care has problems helping the child regulate emotion *or* protecting the child from stressors or reminders. Frequently these two go together. If there are few stressors or traumatic reminders in the environment but the family and others are not attuned to the child's emotional states and have limited capacity to help the child regulate emotion, then the social environment/system of care would still be considered distressed. The ability to help the child regulate emotion is a critical task of parenting and indispensable for child development. Certainly parents who are not able to help their child regulate emotion may not be able to protect their child from future stressors that might arise.

> Certainly parents who are not able to help their child regulate emotion may not be able to protect their child from future stressors that might arise.

3. **If there are many reminders of the trauma in the child's home and parents are not able to change this fact, but the child is receiving good services and is in good psychotherapy, would this be considered a stable social environment?** No. It all depends on what is meant by *good*. We define good services, including psychotherapy, as that which can serve to mitigate the stressors and reminders in the social environment. If services for this child are not in the home working to diminish ongoing stressors or reminders or are not considering out-of-home placement if the aforementioned home-based services are not effective, we would not consider the services or psychotherapy as "good."

What about Denise and Lena?

We have just reviewed operational definitions of different levels of stability in the social environment/system of care. What can these definitions tell us about Denise's and Lena's circumstances?

Denise lives in an environment filled with traumatic reminders. She is exposed to ongoing domestic violence. She has no privacy in that she does not have a bedroom door. There is no evidence that her immediate family can help her manage emotion or protect her from traumatic reminders. There is evidence that her peer group is helpful to her in the regulation of emotion, but they have no influence on her ongoing exposure to domestic violence. There is no evidence from the case vignette

Social–Environmental Stability

		Stable	Distressed	Threatening
Regulation of Emotion	Regulated	5	4	3
	Dysregulation of Emotion	4	3	2
	Dysregulation of Behavior	3	2	1

FIGURE 7.4. Denise's TST Assessment Grid.

that the system of care has been accessed and that helpful services are in place. Accordingly, we would say that she lives in a threatening social environment/system of care. We include Denise's TST Assessment Grid in Figure 7.4. As can be seen, Phase 2 treatment will be appropriate for Denise, because her social environment is threatening.

In Chapter 8 we describe the Phase 2 treatment that Denise will receive.

 Lena lives with her uncle. There is a lot of evidence that he is attuned to her feelings and will work to help her regulate emotion and protect her from traumatic reminders. He feels terrible that his conversation led to her episode of behavioral dysregulation and will make sure that she is not present when he speaks of his brother (Lena's father) until she is better able to manage emotion. Although he himself has traumatic stress symptoms, there is no evidence that they negatively affect his caregiving. There is no evidence of other stressors in the social environment. Accordingly, we would say that she lives in a stable social environment/system of care. We include Lena's TST Assessment Grid in Figure 7.5. As can be seen, Phase 3 treatment is most appropriate for Lena, because her social environment is stable. In Chapter 7 we describe the Phase 3 treatment that Lena will receive.

The next chapter reviews how a TST assessment can be translated into treatment planning.

Social–Environmental Stability

		Stable	Distressed	Threatening
Regulation of Emotion	Regulated	5	4	3
	Dysregulation of Emotion	4	3	2
	Dysregulation of Behavior	3	2	1

FIGURE 7.5. Lena's TST Assessment Grid.

CHAPTER 8

Treatment Planning

How to Plan for Child Traumatic Stress Interventions

LEARNING OBJECTIVES

- To understand how to put together a TST treatment plan
- To learn how to identify priority problems to address in treatment
- To learn about the different treatment phases and modules within TST

How should treatment be planned and organized? We've done a lot of talking about the theory of our treatment. The last chapter offered ideas about doing assessment. This chapter focuses on how to **plan** treatment within the TST model. Finally, Chapters 10–16 describe how to *do* the treatment. This chapter picks up the discussion at the end of Chapter 7 by describing how to use the assessment you have done to inform how you plan and organize treatment. In Chapter 7 we continued our discussion of Denise and introduced Lena. This chapter focuses on how Denise's and Lena's treatment should be set up within TST.

Denise's and Lena's Assessments

 Recall that Denise was considered emotionally dysregulated and had a threatening social environment/system of care, whereas Lena was considered behaviorally dysregulated and had a stable social environment/system of care. Their TST Assessment Grids were shown in Figures 7.4 and 7.5 in Chapter 7. As can be seen, according to our assessment approach, Denise needs to start Phase 2 of treatment; Lena needs to start Phase 3. What does this mean?

Overview of the Five Phases of Treatment

Within TST there are five phases of treatment that correspond to different themes of traumatic stress care, depending on the fit between the child's self-regulation capacities and the stability of the social environment/system of care as assessed using the TST Assessment Grid. These phases are:

- Phase 1: **Surviving**
- Phase 2: **Stabilizing**
- Phase 3: **Enduring**
- Phase 4: **Understanding**
- Phase 5: **Transcending**

 We reproduce the TST Assessment Grid in Figure 8.1 with these phases labeled and give their descriptions below.

Regarding Denise and Lena:

Denise needs the **stabilizing phase** of treatment initially. This phase will involve home-based care to work with Denise and her family to minimize the many reminders in her home and will include advocacy involving the housing authority for improved housing. The stabilizing phase will also require use of the psychopharmacological module and the emotion regulation module to help Denise expand her emotion regulation capacities.

Lena needs the **enduring phase** of treatment initially. This phase will involve the emotion regulation module and possibly the psychopharmacology module to help her expand her emotion regulation capacities. Lena's uncle will be a very important part of her treatment. Her therapist will explicitly help Lena's uncle understand how to help Lena regulate emotion. If Lena's uncle is in some

		Social–Environmental Stability		
		Stable	Distressed	Threatening
Regulation of Emotion	Regulated	**Transcending** Phase 5	**Understanding** Phase 4	**Enduring** Phase 3
	Dysregulation of Emotion	**Understanding** Phase 4	**Enduring** Phase 3	**Stabilizing** Phase 2
	Dysregulation of Behavior	**Enduring** Phase 3	**Stabilizing** Phase 2	**Surviving** Phase 1

FIGURE 8.1. The TST Assessment Grid.

way overwhelmed due to his own traumatic stress symptoms, he will be referred for treatment.

Surviving (Phase 1)

The main theme of the **surviving** phase of treatment is to protect the child from threatening environments and dangerous impulses and to set the stage for interventions in other phases of this treatment. The child is (by definition) behaviorally dysregulated and the social environment/system of care is threatening. Therefore home- and community-based interventions are intensively used during this phase to acquire a comprehensive picture of the child's home environment and to assess the degree of threat and danger. During this phase of treatment there is frequently a need to work closely with social service agencies and inpatient psychiatric units. At some point during this phase it is not uncommon for a child to be hospitalized for suicidal or aggressive impulses. It is also not uncommon for a social service agency to be notified of the possibility of child abuse or neglect. Emotional regulation skills training can be started in this phase, when appropriate. Many children in this phase of treatment require psychopharmacological intervention. There is also frequently a need to advocate for additional, or more effective, services.

Stabilizing (Phase 2)

The main theme of the **stabilizing** phase is the creation of a safe social environment. Families who start in this phase usually have significant problems that will not be helped without home-based interventions. There will usually be problems related to family disorganization and stressors that trigger the child in identifiable ways. Similarly, the child's school, peer group, and neighborhood may be unstable and triggering. Interventions are delivered on site at the area of the social environment that is most contributing to the child's traumatic stress. Emotion regulation skills training is usually initiated in this phase to help the child manage very difficult environments and to set the stage for subsequent phases of treatment. Many children in this phase of treatment will require psychopharmacological intervention. Often advocacy for additional, or more effective, services is required. As can be seen in Figure 7.4, this stage is most appropriate for Denise.

Enduring (Phase 3)

The main theme of the **enduring** phase is the development of skills necessary to manage emotion and the establishment of a safe social environment. The child and family must be taught skills that help them endure the impact of trauma so that extreme behavior can be minimized. In order for a child to be expected to endure this impact, his/her social environment must be safe. The primary mode of intervention in this phase of treatment is emotion regulation skills training. If treatment has started prior to this phase, home- and community-based interventions should be almost complete. For children who start in this phase, home- and community-based interventions may be required at some point. Psychopharmacology will usually be required during the **enduring** phase. As can be seen in Figure 7.5, it is this stage that is most appropriate for Lena.

Understanding (Phase 4)

The main theme of the **understanding** phase is the establishment of therapeutic communication about the traumatic experience, so that the child and family are no longer consumed by it. Techniques of cognitive-behavioral therapy are primarily used during this phase of intervention. Emotion regulation skills training should be completed before this phase of treatment so that the child has sufficient skills to manage the processing of trauma-related cognitions. It will occasionally be necessary to use psychopharmacological intervention during this phase, although it is hoped that this type of intervention will not be necessary.

Transcending (Phase 5)

The main theme of the **transcending** phase is the creation of lasting meaning and perspective out of the traumatic experience. The focus is to learn how to live in a way that is less defined by the past than by the future. During this phase of treatment the child, family, and clinician work toward identifying and constructing culturally syntonic activities that may create lasting meaning out of the child's traumatic experiences. This phase also includes helping the child and family say goodbye to the therapist and move beyond treatment.

Treatment Modules

 TST interventions are delivered according to seven modules that are used in various combinations depending on the phase of treatment the child/family is assessed to be in. These seven treatment modules are described in detail in Chapters 10–16. This section introduces the following seven modules and describes how they are selected within a given phase of treatment:

> TST interventions are delivered according to seven modules that are used in various combinations depending on the phase of treatment the child/family is assessed to be in.

- Ready–set–go
- Stabilization on site
- Services advocacy

- Psychopharmacology
- Emotion regulation
- Cognitive processing
- Meaning making

Ready–Set–Go

Many families have difficulties with the process of engaging in treatment. There may be many reasons for these difficulties: The caregiver's trauma history may lead to an avoidance and mistrust of treatment; severe, ongoing stresses may lead to disorganization, missed appointments, and a failure to follow through on treatment plans; or there may be, as described in Chapter 4, significant cultural barriers to engaging in treatment. The ready–set–go module is used with all families at the beginning of TST. It is a way of introducing our treatment approach, assessing families' capacities to engage, and working to surmount barriers to this engagement. In essence, the ready–set–go module is a formalized way of building a treatment alliance with traumatized families. This module is used anywhere from one session (for well-engaged families) to a number of sessions over a 1-month period (with families that are very difficult to engage).

Stabilization on Site

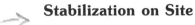

Stabilization on site, or SOS, involves intensive home-based and school-based services that are focused directly on diminishing the sources of stress and traumatic reminders within the child's day-to-day environment. SOS is appropriate for children who are experiencing acute emotion dysregulation and environment instability—for example, those children and families that are in the surviving and stabilizing phases of treatment. SOS can serve as hospital diversion, can be brought in at critical junctures to help stabilize a family, and can provide in-the-moment assistance for emotional and environmental crises. SOS frequently is initiated at the beginning of treatment, but it may also be brought into the treatment plan when a family in ongoing treatment experiences new problems or crises that threaten the stability of the home.

Services Advocacy

Services advocacy involves explicit work with service systems that can offer needed resources to help with emotion regulation and, particularly, social–environmental stability. As described in detail in Chapter 4, a critical problem for traumatized children and families is the presence of severe and very difficult-to-change stressors in the environment. Services advocacy can be essential in the surviving and stabilizing phases of treatment. Often families are entitled to services they are not receiving, and these services can specifically help the child's core traumatic stress problems. Services may include help with education, mental health, social services, housing, or immigration.

Psychopharmacology

Children who have significant problems regulating emotional states, particularly those whose states "spill" into potentially dangerous behaviors, can find psychopharmacological interventions helpful. The psychopharmacology module describes the principles and practice of psychopharmacology as they relate to TST. This module also describes the psychiatric consultant's role on a TST treatment team. The psychopharmacology module is commonly used during the surviving, stabilizing, and enduring phases; it is used less frequently during the understanding and transcending phases. Ideally, psychopharmacology should be discontinued by the end of treatment and children should have sufficient skills to regulate their emotions. Sometimes this goal is not possible, and psychopharmacological agents are continued after treatment ends.

Emotion Regulation

Emotion regulation (ER) is a cornerstone of a child's recovery in TST. The ER module is a semistructured office-based therapeutic approach that helps both parents and children gain greater awareness of emotions and specific skills and strategies for their regulation. In general, the ER module is the primary treatment approach in the enduring phase of treatment. It may also be used in earlier phases under certain conditions. The emotion regulation module is appropriate for children who can't yet talk about, or be reminded of, their trauma without experiencing overwhelming emotions or engaging in inappropriate (or even dangerous) behaviors. The ER module is applied somewhat differently in the earlier phases (stabilizing, surviving) than in the enduring phase.

> Emotion regulation is a cornerstone of a child's recovery in TST.

Cognitive Processing

The cognitive-processing (CP) module is a companion module to the ER module. Once the emotion regulation skills are mastered from the ER module, the child can learn a focused and structured approach that will help him/her talk about the trauma. The CP module involves the child's learning cognitive-behavioral techniques of trauma processing so that he/she will not become dysregulated when faced with stressors or reminders. Using the language of cognitive-behavioral therapy, the CP module focuses on extinguishing the trauma response. This module can only be used, however, when the social environment is reasonably stable and the child has acquired sufficient emotion regulation skills to tolerate talking about the trauma. The use of the CP module anchors the understanding phase of TST.

Meaning Making

Once the CP module has been completed and the child is no longer consumed by the past, it is time to look to the future. The meaning-making module involves finding activities that will help the child and family create lasting meaning about the event. These activities might include a ritual to "mark" the child's moving beyond the trauma, art projects, or activities that involve helping others. Typically, the therapist, child, and family choose activities that are syntonic with the family's cultural and religious background. The therapist guides the child and family toward creating meaning in an active way and thus finally putting the trauma in the past. This module also provides a time for saying goodbye to the therapist and helping the family transition to life beyond treatment. The meaning-making module anchors the transcending phase of treatment.

Putting It All Together

We have five phases and seven modules: How can a clinician keep this straight and remember what goes with what?

The TST Assessment Grid defines the phase,
and the phase defines the types of modules that are chosen.

Key points to remember:

- All children must start with the ready–set–go module.
- All children start with a given phase based on their rating on the TST Assessment Grid. They are expected to transition to more "advanced" phases until their completion of the transcending phase.
- Sometimes children need to go back to a previously completed phase based on a variety of circumstances (e.g., new life stressor).
- If a child is assessed to be in the **surviving phase**, he/she needs the SOS module, the services advocacy module, and probably the emotion regulation and psychopharmacology modules. In this phase, acute psychiatric services and the state social services agency will probably function as important partners in treatment. This phase should last up to 3 months.
- If a child is assessed to be in the **stabilizing phase**, he/she needs the SOS module and probably the services advocacy, emotion regulation, and psychopharmacology modules. This phase should last up to 3 months if the child starts here and up to 2 months if the child completed the surviving phase.
- If a child is assessed to be in the **enduring phase**, he/she needs the emotion regulation module and possibly the psychopharmacology module.

The child may also need the services advocacy module. This phase should last up to 3 months if the child started here and up to 1 month if the child had 3 months of the ER module during the surviving and/or stabilizing phases.

- If a child is assessed to be in the **understanding phase**, he/she needs the cognitive processing module and, infrequently, the psychopharmacology module. The child may also need, though infrequently, the services advocacy module. This phase should last up to 3 months.

- If a child is assessed to be in the **transcending phase**, he/she needs the meaning-making module and, rarely, the psychopharmacology module. The child may also need, though rarely, the services advocacy module. This phase should last up to 2 months.

- Not counting time in ready–set–go, treatment should last a maximum of 11 months for children who start in the surviving phase and 2 months for children who start in the transcending phase.

Figure 8.2 provides another way to understand which modules a child needs in a given phase of treatment.

Back to Denise and Lena . . .

When we said that Denise needs the stabilizing phase and Lena needs the enduring phase of treatment, the meaning should be clear. The decisions regarding which phase of treatment a child is in (and which corresponding modules are implemented) are based on the TST Assessment Grid. All families—including Denise's and Lena's—start with ready–set–go. Once this module is complete, Denise will receive SOS, services advocacy, emotion regulation, and psychopharmacology modules. Lena will receive only the emotion regulation module. As both Denise and Lena complete their modules, the phase of treatment will advance, and they will transition through the TST phases of treatment.

		Phase				
		Surviving	Stabilizing	Enduring	Understanding	Transcending
Module	Stabilization on site (SOS)	***	***	–	–	–
	Services advocacy	***	**	*	*	*
	Psychopharmacology	**	**	**	*	*
	Emotion regulation	*	**	***	–	–
	Cognitive processing	–	–	–	***	–
	Meaning making	–	–	–	–	***

FIGURE 8.2. TST treatment modules used across treatment phases. *Note.* *** = essential; ** = often helpful; * = occasionally helpful; – = not used or contraindicated.

What exactly are the problems to be solved by all these interventions?

TST Priority Problems

Principle Three, introduced in Chapter 6, says: *Create* clear, focused plans that are based on facts.

Chances are, you agree with this idea, but what does it *really* mean? In the assessment chapter and in this treatment planning chapter, we have detailed the facts on which treatment should be based and the types of interventions toward which these facts point us.

What is the focus of treatment within each phase? How do the modules fit together in a focused way? What specifically happens in the different modules? The answers relate to our system of assigning priority—for short, "TST Priority Problems."

If you were treating Denise, on which area, exactly, would you focus? What about Lena?

Determining TST Priority Problems is based on the interface between the child's emotion regulation problems and stressful stimuli in the environment. The clinician is expected to find episodes of emotional or behavioral dysregulation and the stimuli that provoke it. The best way to do this is through the moment-by-moment assessment outlined in Chapter 3. To restate:

- Ask about episodes of dysregulation.
- Understand how the three A's shift during these episodes.
- Find out the precipitants to these episodes.
- Understand how family members (or other members of the social environment) helped or made things worse.
- Find out the cost to the child and family of these episodes.

In summary, the assignment of TST Priority Problems is based on:

- Patterns of links between emotional/behavioral dysregulation and the stimuli that provoke it.
- The role of members in the child's social environment in helping or hindering regulation during these episodes.
- The functional implications of these patterns of links.

The TST Priority Problems must:

- **Clearly reference the patterns of links between emotional/behavioral dysregulation and the stimuli that provoke it.**
- **Assign priority to a given problem based on clinical judgment regarding the amount of dysfunction that the links cause.**

When assigning priority to the problem based on its functional implications, the following guidelines should be used. It is very important to note that these are only guidelines and should be used with a great deal of clinical discretion:

1. Problems that jeopardize physical safety (e.g., suicide, violence, child abuse).
2. Problems that jeopardize engagement in treatment.
3. Problems that jeopardize home placement.
4. Problems that jeopardize school placement.
5. Problems that jeopardize healthy development (e.g., drug abuse, antisocial behavior, sexual activity, eating disturbances).
6. Problems that cause significant distress to the child or to family members.
7. Problems that can be solved relatively easily and are highly meaningful to the child or family members.

Once the TST Priority Problems have been identified, the application of the treatment modules to the problems is very straightforward.

What about Denise and Lena?

It is difficult to provide sufficient detail for treatment planning using brief vignettes. Here we offer a little more information about Denise, followed by a description of her TST Priority Problems.

- Suppose that Denise enters dissociative states regularly—whenever she sees someone who reminds her of her mother's boyfriend—and no one in her family is aware of why she behaves this way. Furthermore, suppose her mother yells at her whenever she seems too "spaced out."
- Suppose that Denise experiences nightmares about sexual abuse on nights that her mother has had a physical fight with her boyfriend. Suppose that she is not able to sleep at night and instead falls asleep in school. Suppose that neither her mother nor her teacher is able to help with the problem and she is failing the year in school.

TST Priority Problems for Denise could be expressed as follows:

1. Denise frequently enters dissociative states when she sees someone who reminds her of her mother's boyfriend (who abused her). Her mother does not yet recognize this link and approaches Denise with anger when she is in this dissociative state. This approach makes things worse.

2. Denise has frequent nightmares after witnessing physical fights between her mother and her mother's boyfriend. These nightmares are contributing to school failure. Her mother does not recognize the role of ongoing family violence in contributing to Denise's symptoms or her failure in school. The lack of a bedroom door and crowded housing make things worse. Denise's mother does not appreciate the impact of family violence on Denise or the privacy problem related to lack of a bedroom door. The school does not understand the reasons behind Denise's inability to do schoolwork and mistakenly attributes her failure to her being "bright but unmotivated."

Okay. Now what do you do?

TST Treatment Planning Form

We have created a Treatment Planning Form for TST (see Appendix). This is the place where the results of your assessment, your description of the TST Priority Problems, and their solutions are recorded. These solutions are the focused, specific plans that address the TST Priority Problems.

The way it usually works is that one clinician on the team (the primary clinician) is designated to complete the Treatment Planning Form with input from the team. The form has six sections, each of which contains important information for carrying out the treatment. We describe each of these sections in turn. Please refer to this form while reading the next section.

1. *Indicate the "players" on the team.* The TST Treatment Planning Form begins with a listing of all providers who will have a role in the treatment, including contact information. The family and all members of the team keep a copy of this form to facilitate communication and treatment focus.

2. *Indicate scores on relevant instruments.* It is often helpful to have the assessment supplemented by quantitative information from measures designed to assess specific areas. We use the Child and Adolescent Needs and Strengths— Trauma Exposure and Adaptation (CANS-TEA), the UCLA PTSD Reaction Index (PTSD-RI), the Trauma Symptom Checklist (TSCC), and the Child Behavior Checklist (CBCL). This type of information can help the clinician and team check to see if their assessment is on the right track. It can also be

used to follow treatment progress in a quantitative way. The TST Weekly Check-In Scale can be very helpful in gathering information from the child every week about emotion regulation and social–environmental stability. This important scale is included in the Appendix.

We have included space within the Treatment Planning Form to indicate the scores on these measures. Other teams may find other measures more useful and should feel free to use those.

3. *Indicate the recommended treatment phase.* The treatment planning form includes a copy of the TST Assessment Grid reviewed above and in Chapter 7. This is a place to summarize the overall level of emotional regulation and social environmental stability and to determine the recommended treatment phase.

4. *Indicate the recommended treatment modules.* Figure 8.4, described above, is reproduced on the treatment planning form. This is the place where the recommended modules of treatment are indicated.

5. *Identify the TST Priority Problems.* A very important part of the Treatment Planning Form is the identification of the TST Priority Problems. As described above, the description of these priority problems puts all the information gathered in the assessment into a clear statement to guide and focus treatment. The team should take great care in the crafting of these statements because, ideally, they will be the focus of all interventions offered within TST. Furthermore, as is described in Chapter 10, they are the beginnings of the discussion to form the treatment alliance with the family. Accordingly, they will need to be constructed in a way that captures both what the team believes is most important and what addresses something that the family is motivated to change.

6. *Identify the solutions to the TST Priority Problems.* The next part of the Treatment Planning Form is devoted to the specific solutions for each of the priority problems, including space to describe strategies for surmounting practical barriers. On this page the clinician describes the solutions to the problems via the intervention modalities of TST and, particularly, who is accountable for what (*insist on accountability, particularly your own*; Principle Six).

The "solutions" section has six columns.

- The first column specifies who or what is the focus of a given solution. This column is organized according to the level of the social ecology that needs intervention, starting with the child.
- The second column indicates which priority problem (PP #) the given solution is meant to address. Some solutions may address more than one priority problem.
- The third column provides space for a clear description of the solution. This description should include how a recommended treatment module will be used to address the priority problem.

- The fourth column provides space to indicate the person or persons responsible for providing the recommended solution (*insist on accountability, particularly your own*).
- The fifth and sixth columns are used to indicate when the problem/solution was noted and when the problem is resolved.

The TST Treatment Planning Form is completed as a team activity (with the primary clinician as the lead). The form is initially considered preliminary because it must be reviewed with the family. Indeed, it serves as a springboard for building a treatment alliance with the family based on negotiation and agreeing on the problem and solution. This process of *agreeing on the problem and solution* is a critical part of alliance building and is detailed in Chapter 10. Once this agreement is reached, the plan is considered final. It can—and should—be updated, however, to reflect new information. The preliminary plan is the team's recommendations to the family. The final TST Treatment Plan is considered a contract between the family and the team, with rigorous expectations of accountability (Principle Six). Copies of the treatment plan are distributed to all the players on the team to create a transparent and accountable process within the team and with the family. As is reviewed in Chapter 10, divergence from the plan must be actively discussed and reconciled.

Back to Denise . . .

Recall that Denise is considered in the stabilizing phase of treatment based on her emotion dysregulation and the threats in her social environmental. In this phase Denise has access to home-based, advocacy, emotion regulation, and psychopharmacology intervention resources. Any of these intervention resources may be devoted to one or both of the TST Priority Problems identified above. The team decides how these resources will be allocated for Denise (*put scarce resources where they'll work*, Principle Five).

Figure 8.3 is Denise's TST Treatment Plan, illustrating how this document can focus and specify care.

CHILD NAME _Denise Vasquez_   DOB _8/13/99_   RECORD # _24680_   DATE _2/8/05_

TST TREATMENT PLANNING FORM

1. Indicate the "players" on the Team

The Team	Name	Ways to reach	Signature
Child or adolescent	Denise	444-4444	Denise Vasquez
Family	Mrs. Vasquez	444-4444 cell # 555-5555	Donna Vasquez
Therapist	Dr. Ellis	666-6666	B. H. Ellis
SOS clinician	Ms. Chapman	777-7777	Carolyn Chapman
SOS clinician			
Legal advocate	Ms. Tames	888-8888	Pamela Tames
Psychiatric consultant	Dr. Saxe	999-9999	Glenn Saxe
Others*	Mrs. Lester (teacher)	333-3333	Mrs. Lester

*Godparents, involved neighbors, extended family, mentors, social service providers, pediatricians, religious leaders.

2. Indicate scores on relevant instruments

	TR HX	TSS SX	E Reg	B Reg	Soc Env	Str	Fn
CANS-TEA	3	12	10	5	18	4	
UCLA PTSD-RI	2	17					
TSCC		23					
CBCL			Int:	Ext:		Comp.	

3. Indicate the recommended treatment phase

	Stable	Distressed	Threatening
Regulated	Transcending Phase 5	Understanding Phase 4	Enduring Phase 3
Dysregulation of Emotion	Understanding Phase 4	Enduring Phase 3	Stabilizing Phase 2
Dysregulation of Behavior	Enduring Phase 3	Stabilizing Phase 2	Surviving Phase 1

(continued)

FIGURE 8.3. TST Treatment Planning Form for Denise.

4. Indicate the recommended treatment modules

	Surviving	Stabilizing	Endurirng	Understanding	Transcending
Stabilization on site (SOS)	***	(***)	—	—	—
Services advocacy	***	(**)	*	*	*
Psychopharmacology	**	(**)	**	*	*
Emotional regulation	*	(**)	***	—	—
Cognitive processing	—	—	—	***	—
Meaning making	—	—	—	—	***

Note. *** = essential; ** = often helpful; * = occasionally helpful; — = not used or contraindicated

5a. Identify the TST Priority Problems

TST Priority Problems:

1. Identify patterns of links between social–environmental stressor and emotional/behavioral dysregulation.
2. Prioritize those patterns ot links that most interfere with the child's functioning. (Use point 5b to help decide on the level of priority. It is very important to note that point 5b offers only rough guidelines and should not override clinical discretion.)

Priority Problem 1	Priority Problem 2
Denise frequently gets spaced out when she sees someone that reminds her of someone who hurt her. Mrs. Vasquez sometimes does not see how getting spaced out can be related to seeing someone who looks like a man who hurt her. Sometimes Mrs. Vasquez gets upset during these times because it appears that Denise is "going away" and "not trying."	*Denise often has nightmares when her mother and her mother's boyfriend fight. On nights she has nightmares, it is hard to focus at school the next day. The fighting between Mrs. Vasquez and her boyfriend has become a problem for Denise's sleep and school performance. The school has not seen how Denise's fears and poor sleep have interfered with her performance. Denise's lack of privacy also makes her level of stress worse at home.*
Priority Problem 3	Priority Problem 4

5b. Guidelines for assigning priority to a problem identified in point 5a

1. Problems that jeopardize physical safety (e.g. suicide, violence, child abuse).
2. Problems that jeopardize engagement in treatment.
3. Problems that jeopardize home placement.
4. Problems that jeopardize school placement.
5. Problems that jeopardize healthy development (e.g. drug abuse, antisocial behavior, sexual activity, eating disturbances).
6. Problems that cause significant distress to the child or family members.
7. Problems that can be solved relatively easily and are highly meaningful to the child or family members.

(continued)

FIGURE 8.3. *(continued)*

6. Identify the Solutions to TST Priority Problems

Who/What does solution address?	PP #	Description of solution	Person responsible	When noted	When resolved
Child (indicate skill module and/or psychopharmacology)	1	Emotional regulation skills to help calm down when you see someone who reminds you of person who hurt you.	Dr. Ellis	2/8	
	2	ER skills to help focus on school when feeling very upset.	Dr. Ellis	2/8	
	1, 2	ER skills to help you talk with your mother without needing to leave.	Dr. Ellis	2/8	
	1, 2	Medications to help with sleep, nightmares, and calming down.	Dr. Saxe	2/8	
Social environment					
Caregiver (e.g., emotional and/or substance abuse, monitoring/supervision, knowledge, family violence)	1, 2	Referral to psychiatric assessment for possible depression.	Dr. Saxe	2/8	
	2	Home-based assessment and intervention in triggers related to violence and privacy.	Ms. Chapman	2/8	
	1, 2	Give Mrs. Vasquez more information on trauma, emotion regulation, and dissociation			
	2	Give Mrs. Vasquez information on domestic violence and shelter contact info			
Siblings					
Housing	2	Needs bedroom door, possibly less crowded apartment.	Dr. Ellis with help from Ms. Tames	2/8	
Resources					
School	2	Work toward IEP that integrates interference in school performance related to nightmares/sleep, anxiety/dissociation in school.	Dr. Ellis with help from Ms. Tames	2/8	
Appropriateness of placement					
Neighborhood					
Peers					
Other					

(continued)

FIGURE 8.3. *(continued)*

Barriers (Describe practical barriers that may interfere with solving priority problems; describe strategies to surmount barriers.)					
Description: Mrs. V. reports that it is very hard to bring Denise to appts. due to work schedule.	1, 2	Strategy: Work on flexibility in appt. times, troubleshoot mom's work schedule and whether mom can get aunt to bring to every second appt. Home-based care (SOS) should help.	Dr. Ellis Ms. Chapman Dr. Saxe	2/8	
Strengths (Describe strengths of child/assets in social environment that may be engaged to help with solutions to priority problems.)					
Description: Denise is very bright and engaging.	1, 2	Strategy: Denise's intelligence may help offset emotional reasons for school failure. Social skills can be used to elicit help from friends, teachers, and relatives.	Dr. Ellis	2/8	

FIGURE 8.3. *(continued)*

CHAPTER

9

The Treatment Team

How to Build a Multidisciplinary
Treatment Team (and Keep It Going!)

LEARNING OBJECTIVES

- To understand why a treatment team is a necessary part of TST

- To learn how the treatment team contributes to treatment fidelity

- To learn how to use the treatment team to support members

If it takes a village to raise a child, it at least takes a team to provide intervention after a trauma. TST, by design, is not a treatment that can be accomplished by one lone therapist in an office. We think treatment is best done by a web of providers who together form a net to support kids and families during the toughest times. Not only that, but our net of providers helps *each other* during tough times. There's a Somali proverb that says if you have five sticks and hand them to five people, each person can break the stick. If you have five sticks in a bundle and hand them to one person, the sticks will not be broken. So it is with the TST team. Providers are stronger and better able to hold onto hope and patience during the difficult periods of treatment when they aren't standing alone.

This chapter discusses the importance of building and maintaining an interdisciplinary team that can serve to support both families and team members.

The Burnout Mode

Marlene is a 32-year-old social worker who was feeling tired at work and then noticed that she'd started having a glass of wine every night when she got home—something she didn't used to do. She was having trouble sleeping and thought she might be getting depressed. Sometimes she would wake up in the morning with a feeling of dread, and it would be very hard to get herself out of bed to go to work. One night she dreamt that her daughter had cut herself all over her arms, and no matter how hard Marlene tried to help her, it was as if she were in a glass box: She couldn't make any sound and couldn't reach her daughter. The next day at work, Marlene told her supervisor that she thought a high-risk client she had been working with for several months needed a new therapist because they just weren't making any progress.

What is going on here? Is it possible for a therapist to dread going to work? Marlene should be looking for a new profession, right? Perhaps Marlene's story hits close to home. Perhaps you have sometimes felt like staying away from your work with traumatized children. Maybe you've never experienced just what happened to Marlene, but chances are that if you work with traumatized kids long enough, *some* of these will ring true: feeling depressed, losing hope for a client, feeling like a failure, having nightmares, using unhealthy coping strategies, or having trouble separating work from home life.

We can make a pretty good guess that Marlene's difficulties are making it hard (if not impossible) for her to give the best care to her clients. We can also guess that her clients' multilayered difficulties are at least part of what is affecting Marlene. This all-too-common scenario is a perfect recipe for burnout. These problems have been called countertransference, vicarious traumatization, or just plain hopelessness and are very common in working with traumatized children. Why? Because we are human! Add in a few dealings with ineffective service systems or a resource-poor agency, and it is downright amazing that we don't *all* burn out!

The Balance between Product and Process

There are two overarching goals on the TST team:

1. To provide effective care for traumatized children and families (TST Principle One: *Fix a broken system*).
2. To take care of the people who are providing this care (TST Principle Eight: *Take care of yourself and your team*).

Both of these goals must be priorities within the treatment team. If the team does not attend to the structure of effective care (Is TST assessment and intervention done adequately?), then the team might as well be meeting to talk about last night's hockey game. If the team does not attend to the emotional needs of its members, the team conference room will be empty before too long. Effective care is the TST product. Providing

Effective care is the TST product. Providing this care in a sensible way is the TST process.

this care in a sensible way is the TST process. There are no hard and fast rules dictating how to achieve this balance. The team leader and team members must always be mindful of this balance. It often helps during a team meeting if some of the following questions are asked:

- Are we doing TST correctly?
- Are we sticking to TST principles?
- Are we holding ourselves accountable for what we said we'd do?
- Are we following the treatment plan?
- If not, is there new information that needs to be incorporated into the treatment plan?
- Is our treatment working?
- If not, what are we missing?
- What can we do to make our treatment better?
- How is everyone doing?
- Are we taking care of ourselves and our team?
- What could we be doing to support our therapists better?
- Are people remaining hopeful?
- Is the meeting too heavy?
- Is there anything else we can do to make the meeting more bearable?
- What's going well?

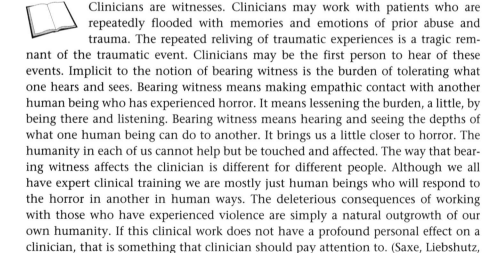 Clinicians are witnesses. Clinicians may work with patients who are repeatedly flooded with memories and emotions of prior abuse and trauma. The repeated reliving of traumatic experiences is a tragic remnant of the traumatic event. Clinicians may be the first person to hear of these events. Implicit to the notion of bearing witness is the burden of tolerating what one hears and sees. Bearing witness means making empathic contact with another human being who has experienced horror. It means lessening the burden, a little, by being there and listening. Bearing witness means hearing and seeing the depths of what one human being can do to another. It brings us a little closer to horror. The humanity in each of us cannot help but be touched and affected. The way that bearing witness affects the clinician is different for different people. Although we all have expert clinical training we are mostly just human beings who will respond to the horror in another in human ways. The deleterious consequences of working with those who have experienced violence are simply a natural outgrowth of our own humanity. If this clinical work does not have a profound personal effect on a clinician, that is something that clinician should pay attention to. (Saxe, Liebshutz, Edwardson, & Frankel, 2003, p. 157)

TST is designed to provide treatment to some of the toughest cases out there. TST is for kids who have experienced horrific traumas, and often lots of them.

It's for families that have trouble engaging in treatment. It's for service systems that aren't able to help and might, in fact, be hurting. TST is conducted by therapists who must bear witness to all of these things. TST demands a lot of its therapists—that you think (and work) beyond the office and beyond the 50-minute hour. So TST needs to also be concerned with how to keep its therapists going.

The good news is that TST has built into it some pointers that make doing therapy in a tough world a little bit easier. It's got systems for facilitating communication between agencies. It's got guidelines for advocating within systems. But most importantly, it's got a TST *team*.

How Does the TST Team Work?

The TST team meets on a weekly basis. Unlike the Family Collaborative Meeting, detailed in Chapter 10, which pulls together providers from the larger TST team who are focusing on a single family, the TST team meeting is for all the TST providers who see any TST family. This is a chance for all TST providers who see different families to come together and talk about their various experiences. Team meetings last 1–1½ hours, depending on how many cases need to be discussed. The team should have one or more leaders identified who have the responsibility of both ensuring that the team is *doing* TST, and also that the team members are taken care of and able to keep up the hard work. The leader

> The leader of the TST team meeting should be a senior clinician who has strong clinical skills, is well versed in TST, and is attuned to the team members.

of the TST team meeting should be a senior clinician who has strong clinical skills, is well versed in TST, and is attuned to the team members. In sum, the team leader needs to be both a teacher and a cheerleader. The team itself may consist of social workers, psychologists, psychiatrists, nurse specialists, home-based clinicians, advocacy attorneys, and trainees.

This format probably sounds very familiar to many clinicians. We, of course, did not invent the multidisciplinary treatment team meeting. Our point here is to highlight the team format as a necessary condition for effective treatment. We have thought a lot about how this type of team can be structured to fit within TST.

TST team meetings follow this basic structure:

1. Set the agenda.
2. Discuss new intakes.
3. Discuss ongoing cases (crises and updates).
4. End with something good.

Here we talk about what happens, practically, during each section of the meeting—the content. Then we talk more generally about how to make the meeting supportive—the process.

Setting the Agenda

This is a straightforward part of the meeting: Who has new intakes? Who has an ongoing case? Who has something good to report? The practical side of agenda setting is to make sure that the meeting is paced to allow for all topics to be covered. But this is also an important time to take the pulse of the group. Some days people have lots to say—and this is usually a good sign. Team members are actively working on their cases, ready for and open to input, and willing to share with the group. Usually this behavior means that they have some energy for new ideas and feel supported by the group. *Bingo*—that's what we want our therapists to feel.

Some days, however, it's ominously quiet when it's time to set the agenda. It could be, of course, that there were no new intakes and everyone's cases are just cruising along with no problems and therefore nothing to discuss. Unfortunately, however, this is rarely the case. Instead, one team member may be thinking, "I've tried everything with Kenny, and I just can't hear another suggestion. They don't get it—nothing works." Or "If I talk about Lori and this school issue, they're going to tell me to get in contact with the teacher. I just don't have time for that this week!" Or maybe even "I've done such a bad job of this, I'm too embarrassed to tell people. I mean, I just don't even know what the problem is."

So pay attention during agenda setting. If the room starts to have that weirdly quiet sound and people are carefully looking away from the eyes of the agenda-setter, it may be time to take stock of the team culture. It could be time for the team leader to provide some cheerleading, or bring in pizza, or check over the level of support that people have been getting in response to their case presentations (more on these matters later). Just as therapists need to take some responsibility for getting their clients to engage in treatment, a team leader needs to take some responsibility for getting members engaged in the TST team meeting.

> Just as therapists need to take some responsibility for getting their clients to engage in treatment, a team leader needs to take some responsibility for getting members engaged in the TST team meeting.

New Intakes

A new family comes in for an intake. You sit with them for an hour or 2 or 3, depending on your intake model, and are supposed to come out at the end with a clear sense of the problem and treatment plan. Chapter 8 covers the details of how we do this under TST. But although our therapists know the material in

Chapter 8 really well, we all discuss every single new case that comes to our clinic on the TST team. We do this for several reasons.

First, a clinician is only one person with one perspective. A good clinician presenting a case will most likely have an excellent sense of a child's development, mental health symptoms, and which treatment approach seems appropriate. A legal advocate listening to the case presentation may pick up on the fact that the housing is substandard and that there are resources for improving this situation. As the advocate points this out, the clinician begins to think about how the quality of the home may be contributing to the child's posttraumatic symptoms. An SOS clinician notes that he's familiar with the neighborhood and that there is a lot of gang activity near the family's current home. The team concurs that the environment is distressed, so advocacy for better housing in a safer neighborhood becomes a priority. A psychiatrist wonders whether a medication evaluation could potentially provide some immediate change in behavior to help stabilize the child while the longer-acting advocacy is taking place. And so it goes, with the different perspectives gradually building a well-rounded treatment plan.

> Once a client is discussed by the TST team, he/she is part of the family, and we participate in the struggle through the challenges and in celebrating the successes.

Another reason all new cases are discussed during TST team meetings is that it is a way of introducing them—a sort of "We have a new member of the family" approach. Down the road, a new complication may come up with treatment, or some great progress will be made, and when the clinician says "Hey, remember that boy I talked about who came in with the bee-bee lodged in his head?" team members nod, curious, and say "What *did* happen with him?" Once a client is discussed by the TST team, he/she is part of the family, and we all participate in the struggle through the challenges and in celebrating the successes.

Finally, and perhaps most importantly, we have an idiom on our team that we stand firmly behind. It's something that a supervisor once told a trainee, who became a supervisor and then told it to a trainee, who then became a supervisor and . . . it's this:

                    Never worry alone.

Pretty simple, but very important. With a treatment such as TST, you are bound to be working with some very high-risk cases. TST does a lot to keep kids out of the hospital and to provide intervention in the least restrictive environment. We think this is great for kids, but it also means that providers need to be very watchful, curious, and concerned about how clients are doing. The better you know a family, the better able you are to sense when things are heating up or seeming unusual and worrisome. But new intakes have lots of unknowns and can be difficult to judge for safety. The last place we want a TST clinician to be is staring at the ceiling in the middle of the night, worrying about a decision that he/she made. All intakes are reviewed by the entire team to make sure that we've thought through the risk level carefully and that the clinician is not worrying alone.

> All intakes are reviewed by the entire team to make sure that we've thought through the risk level carefully and that the clinician is not worrying alone.

Ongoing Cases

Once a case becomes "part of the family," it's important for the team to stay up-to-date on major changes, complications, or progress. Sometimes TST team meetings become their own mini-series, with weekly updates full of drama and intrigue. However, with a mini-series you can just watch—when you're on the team, you are an active participant in solving the problems and supporting the therapist.

High-risk cases should be discussed on a regular basis. As with new intakes, this protocol helps bring many perspectives to bear on a critical case. It also helps to have more than one set of eyes on the risk level. Remember . . .

Never worry alone.

Finally, another key reason for discussing high-risk cases on a regular basis is that frequently these cases have the most providers involved. Communication between providers and agreement on goals and treatment plan are essential to making TST work. Being able to use 5 minutes of the team meeting to say "Hey, I got a call this morning from Mom, who thought that I was dealing with the housing issue . . . " can make all the difference in providing integrated, focused care.

Something Good

Picture this: Three new intakes—a 16-year-old girl who was raped, a 14-year-old Somali boy who saw his father murdered in the war, and an 8-year-old boy who just reported that his mother was beat up by her boyfriend last night. Two ongoing cases—that one with the gang-involved adolescent, and the other one with the girl who witnessed her mother's rape. Feeling good yet? Ready to head out of the meeting and greet the world?

Probably not. And week after week of leaving the TST team meeting with your tail dragging and head down is not going to help anyone feel inspired to keep fighting the good fight. So reserve a little bit of time at the end of the meeting for *something good*. If people have a good story about a case, great! Put it on the agenda as a way to end the meeting. If nobody has a case that is uplifting just then, not to worry—have somebody share something from outside of their

> Bring in readings, make a note of good movies or books that the team might be interested in, or just get the team thinking about some little tidbit of good news.

work. Just make it good. Bring in readings, make a note of good movies or books that the team might be interested in, or just get the team thinking about some little tidbit of good news. We don't mean to invite Pollyanna onto the team, but neither do we want to have the Grim Reaper holding court.

What Separates the TST Team from the Spanish Inquisition?

In addition to providing support and ideas for clinicians, the TST team has a very important function of making sure that the interventions offered are faithful to the TST model. Adopting TST on a treatment team means changing a culture. There's a language that goes with it, a way of doing things, and a list of things that are, and are not, TST.

For the team that is trying to adopt the TST treatment, it can be helpful to rate cases based on how closely they adhere to the 10 core principles and to behavioral indicators of these principles. Our Fidelity form is included in the Appendix. While a clinician presents his/her case, a team member ticks through the list of actions to make sure that what is supposed to be done is being done.

We started doing this on our team but quickly ran into a problem: Who wants to present a case when you're about to be judged? The very environment that was supposed to feel supportive to a therapist suddenly was charged with criticism and corrections. Uh-oh. The therapist burnout index just went up.

When we thought about it a little bit more, we realized that if the intervention wasn't consistent with TST or if the therapist wasn't feeling supported, then that was a problem with the *team*. Are team members listening actively? Are they noting the progress of the case or positive actions of the therapist? Are they coming up with concrete suggestions that are consistent with TST? Are they acknowledging the very real challenges the therapist is facing?

The culture of the TST team is what makes or breaks the TST treatment. If the team is supportive, understanding, and well-versed in how to make TST work, then the therapist on that team is going to be able to provide good treatment.

 A team leader can do a lot to encourage a culture of support on the team. Here are a few ideas:

- Be quick to point out the successes and achievements.
- Mark successes or accomplishments with a celebration (food never hurts).
- Be ready to remind people of the larger context in which the work takes place—the possibility of making a real difference in a kid's life.
- Don't be afraid to acknowledge how hard it is and how much we are asking of people. Admitting that, at times, you get discouraged or feel burned out too can encourage more open discussion.
- Lighten things up a little, using humor if possible.
- Strike the right balance between *product* and *process.*

Final Thoughts on the TST Team

The TST team functions as a container. If the team is organized right, team members will feel *contained.* That means that they will feel that they have a safe place to go to discuss their work; they will feel that there is a clear structure that supports effective service. We must never forget: Team members are being asked to manage powerful posttraumatic emotions. Such emotional intensity can be destabilizing not only for kids but for clinicians, supervisors, teams, and agencies. Indeed, the same type of care that is necessary for working with traumatized families is also necessary for the clinical teams that work with these families. In essence, teams need safety, containment, and structure. If these are in place, the work becomes not only manageable but also effective.

PART III

Doing Trauma Systems Therapy

Ready–Set–Go!

How to Engage a Family in TST

LEARNING OBJECTIVES

- To identify key barriers to treatment engagement
- To identify key motivators for treatment engagement
- To learn to develop an alliance around treatment goals

After reading Chapters 1–9, you should have a good sense of how TST addresses the problems of traumatized children, the general course of treatment, and the importance of factors such as a stable environment and good regulation skills. Perhaps you even feel hopeful that beginning treatment with a family can make a difference. Great! So, are we ready to get started?

Not so fast! Remember Principle Four?: "Don't 'go' before you are 'ready'!" This chapter explores what that principle means. How do we get ready to go? How do we prepare for treatment? Ready–set–go helps you to help family members do what they need to do to help the child recover.

As noted, no matter what treatment phase a family is in, we start with this module, which we call ready–set–go. For families that come in with a fairly clear understanding of how trauma affects kids and how a treatment such as TST could help them, the ready–set–go module might just take one session. For other families, it may take about a month. The ready–set–go module focuses on building a relationship with a family, setting common goals for treatment, and agreeing on how you are going to work toward those goals. This chapter describes some of the fundamentals of how to accomplish these tasks.

Why Not Just Get Started?

The reality for many mental health settings is that if a family doesn't come to treatment, that's the end of treatment. Three no-shows and the letter goes out, *case closed*. In TST, though, that's where we begin. Take, for example, this all-too-common scenario:

 Duncan is an 8-year-old boy referred to treatment for aggressive behaviors at school. He has gotten into several fights with classmates and was recently suspended for using vulgar language in the school library. Duncan's mother brings him to an intake evaluation appointment, along with a letter from the school saying that he cannot return to school until he receives a psychological evaluation. In the course of this first meeting, she becomes tearful as she describes the violent relationship she has had with Duncan's father, the financial difficulties she has faced since she moved out on her own 2 months ago, and her feelings of being overwhelmed by "having to handle Duncan" all on her own. She works at an office in the filing department but has had to leave work to get Duncan from school when he misbehaves so many times that she is afraid that she will be fired. In fact, she says that she missed work again to come to this appointment today.

Following the intake appointment, the therapist schedules a weekly meeting. They miss the first appointment. After a phone call from the therapist, they reschedule for the following week. They again miss the appointment.

When family members repeatedly miss appointments or don't come back after an evaluation, it's easy to dismiss them as "resistant" or "not ready for treatment." Unfortunately, however, often the very families that are not able to commit to regular treatment are the ones who are in the greatest distress.

Duncan's mother, for example, is clearly overwhelmed—in part because of Duncan's behavior problems. Duncan himself is dealing with a history of witnessing serious violence at home, the recent transition of having moved out from living with his dad, and significant stressors in the financial and emotional environment at home. From this vantage point, safely behind this book we're reading, it seems pretty clear that TST could really help this family. But what does it look like from Mom's point of view? One more meeting (or more!) a week, missing more work, paying money to take the bus to the clinic . . . basically a lot of stress and hassle and work, and it's all for Duncan—with whom she's pretty angry anyway ("Why can't he just behave at school?!").

Until Mom shares our understanding of why treatment could help, and until some of her very real problems are solved (how *do* you get a kid to appointments without losing your job?), we can't begin treatment. Or, more to the point, addressing these issues *is* the way to begin treatment.

As noted previously, before a family will participate in treatment, two key conditions must be met:

1. The family and the therapist must "agree on the problem." This means that the family and therapist identify an important source of pain for the family that will be addressed in treatment.

2. The family and the therapist must "agree on the solution." This means that the family and the therapist must believe that, should they engage in treatment, then it is likely that this source of pain will be relieved.

Given the considerable barriers to treatment encountered by families such as Duncan's, it is very hard (perhaps impossible) to engage them in treatment until the above two conditions are met. This chapter focuses on meeting these two conditions. The way in which the therapist and family work toward agreeing on the problem and solution constitutes the process of forming a treatment alliance.

Goals of Ready–Set–Go

The basic goal of the ready–set–go module is simple: Engage the family in treatment. More specifically, accomplish the following:

1. Establish a treatment alliance with the family.
2. Educate and provide information about trauma and TST.
3. Troubleshoot practical barriers to families accessing treatment.

In short, this module is intended to put the team's ideas about the problems and solutions into a useable framework for the family.

Each of these specific goals, along with ideas about how to accomplish them, are detailed in this chapter. These goals and ideas completely line up with our treatment planning process, described in Chapter 8.

Ready–Set–Go: The Bridge between Treatment Planning and Treatment Doing

The ready–set–go module can be seen as a bridge that takes the team's ideas about what is needed and transforms them into a series of effective interventions. We ended Chapter 8 with the process of completing the TST Treatment Planning Form. This document identifies the priority problems that the team must work toward solving. As noted in Chapter 8, these priority problems must focus on the patterns of links between environmental stressors and episodes of emotional/behavioral dysregulation. The Treatment Planning Form records the team's ideas about solutions to the priority problems. The presentation of these problems and solutions at the "family collaborative meeting" is the preliminary treatment plan. The treatment plan is only considered final when the problems and solutions are agreed upon by the team and family. This process involves a lot of discussion about the families' perspectives on the problems and solutions. An important milestone for this discussion is the family collaborative meeting, which marks the start of the ready–set–go module. This meeting is our chance to begin this discussion with everyone in the room (especially the family).

The Family Collaborative Meeting (FCM)

The family collaborative meeting (FCM), as we described, is the occasion when the treatment team shares with the family its initial ideas about the problems and solutions. After the assessment is completed (usually after two sessions with the child and family), the team completes the TST Treatment Planning Form. A meeting is then set with the family (the FCM), and everyone involved in the child and family's treatment is expected to attend: the child, the parent, the clinicians. It also includes the psychiatric consultant and the legal advocate if they will be involved in treatment. The FCM can include other family members and other supportive adults. It should be introduced at the very beginning of treatment—when a clinician first meets a family.

There is an art to conducting the FCM. The family's *and* the team's perspectives should be front and center. In practice a sort of tightrope is walked. If the team dogmatically insists on its perspective on the problems and solutions, the family is unlikely to agree and form a solid treatment alliance. Similarly, if the team does not present a clear perspective, the family will never be sure to what it is agreeing. It is very important for the team to enter this meeting with a clear idea of the problem and its solutions (the preliminary treatment plan) but to be open to changing the plan based on the family's ideas.

During this discussion always remember to present plans that are clear, and based on facts (Principle Three). What will help you keep your balance is to remember that the alliance with the family is always constrained by the alliance with reality (Principle Seven).

In TST, we start talking about the FCM from day 1. When a family comes in and is handed some questionnaires to fill out, one of us says, "We'll be able to look at these scores in the FCM and get a sense of how your child is doing emotionally." When the family talks about an important source of its pain, one of us says, "I'm really glad you brought that up with me. I'm hoping you feel comfortable sharing that at the FCM, too."

In TST we make a big deal of the FCM. Why? Because we think it *is* a big deal. The FCM is the beginning of fixing a broken system (Principle One). It is also a way of communicating accountability with the family. Everyone involved in the care is present and will "sign off" on the Treatment Planning Form. This is an important foundation for Principle Six: Insist on accountability, particularly your own.

It may be necessary to delay the FCM for a little while in order to prepare the family. For reasons that we cannot possibly imagine, families are sometimes intimidated by meetings with rooms full of professionals. Reasons for delaying the FCM include (1) evidence that the family and team see the problem as so different that a "meeting of minds" is unlikely to be possible (align with reality, Principle Nine); (2) an ongoing DSS investigation where it is unclear the role the family will play; or (3) an incapacitation on the part of a key family member that suggests collaborative problem solving is unlikely to be effective (e.g., psychosis, severe depression, substance abuse).

It is important for families to be prepared and for clinicians to do everything possible to minimize surprises during this meeting. The FCM should be conducted as early as possible after the two-session evaluation. Clinical judgment should be used regarding when this meeting should be scheduled.

Accomplishing Ready–Set–Go

As we described, the ready–set–go module has three main goals.

1. Establishing the treatment alliance with the family.
2. Educating and providing information about trauma and the TST treatment.
3. Troubleshooting practical barriers to families' accessing treatment.

We begin to work on these goals with the family as we prepare for the FCM. These goals are pursued following this meeting until they are sufficiently met. We describe each of these goals in turn.

The Treatment Alliance

If there's one element that stretches across all treatment modalities in therapy, it's the alliance. Everyone acknowledges that a clinician has got to have it. How to build it is another matter. Many elements go into building an alliance, and detailing all of them is beyond the scope of this chapter. Instead, we've isolated a few key elements that we think are essential to alliance building in TST and necessary (though probably not sufficient) to the ready–set–go module.

 It is important to understand that the treatment alliance is much more than just "good feelings" between the therapist and family. It is much more than the therapist and family liking each other and wanting to work together (although these should be a natural outcome of forming a solid treatment alliance). The TST perspective of the treatment alliance is very specific: The therapist and family agree on the specific problem that must be addressed *and* they agree to a plan for how to solve this problem. In order for this agreement to occur, the therapist must communicate clearly to the family and with a great deal of respect and genuineness.

> The TST perspective of the treatment alliance is very specific: The therapist and family agree on the specific problem that must be addressed *and* they agree to a plan for how to solve this problem.

For families to be able to do the work that we ask them to do, they need to know upfront specifically what this work will require and that they are being asked to do it by a real person who cares about them and respects them. Anything less will not work.

Agreeing On the Problem

Caregivers bring children to treatment for many different reasons. Sometimes they come because they are worried about their child. Sometimes they come because they are being driven crazy by their child. And sometimes they come because someone else is making them. What the caregivers see as the "problem" might look really different depending on why they are coming for treatment. Is the problem that their child is sad a lot? Or that the furniture in the house keeps getting broken? Or that the Department of Social Services won't get off the family's back?

> You are not likely to get too far if you are heading down the road in search of a solution to a problem that the parent doesn't see, and meanwhile ignoring all the red flags the parent is waving to get help for what he/she sees as the "real" problem.

As a clinician, you will be formulating your own ideas about what the problem is. Whatever it is, you are not likely to get too far if you are heading down the road in search of a solution to a problem that the parent doesn't see, and meanwhile ignoring all the red flags the parent is waving to get help for what he/she sees as the "real" problem. So the first step is to come to some agreement.

Often this isn't as hard as it initially sounds. You don't have to give in and say "OK, OK, social services are the problem! We'll get rid of them!" (Principle Seven: Align with reality). Instead, maybe you can come to this agreement:

"It sounds like you'd really like to have your family back to yourselves—without a lot of outside involvement. So a goal of our work could be to help get things to a place where so many people don't need to be involved. Right now, it seems like Johnnie's sexualized behavior at school is worrying a lot of people, so maybe we can start by thinking about why he does this—and how to help him not do it."

When working toward agreeing on the problem, it's important to find out the answers to these questions:

1. What does the caregiver see as the problem?
2. What does the child see as the problem?
3. What would the caregiver and child like to see change in the family/in their life?

Once you've gotten clear answers to these three questions, you're in a better position to suggest a change that feels true to what each of you thinks is the problem. Generally, it's best if you can agree on a problem that is specific and nonblaming. For example, you might agree that the problem is that being teased at school leads to Susie hitting other classmates and her mom having to leave work to pick her up when she is subsequently suspended. What Susie sees as the problem (being teased) is thus linked to what Mom sees as the problem (leaving work to pick her up), and the whole chain of events can be addressed as part of the same problem.

Sometimes it is hard to reach agreement about the problem right away. Providing parents with more information and education about trauma and how it affects children can be helpful. It is also important to realize that caregivers and children (particularly adolescents) will sometimes not agree on the problem ("You have too many rules!!" . . . "But I never know where you are or who you're with!!"). It is ideal for the clinician, family, and child to agree on the problem and solution, but sometimes this is not possible initially. It is important, however, for the clinician to establish a treatment alliance with both the child and caregivers in which there is at least an agreement with each, respectively, on an important problem to work on and a solution that will help.

Agreeing On the Solution

Agreeing on the problem is a good start, but now you've got to agree on the solution. Let's take Johnnie and his sexualized behavior. What if the parents think the solution is to take Johnnie out of school or to punish him more harshly? They will be highly motivated to do those things. What if the parents think that therapy is useless? They will not be motivated to engage in treatment. Families will be motivated by what they think will help fix their problems.

Part of your task in building
the alliance is to instill hope.

Part of your task in building the alliance is to instill hope in family members that you, and TST, will be able to help them with their problem. Sometimes families seek mental health treatment as a last resort—they've tried everything, and nothing has worked. Will this be any different?

Hope can be offered to families in different ways. Of course, no one can predict the future of any given child. But we *do* know a lot about kids generally and how they can recover from trauma. We know that, with enough time and energy and support, treatment really works! Part of the education you provide to parents about TST will help ignite this hope.

Once parents have a sense of hope that you and TST may be able to do something to help, you can get more specific about *how* you will be working together to fix things. Parents need to know, and agree up front, what goes into the treatment. If SOS will be involved, spend some time talking with the parent about how it might help. If you are making a psychopharmacology referral, share your rationale and learn what the parents' attitude(s) toward medication is/are.

As you and the parents talk
about how treatment can help,
spend some time talking with
them about why consistency
matters.

Finally, no matter which phase of treatment you will be starting in, *consistency* is critical. As you and the parents talk about how treatment can help, spend some time talking with them about why consistency matters. It's not just that three missed appointments results in a case-closed letter—it's that three missed appointments can really set a kid back from the (admittedly slow) process of learning and healing.

Don't Forget to Be Genuine!

Above all, don't forget that you're a real person meeting with real people. It can be easy to get trapped in a maze of goals, flow sheets, terminology, bulleted do's and don'ts, and academic arcanity. (We know, because we've included a bunch in this book!) But if, after the day is done, family members don't feel that you were a real person who saw them as real people, then forget it. Forget all the bulleted do's and don'ts, etc., because the family won't come back. And they *shouldn't* come back.

On the other hand, if you can really listen and convey respect for family members, you've just wildly increased your chances that they will respect *you* and the work you are trying to do. There well may be difficult times in treatment when it seems as if no progress were being made, and having a trusting relationship can help you and the family hang in there through those times.

Being genuine is the start of communicating to the family that you are a trustworthy person. This type of communication is extremely important but, in practice, can be very difficult because of the degree to which it can be tested. We discuss the critical issue of trust in detail in Chapter 5. The issue of trust is contained in Principle Six: Insist on accountability, particularly your own. The building of trust requires very close attention to accountability; doing what you say you will do and accepting your lumps when you fail is as important a part of the work as anything.

> The building of trust requires very close attention to accountability; doing what you say you will do and accepting your lumps when you fail is as important a part of the work as anything.

Providing Education and Information

The ready–set–go module is a time to find out what a family knows about trauma, the effects of trauma, and what to expect from TST. Chances are there will be at least a few, if not many, gaps in the family's knowledge of these areas. After all, it's *your* job to know all that stuff. But it's also your job to share that knowledge with family members so that they can be empowered to understand what's going on with, and what will help, their kid.

The following basic areas of psychoeducation should be covered:

1. How trauma can affect a child's emotional nervous system.
2. How the social environment can help/hinder a child's emotional regulation.
3. What TST looks like.

These three areas are covered in detail in prior chapters of this book. But even though we think Chapters 1–5 are great, we don't think parents should have to read them. Below is the "CliffsNotes" version of what you might want to share with parents.

1. Trauma affects a child's ability to regulate emotions.
   - Sometimes emotional responses can feel more intense, and be harder to regulate, for kids who have been traumatized.
   - Sometimes their behaviors are attempts to handle these intense feelings, and they need help learning other ways of handling these feelings.

2. The social environment is a big part of what leads kids to have these intense emotions.

- Traumatic reminders can quickly catapult the child into a different emotional state, wherein emotions are more intense and harder to manage.
- Traumatic reminders can lead to changes in how a child feels, acts, and relates to the world.

3. TST helps by simultaneously giving kids and families better ways to regulate emotions, as well as decreasing traumatic reminders in the social environment. TST involves a whole treatment team (including the family) working together and really committing to helping the child.

As parents learn more about how trauma affects kids and what they can do to help, they are likely to feel more empowered. Have you ever heard a parent say "I don't know what happens—it's like somebody flips a switch and then suddenly Gregory is out of control!" As parents begin to get a sense of how and why traumatic reminders "flip the switch," this kind of behavior will feel less "out of the blue" and more predictable. And once something is predictable, you're on your way to preempting it or at least being able to prepare for it. As a parent, that feels better already.

 Let's think about Duncan's mom for a minute. She's talked about Duncan being "difficult to handle." She's also talked about some traumatic events in his life, such as witnessing violence. Is she connecting these two areas? If not, it would be helpful to educate her about how trauma affects kids. She has mentioned a lot of life stressors that might be exacerbating the situation. We know that she's aware of how being financially stressed has made her feel overwhelmed, but is she aware of how that home-based reality is affecting Duncan? And what about Mom being less available because she has to work—did his social environment just get less supportive, and is this diminishment of support affecting his ability to regulate emotions? If Mom begins to see the connections between trauma, the social environment, and Duncan's behavior, she might react differently. She may be less angry at Duncan and blame him less. She may feel that there are concrete things she can do to help her son. In brief, she may be able to become Duncan's ally in helping their family to survive and move beyond the trauma.

Troubleshooting Practical Barriers

No matter how committed a family may be to treatment, very real barriers can still impede their engagement. If we, as helpers, don't recognize and deal with these real-life barriers, then we send a message that we don't really care. Not only that, but we lose our shot at providing good, consistent treatment to the family.

We can't solve all of the barriers, but we *can* find out what they are and brainstorm with the family about how to solve them. Or we can make compromises in our own ways of doing things to make it easier for the family.

We can't solve all of the barriers, but we *can* find out what they are and brainstorm with the family about how to solve them.

We talk about specific situations here. Solutions will vary depending on the resources of your agency, the family, and the community. The key is to pick up at least part of the responsibility of recognizing, and trying to diminish, barriers to treatment.

Transportation:

"I'd love to have my kid in treatment, but how do I get her there?"

Good question, and the answer is not as simple as "Go straight down Massachusetts Avenue and left at the light." Cars and public transportation take money. A single parent with three kids might have to take *everyone* to the appointment. Throw in the fact that Susie's school is on the other side of town, and you've got a real pickle. What to do?

- Ask the parent if he/she has a way to get here; acknowledge the problem if there is one.
- Brainstorm about other transportation. Has he/she tried public transit? Will the school bus drop the child off at the clinic? Is there a godfather, or someone else, invested in the child's care who could help?
- Identify any related barriers such as finances or social phobia. If the family doesn't have money for public transit, can you initiate advocacy to get the family more financial resources? If social phobia is preventing the parent from bringing the child, work on getting treatment for the parent.
- Consider other modalities/locations of treatment. Could your clinic do home-based individual therapy? School-based?

Scheduling:

"I have to be at work until 5:00, so there's no way to get here in time."

Sometimes scheduling conflicts are a reflection of the fact that other matters hold higher priority than treatment. If you find that the child's favorite TV program is bumping therapy from the schedule, it might be time to revisit "agreeing on the solution" in the first part of this chapter. But scheduling conflicts are often very real.

Let's take Duncan's case again. Mom is working hard to make ends meet so that they can be independent from the abusive father. This is obviously an important goal. And it could very well be true that if she left work early once a week to take Duncan to therapy, she would lose her job. This scenario would be bad for everyone involved. So what can you do?

- Examine your appointment hours. Could you shift your schedule a half hour later to accommodate the family? Is there a better day of the week for them? Demonstrating a little flexibility is a big gesture and a big help at times. (On the other hand, being late for your *own* child-care commitments or coming in on a Saturday could quickly lead to resentment, so be careful that you don't make concessions that are going to tax you.)

- Brainstorm with the parent for other people in the child's life who might be able to help. Could Grandma Jane bring Duncan to therapy some days? Is Grandma Jane willing to be a part of the treatment team?

- Try to double-up appointments. If the child needs to come for psychopharmacology appointments and therapy appointments, and Mom needs to meet with a legal advocate, that's a lot of meetings! One trip with back-to-back meetings cuts down on the time for the family.

- Encourage creative problem solving. Could Mom go to work early on Thursdays so that she could leave early? Does Mom feel comfortable talking to the boss so that he/she is aware of the situation and doesn't penalize Mom for leaving early on appointment days?

- Initiate advocacy so that the parent can fulfill his/her obligation to care for the child. The Family Medical Leave Act protects a parent from being fired if a child is in serious need of care, such that a parent needs to be able to go to multiple appointments during the week and/or provide constant supervision.

Child Care:

"That's great that you'll meet with Jan, but what should I do with the rest of the Brady Bunch?"

This is a thorny problem, particularly if you want the parent to be involved in the treatment. We've seen our waiting room ripped to shreds by siblings while the mother is in the room with the therapist and the child. Some suggestions:

- Initiate a volunteer program or glom onto an existing volunteer agency and get someone to staff your busiest waiting room hours.

- Brainstorm other community resources or family members who could help.

- Schedule appointments at a time when some of the kids are in after-school programs, or Dad is home, or . . .

Language:

"¡Estoy tan contento finalmente haber encontrado alguien que entiende realmente!"

Huh? Now try saying "The declarative memory system is largely mediated by the hippocampus. . . . "

We are an incredibly diverse country, with the proportion of non-English speakers increasing daily. Immigrants and refugees are, or are going to be, part of the clientele we serve no matter where we are and which languages we do (or don't) speak. So what do you do if the parent, child, or both don't speak the same language as you do? Some suggestions:

- Work toward system-wide change in your clinic; advocate for the hiring of multilingual staff.
- Build partnerships with community agencies who *do* provide some types of services in different languages.
- Work with an interpreter. *Don't* use the child as the interpreter. In a pinch, you can use a nationwide phone interpreter system.
- Remember that body language is very communicative. Maybe you didn't learn until the first appointment that the family only speaks Somali. Even though you can't get a translator on such short notice, you can still communicate respect and caring for the family. Make eye contact, speak sincerely, and then do everything possible to get an interpreter there for the next session.

Parent Limitations:

"Sure I'll bring Tony to treatment (unless, of course, it means I have to leave the house)."

Trauma often affects a whole family. Parents may themselves have significant mental health needs or other problems that make it difficult for them to follow through with treatment for their child—despite their best intentions. Parental PTSD might lead to avoidance of talking about past traumas—and, naturally, avoidance of their child's appointment. Drug or alcohol use might render the parent incapable of getting the child to appointments. Depression might affect a parent so deeply that he/she doesn't get out of bed. Cognitive limitations or disorganization might lead to habitual forgetting of the appointment.

All of these problems not only prevent the child from getting treatment but also contribute to a distressed social environment. In short, they are *big red flags* that the family really does need help. Some suggestions:

- Work to get the parent into his/her own treatment.
- Try to have the parent see you as a source of support, not as someone who is critical and shaming because Mom or Dad is (yet again) failing his/her child.
- Consider SOS as a way to get treatment started for a family who can't make it to the office.

Stigma of Mental Health Services:

"I don't want my child to be branded as a nuts-o!"

The stigmatization of mental illness is an unfortunately prevalent phenomenon. Find out if the family is worried about this and do your best, via psychoeducation, to whittle away at the myth that receiving mental health services means that you're crazy, weak, or otherwise less than someone else.

Fear of Social Services:

"If I bring my child here, you're just going to file a report to the Social Services Agency. I don't want anything to do with you."

This barrier would be a lot easier to handle if we could just say "No, I promise, I won't file!" But we can't. We're mandated reporters. And we have a duty to protect kids.

But we can do a lot to help parents understand exactly when and why we would report child abuse to the authorities. And if we have to make a report, we can do our best to work *with* the parents while doing it. You can certainly emphasize the strengths—"The family is engaging in treatment, is here with me in the office, and we agreed to call this in together. The mom is open to support around parenting. . . . " And hopefully, if social services gets involved, you can bring them into the treatment team so that they are part of the integrated system of care under TST.

Using the TST Treatment Planning Form to Accomplish the Goals of Ready–Set–Go

The basic format of the TST Treatment Planning Form provides a more detailed analysis of the problems and solutions and gives a clear description of who is accountable for what. We use this form to guide discussion at the FCM and subsequent meetings with the family, to get a close-enough agreement on the problems and solutions before moving to the *go* stage. As is described below, even then the Treatment Planning Form continues to guide treatment by making very clear and concrete what the treatment is all about.

The detail of how this form should be completed is given in Chapter 8 and the form appears in the Appendix. The most important areas are the clear statement of the TST Priority Problems (section 5a) and the recommended solutions (section 6). In order to maximize the likelihood of forming an agreement, the following guidelines should be used:

1. Identify the TST priority problems and their solutions clearly and simply. Use language that you think the family will understand and accept.

2. Be clear but not dogmatic. Step back when you see that the family either does not understand or strongly disagrees with what you have written.

3. Listen carefully to what the family members want. Do everything you can to integrate what is most important to them in the Treatment Planning Form.

4. If you are convinced by the family that you have missed something, modify the problems or solutions accordingly.

5. If you are not convinced by the family that you have missed something, modify your approach to the discussion of the problems or solutions. As we described in the treatment alliance section (pp. 157–161), make sure that the problem is described in a way that addresses something the family is highly motivated to change (i.e., addresses their pain).

6. Once agreements are reached, get signatures from all the players and make copies of the form for all members on the team (especially the family).

7. Take out the TST Treatment Planning Form at all subsequent encounters during treatment to "check in" about progress on priority problems. Use this discussion to get information on whether each member of the team is doing what he/she has agreed to do.

8. Give family members a lot of credit for doing what they have agreed to do.

9. When family members have not done what they agreed to do, the reasons must be discussed and understood. There may be many reasons why a family has not done what was agreed. Each reason requires a different clinical approach. Some of the common reasons are detailed below:

   a. **The family did not really understand what you meant by the problem and solution.** Families express agreement for many reasons other than that they really agree. Has the family really understood what you were talking about? If family members are not doing what they said they would do, it is important to recheck whether they understood. If there are important misunderstandings, simpler language must be used. More psychoeducation can also help.

b. **The family really disagreed about the problem or solution.** Did family members say yes so that you would get off their back? Did they say yes because they were afraid to say no? Any time a family is not following through on agreements, this possibility must be rechecked and, possibly, renegotiated.

c. **There is a practical barrier interfering with following through on agreements.** Perhaps the family understands and agrees but did not sufficiently anticipate such things as scheduling or transportation barriers. This area should be rechecked.

d. **The family believes that you have not kept your agreements.** Have you? Please check!!

What if you can't agree?? There are times when the clinician and the family just don't agree on what the treatment priority should be. For instance, Mom may not see herself as depressed or may not think that her depression affects her kids. In this situation, clinicians should do their best, using psychoeducation, to help Mom see why they think something is a priority for treatment. When you just can't reach agreement, it might be necessary to acknowledge differences and strike a compromise.

> When you just can't reach agreement, it might be necessary to acknowledge differences and strike a compromise.

"It seems like we see things a little differently—you see that living in a cramped house is really making it hard for you to take care of your kids the way you want to, and I see that some of your sadness might be adding to this difficulty. You know, it could be that we're both right. It seems like, given how important it is to get Denise some help right now, we should go down all roads. How about we agree to try both things—I'll start working on advocating for housing, and you agree to talk to a therapist about some of the sadness and sleeplessness you've been experiencing."

How Do You Know When You Are Ready for the "Go"?

Ready–set–go is a critical module with which every family starts, no matter what the phase of treatment. Because families are going to enter treatment with different bases of knowledge, histories of treatment experience, and expectations, this module is highly individualized. Some families are ready to go after day 1, other families will need a lot more time. So how do you know when a family is ready to move out of the starting blocks?

Family members are ready to move on from the ready–set–go module when:

- They show behaviorally that they are ready by attending appointments regularly.
- There is a general agreement on the problem and solution (the beginnings of a treatment alliance).
- They have a basic working knowledge of how trauma affects kids.
- They are familiar with how TST works and what their involvement in TST will look like.

Even after they've moved on to other modules of treatment, there may be times when they need a "booster" session of ready–set–go. Maybe a new barrier emerges, maybe their hope begins to flag, maybe they enter a new phase of treatment with which they are unfamiliar. If a family seems to be disengaging from treatment in some way, take a session or two to troubleshoot problems and boost motivation. Sometimes another FCM can help to pull the team back on track.

The work done during the ready–set–go module lays the foundation for all the modules to come. If you've succeeded at this stage, you've just made the rest of your job easier.

Stabilization on Site

Community-Based Care to Help Kids Stay in Their Homes and Schools

---

LEARNING OBJECTIVES

- To help stabilize the family so that a child may stay safely in the home
- To increase the family's ability to support the child's emotion regulation
- To stabilize the environment through advocacy and parenting support

---

Stabilization on site, or SOS, involves intensive home-based and school-based services that focus on directly diminishing the sources of stress and traumatic reminders within the child's day-to-day environment. SOS is appropriate for children who are experiencing acute emotion dysregulation and environmental instability—for example, children in families who are in the surviving or stabilizing phase of treatment. SOS can serve as hospital diversion, can be brought in at critical junctures to help stabilize a family, and provides in-the-moment assistance for emotional and environmental crises. SOS frequently is initiated at the beginning of treatment but may also be brought into the treatment plan when a family in ongoing treatment experiences new problems or crises that threaten the stability of the home.

Isn't It Just Therapy in the Home?

Although SOS shares many elements common to office-based therapy, there are some important differences. No matter how egalitarian a therapist makes an office-visit session, it is still taking place in the *therapist's* office. That location

---

We would like to acknowledge the contributions of the following people in the development and writing of this chapter: Carolyn MacDuffee Chapman, Theresa Cain, Kendra Johnson, Joel Goldstein, and Tom Faxton from the Home for Little Wanderers, Boston.

170

Home therapy – families in charge [handwritten annotation]

automatically puts the therapist in charge. And the other side of the coin is that no matter how much a therapist knows, when he/she shows up in a family's home, the *family* is in charge. This can be a really wonderful part of SOS. Family members may feel more involved and invested in treatment that happens in their home. They may take more responsibility for making changes. They may also throw you some curveballs, such as watching TV while you try to talk, or inviting a neighbor to join the session. All of these eventualities set SOS apart from office-based therapy.

SOS creates a lot of opportunities that don't exist in office-based therapy. Clinicians can see what a home looks like and assess safety and triggers in a way that office-based therapists can't. SOS clinicians learn a lot about how a family functions just by seeing it in action. They often are able to attend school meetings or go with a family to the public housing office.

> Clinicians can see what a home looks like and assess safety and triggers in a way that office-based therapists can't.

SOS also creates a lot of challenges. What do you do if the neighbor's child is over to play? What if the phone keeps ringing? What if you hear a gunshot as you are driving to a home visit and find yourself feeling really scared? Part of SOS is learning how to make sure that treatment is moving forward even when unexpected and unpredicted events happen. SOS isn't just therapy in the home. It's being willing to enter a family's world for a little bit of time. Learning how to take advantage of some of the opportunities this presents *and* avoid the pitfalls is the subject of this chapter.

When Is SOS Appropriate?

Three factors must be considered before implementing SOS:

1. Safety of the environment for the clinicians implementing SOS.
2. Immediate safety of the environment for the child.
3. Willingness of the family to engage in home-based services.

If each of these criteria is met, then proceed with identifying children who are experiencing acute problems with emotion regulation and environmental stability (kids in the surviving or stabilizing phase of treatment) as good candidates for SOS treatment.

Safety of the Environment for the SOS Team

Unfortunately, some of the same environmental reasons that make it unsafe for a child to be in the home also create an environment that is not safe for service providers to make home visits. For instance, if a gang-involved family has been threatened, visiting the home may place the clinician in jeopardy. Similarly, if a clinician has been involved in supporting a mother who called the police on an abusive partner, the clinician may become a target for the abusive partner's anger. In these situations, the clinician implementing SOS may meet with the family in a clinic or elsewhere in the community. Initiating advocacy to help the family achieve safer living conditions may be the most important step.

Immediate Safety of the Environment for the Child

If there is ongoing abuse or domestic violence in the home, SOS is not appropriate. The state social service authorities must be informed and immediate steps taken to provide the child with a safe environment. In this circumstance, the clinician's role is to advocate for the child with the social service authorities to ensure that he/she goes to a safe place. This action follows Principle Two: Put safety first.

In some states, child protective services use home-visit teams to help families who are having trouble providing appropriate care for their children. In these situations, SOS can work with the family and social services to help create a safe home to which a child can return.

Willingness of the Family to Engage in Home-Based Services

Home-based services require the active participation of family members. Having clinicians visit the home several times a week can feel threatening or invasive to some families. Some families may feel that the problem is the child's rather than a family issue. In this situation, the individual clinician can work with family members to understand their concerns and see if these can be addressed. If the family prefers not to have someone come to the home, then meetings could occur in a clinic setting. If the family perceives the problem to involve the child alone and not the wider context of the family, then continued work on framing the problem, as reviewed in the ready–set–go module, would be indicated.

 Another common problem is that families feel overwhelmed with services, in general. Why would they want another provider? If, in fact, SOS is just added on top of other services, this problem is very real. On the other hand, if SOS care is woven into other systems of care—through careful communication and integration with individual therapy, social services, etc.—then the involvement of SOS will actually speed a family toward needing *fewer* providers in their lives.

If SOS care is woven into other systems of care—through careful communication and integration with individual therapy, social services, etc.—then the involvement of SOS will actually speed a family toward needing *fewer* providers in their lives.

The clinician's job is to help family members understand why such intensive home-based interventions are recommended and what they can potentially gain from these services. This is partially a matter of building a treatment alliance with the family so that everyone agrees on what the problem is and how to fix it. It may be helpful to let families know that most families really like SOS services and find them more helpful and convenient than anything else.

Typically, the primary clinician introduces the idea of SOS to a family. This idea should be presented early in the assessment process, as soon as there is sufficient information to suggest that the child is in the surviving or stabilizing phase of treatment and that SOS is, accordingly, indicated. The first meeting between the SOS clinicians and the family can occur as part of the family collaborative meeting (FCM). As we described in Chapter 8, treatment planning and the FCM provide an opportunity to:

1. Agree on the priority problems.
2. Agree on the solutions.
3. Determine who is accountable for what.

This can be an important time to come to a preliminary agreement about what, exactly, the SOS clinicians will do. Because being in the home often leads SOS clinicians to learn important information that can impact treatment planning, the treatment plan often needs to be revised based on this new information.

Treatment Structure

SOS treatment typically lasts from 3 to 4 months. Initially, treatment is more intensive (two or three times/week). Over time, the frequency of visits decreases to once a week. Throughout this period, an emergency SOS clinician is always available by phone or pager so that families can receive verbal assistance during crises. Treatment usually occurs in the home, unless safety or family preferences indicate otherwise. For safety reasons, an SOS visit usually involves two clinicians.

Assessment Phase

When SOS is initiated, there's usually at least a little information about the problem at hand or the treatment goals. But chances are there's no information about what the family's living room is like. OK, so maybe it doesn't really matter how the family has decorated. But what *does* matter are the subtleties of how a family works. Who is in the living room? Is the TV on, and if so, why?

Does it help calm the kids, or is it distracting everyone and making them talk louder? Is this a smoking house? Is it important to let Mom self-soothe in meetings by smoking, or is drug use one of the problems you are addressing—and thinking about reducing cues for using is a good goal? Is the family environment chaotic and noisy and potentially triggering for traumatized kids, or is this just a lively, rambunctious household?

The first three or four visits with a family are a chance for the family to get to know the SOS clinicians a little bit, and for these clinicians to learn what makes the family tick. These visits may not have any specific structure to them—remember, family members are in charge and your job is to take their lead in how they want to let you into their home and lives. During this assessment period, however, your goal is to build on the treatment alliance developed in the FCM by:

1. Agreeing on a problem and discuss how SOS is part of the solution (see the ready–set–go module for more on this area).
2. Agreeing on a way to work together (including the big picture of what you're working on, as well as the little picture of how home visits will, hopefully, run).

The Little Picture: How Home Visits Will, Hopefully, Run

We title this session *how home visits will, hopefully, run* because visiting a family is anything but predictable. You didn't know it was Clarissa's birthday? No problem! You're here just in time for cake. Just put on this party hat. . . .

So when we talk about what sessions should look like, bear in mind that there will be a lot of times when they won't be that way at all. It wouldn't help anyone if you refused to put on a party hat at Clarissa's birthday and instead pointed out that you had a "no eating during session" rule that clearly excluded cake. On the other hand, it wouldn't be all that helpful if you showed up for a session with a haphazard "Oh, maybe we'll get something done—and maybe we won't!" attitude. So we offer a suggested structure for sessions in the hope that it can help steer your interactions toward more predictable, and more productive, work with the family.

Sessions are typically about 1 hour long. Because sessions usually occur in the home, routines that help establish the beginning and end of the session are especially important. Once the family and clinician have agreed on what signals

the beginning and end of a session, it is also important to agree on ground rules for what can occur
during the session time. Is it OK for someone to
answer the phone? Can the radio be on? Who
should be part of the sessions? What happens if a
neighbor drops by?

> Once the family and clinician have agreed on what signals the beginning and end of a session, it is also important to agree on ground rules for what can occur during the session time.

Although it makes a lot of sense for office-based
therapists to start with the rules in the first session, this doesn't necessarily work
in SOS. For one, you are a guest in someone else's home. Imagine your mother-
in-law coming into your home and telling you to turn off your music, stop
eating in the kitchen, and—oh, you need new window treatments, too. Unless
you are a better person than we, you might think twice about being home the
next time she comes to visit.

Starting a session off with ground rules about what family members can and
can't do *in their own home* can feel pretty jarring. Not to say some rules aren't
important—just that part of your job is to figure out which ones are really necessary and hopefully arrive at them *together*.

Home visits from SOS clinicians should help the family feel empowered and in
control of their home, rather than the opposite. This is not to say that the SOS
clinicians must accommodate all of the family's wishes and attempt to conduct
sessions over the blaring radio and while dinner is
being cooked. Rather, by sharing their rationale for
various ground rules (e.g., no TV or radio on during
session), team members can model effective communication and convey the value they place on
being able to hear and focus on what the family has
to say. Topics and ground rules to discuss at the
beginning may include (but are not limited to) the
following:

> By sharing their rationale for various ground rules (e.g., no TV or radio on during session), team members can model effective communication and convey the value they place on being able to hear and focus on what the family has to say.

1. Policies around TV, radio, or other ongoing sources of noise.
2. Which family members attend and whether it is OK for people to be
   home without being involved.
3. Where sessions should take place.
4. Whether there are rooms or times that are "off limits" for the SOS team
   to visit.
5. How to handle telephone calls and doorbells.
6. Whether other activities (e.g., sewing, note taking, playing video games,
   eating, smoking) can take place during a session.

Ground rules should apply to both SOS clinicians and the family. If there need to be exceptions to rules—for example, the SOS team needs to be able to answer emergency phone calls—this should be spelled out in the beginning.

There is no hard-and-fast set of rules that will work for all families. For instance, whereas it might sound reasonable to make a rule that TV must be off for all families, that's not necessarily the case. Take, for example, a situation in which there is a 3-year-old who would be running wild around the room unless he was watching a video. Maybe the video in the corner of the living room is helping people to focus! Or take the example of a mom who has a really tough time tolerating any silence; having the TV off would raise her anxiety through the roof. Of course, you can't know these things when you start working with a family— that's why the first few sessions are designed to let you observe and find out a little bit more about why the family does things the way it does.

A discussion of the ground rules can also be a time to agree on a structure for the sessions. Sessions should include these basic components:

- Settling in
- Checking in
- Problem solving/strength building
- Closing ritual

Just how you structure these different stages of the session can be based on the family's routines. For instance, if you find during the assessment phase that Mom likes to offer everyone something to drink when they first arrive, then pouring coffee and chatting can become the "settling" routine. Maybe the youngest child has a stuffed animal that she brings out to cuddle with on the couch—in this case, asking her to go get the stuffed animal could be the settling signal. You could even use that stuffed animal later to signal who gets to talk by passing it around. *What* the routine is doesn't matter; *that* you develop one does.

A sample session is illustrated in Figure 11.1.

Sessions often require flexibility. For instance, SOS clinicians may happen upon an argument in the family or witness a child's dysregulation during the session. In these instances, maintaining a balance between retaining the structure and responding to the current tenor of the home is necessary. Clinical judgment will determine just where the balance falls. For instance, if SOS clinicians enter the home while the child and parent are screaming at each other, the clinicians will need to quickly assess safety and the feasibility of starting with the usual routine. The "On-the-spot decision tree" (Figure 11.2 on page 181) can be used to help clinicians determine how to handle crisis situations.

10 minutes	**Stage:** Settling time
	Signaled by: Arrival of SOS clinicians
	Activities: Family members get coffee/soda, turn off TV, take phone off hook, call kids in from outside, engage in small talk
20 minutes	**Stage:** Checking in
	Signaled by: Youngest child gets his stuffed parrot
	Activities: Check in about recent events, update Emotion Regulation Guide (described later in this chapter). Pass the stuffed parrot to make sure everyone gets a chance to talk. SOS clinicians assess ongoing safety of home/child.
25 minutes	**Stage:** Active problem solving/strength building
	Signaled by: Intervention section of Emotion Regulation Guide
	Activities: Using Emotion Regulation Guide, SOS clinicians work with family to identify ER strategies or areas of advocacy around home instability.
5 minutes	**Stage:** Closing ritual
	Signaled by: Parrot put away
	Activity: Parallel closing ritual used by individual therapist (e.g., a special handshake) and confirm next appointment.

FIGURE 11.1. Sample within-session structure.

The Big Picture: What You're Working On

Treatment Domains and Goals of SOS

The specific goals of SOS vary depending on the family, but overall the goal of SOS is to stabilize the family so that a child may stay safely in the home. The stability of the home placement may be threatened by the child's dysregulation, environmental instability, or (more commonly) a combination of both.

> The stability of the home placement may be threatened by the child's dysregulation, environmental instability, or (more commonly) a combination of both.

SOS is typically conducted with families under a lot of stress. To engage families, it is extremely important to form a treatment alliance around a clear set of problems that are causing pain for family members. As we discussed in Chapter 10, the child and family must help set and value the treatment goals for such an alliance to form and for treatment to work. For the family to "buy into" the treatment, they must believe two things:

1. If the treatment works, it will relieve a considerable source of pain and distress.
2. Treatment *can* work.

To restate our mantra:

> If there is no alliance, there is no treatment.

SOS during the Surviving Phase

The surviving phase is defined by a child who is behaviorally dysregulated (engaging in potentially dangerous behaviors) and a social environment that is threatening (there is a risk of harm to the child). Obviously treatment in this context is fraught with peril. During this phase, TST clinicians can expect to have a lot of interactions with such professionals as emergency room staff, inpatient psychiatric clinicians, social service workers, and police officers. The situation of a child who is engaging in dangerous behaviors and a home life that poses danger to the child is among the most tenuous of clinical situations, yet this is the situation that mental health clinicians frequently encounter when working with traumatized children. When we call this phase "surviving," we mean it literally.

> When we call this phase "surviving" we mean it literally.

Children engaged in potentially dangerous behaviors must be regularly assessed for safety (e.g., for suicidality, aggressive or sexual impulses toward other children in the family or neighborhood). In this situation, the primary goal of SOS is to assess the risk of harm and, if the child does not need to be assessed in an emergency room, to provide the family with in-the-moment assistance in helping the child to regulate his/her emotions, and to immediately remove triggers and stressors in the home life.

If the home is not a safe environment—that is, an environment that can contain the child's dysregulation and in which there is no threat of harm to the child—then the home placement may be threatened. By being in the home, SOS clinicians are likely to observe many things that people outside the home couldn't know. During the surviving phase of treatment, SOS clinicians need to frequently assess the risk of harm to the child and, if necessary, involve the state social services agency. Obviously there is a risk of disrupting the treatment alliance with a report to the social service agency to investigate abuse or neglect. Nevertheless, if evidence suggests that abuse or neglect is occurring, clinicians must fulfill their professional obligations and report their concerns. In our experience the treatment alliance is disrupted far less than one might expect. Most caregivers who are out of control know, at some level, that they are out of control. Many caregivers with whom we work have their own trauma histories and consequent emotion regulation difficulties. They love their children but have a hard time controlling their own behavior. A professional who

> A professional who stands for safety and the care of their child can be containing for such caregivers by clearly modeling safe and caring behavior.

stands for safety and the care of their child can be containing for such caregivers by clearly modeling safe and caring behavior.

"On-the-Spot" Decision Tree

To help SOS clinicians assess crisis situations, we created an "on-the-spot" decision tree. This tree should also be used in the stabilizing phase. We describe it in the surviving phase because of its utility in crisis.

What it is: A tool to guide clinical judgment about crisis situations in the home.

When to use it: During home visits when a family is in crisis or otherwise unsafe.

Target goals: Maintain safety for SOS clinicians and family.

One of the greatest assets of SOS clinicians is that they are present in the home and can provide intervention when and where dysregulation is most likely to occur. However, this asset also presents the challenge of knowing what to do when they encounter families in moments of crisis. SOS clinicians entering a home in a state of crisis must be able to rapidly assess the situation, evaluate safety, and decide on a course of action. Maintaining too rigid a structure in times of crisis may be ineffective or, at worst, even dangerous. On the other hand, always responding to the crisis by abandoning routine and focusing just on the crisis of the moment can lead to clinicians' being pulled into the family's perpetual crisis state. The on-the-spot decision tree can be used to guide SOS clinicians when they encounter a crisis in the home.

> SOS clinicians entering a home in a state of crisis must be able to rapidly assess the situation, evaluate safety, and decide on a course of action.

The following material describes how this decision tree should be used. It is followed by the "tree" itself (Figure 11.2).

1 The first questions to ask upon arrival at a home are "Is something unusual happening? Does it appear to be a crisis?" If clinicians feel that something is out of the ordinary and the family seems to be in a crisis, the next immediate question is asked: "Is it physically safe for SOS to enter?" If domestic violence is occurring, SOS clinicians should not attempt to intervene directly. If there is any direct threat to clinicians' safety, the team should leave the immediate area and call 911.

> "Is something unusual happening? Does it appear to be a crisis?"

> "Is it physically safe for SOS to enter?"

Assess the family and child's
physical safety.

2 If it is safe to physically enter the home, the next step is to assess the family and child's physical safety. If the child is threatened in some way, clinicians should make every attempt to get the child to safety. This may be through an emergency call to 911 or the social services authority, if it is not possible to intervene directly.

Determine whether the structure
of the therapeutic session should
be implemented or if crisis-
focused intervention is required.

3 If everyone present appears physically safe, the next step of the decision tree is to determine whether the structure of the therapeutic session should be implemented or if crisis-focused intervention is required. Is the family responsive to the SOS clinicians' entry, and are they able to modulate their activity in response to the clinicians' requests? If the entrance of the clinicians provides a break in the crisis activity, then initiating a session may itself become an intervention. The comfort of routine and the reassurance that the current incident of emotion dysregulation has not disrupted everyone and everything can, in itself, provide important calming and perspective. In this instance, the crisis is not ignored—rather, a discussion of the precipitants, emotional responses, and possible interventions fits within the structure of reviewing the Emotion Regulation Guide (explained later in this chapter and in detail in Chapter 14). Indeed, these moments may be especially helpful to the therapy process; children are helped to slow down and identify, in the moment, what they are thinking and feeling.

At times, however, the family is not responsive to the SOS clinicians' attempts to initiate structure. In this case, rather than battle with the family for attention, SOS clinicians can initiate a crisis intervention by asking a parent's permission and then using the Emotion Regulation Guide either to coach the parent or directly model the intervention. By articulating, out loud, their thought processes, the actions of the clinicians can be used to both intervene with the situation and model more constructive behavior for the parent and child. For instance, a clinician might identify, out loud, that the child appears to be feeling really upset, but that he/she is still able to stay in control (thus providing some praise for the child and at the same time, identifying the appropriate phase of the guide to use). The clinician can then point out some of the interventions listed under the "mutual regulation" section of the guide and encourage the parent and/or child to engage in one of them.

Throughout this on-the-spot assessment, SOS clinicians need to communicate with each other about each person's comfort level. Asking the first question, "Is something unusual happening here?" is easy enough to do by having a conversation when standing outside the front door. Once you are in the home, however, nonverbal communication may be very important. One clinician may pick up on a danger the other is not noticing or has a different comfort level with what is going on. If you are new to working together, it is a good idea to spend a little time discussing how you will communicate concern to each other nonverbally. It is also a good general rule to abide by the lower threshold when deciding how safe things are; if one person feels that the situation is high risk, then it is treated as high risk.

It is also a good general rule to abide by the lower threshold when deciding how safe things are; if one person feels that the situation is high risk, then it is treated as high risk.

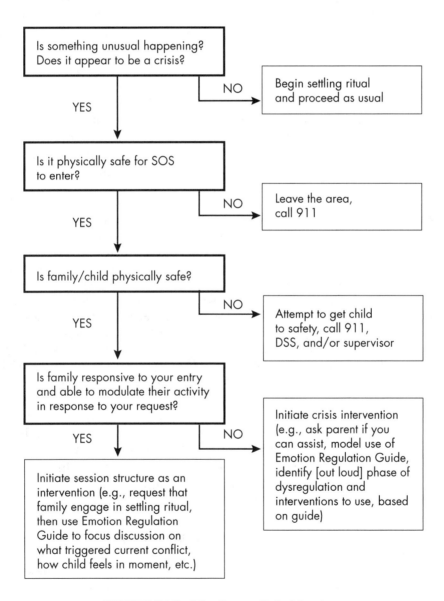

FIGURE 11.2. "On-the-spot" decision tree.

Of course, the process of deescalating the crisis is likely to be much more complicated than simply picking an intervention off the list. The process may require flexibility, trying alternatives, and maintaining patience. For a parent who has struggled with trying to manage his/her child's emotion dysregulation, witnessing a clinician attempt different strategies before successfully helping the child to regulate can be validating and more helpful, in many ways, than seeing a clinician experience instant and seemingly mystical success.

 The goal of a home visit is always to maintain as much routine in the session as possible. Thus, if a family successfully resolves a crisis, the SOS clinicians can initiate the usual routine (using the incident as a springboard for discussing which interventions worked, etc., and revising the Emotion Regulation Guide).

SOS during the Stabilizing Phase

SOS is more commonly conducted during the stabilizing phase of treatment, when there isn't such a risk of the child perpetrating harm or harm being perpetrated on the child. Many of the tools described below can also be used during the surviving phase when the child or family is not in immediate crisis.

 The case of Denise, described in Chapters 3, 7, and 8, continues to be illustrative. Denise's home contains several destabilizing elements; she sleeps on a mattress in the bedroom, where the lack of privacy may contribute to feelings of shame and fear related to the rape. In addition, her brother's drug use and sexually provocative comments further contribute to a home environment in which she may be reminded of, and feel threatened by, sexual trauma. In this situation, SOS would identify these problems and initiate advocacy to move the family to better living conditions where Denise could have a room with a door. SOS may be further involved in working with the family to help them see that the brother's behavior is hurting Denise, and that the brother himself may require treatment. Finally, if financial strain is requiring the mother to hold two jobs and preventing her from being at home to monitor the children, advocacy consultation regarding other financial supports could be helpful.

> Overall the goal of SOS is to stabilize the family by either increasing members' ability to support the child's emotion regulation, increasing the stability of the environment, or a combination of both.

The specific goals of any given situation will vary. However, overall the goal of SOS is to stabilize the family by either increasing members' ability to support the child's emotion regulation, increasing the stability of the environment, or a combination of both. Specifically, SOS identifies elements of the day-to-day environment that trigger a child's dysregulation and eliminate, or at least reduce, these triggers. Home or school—the two places kids spend most of their time—are likely locations of these triggers. SOS can work in either or both of these places to help reduce the likelihood that the child will encounter triggers in the course of the day.

working document (handwritten)

Treatment Tools

 SOS is typically implemented along with other services, including the emotion regulation, services advocacy, and psychopharmacology modules. Close communication and service coordination are critical to treatment success. The Emotion Regulation Guide and the TST treatment plan are two tools designed to help all of the different players communicate: Think of them as paper and electronic versions of the halftime huddle. The treatment plan (described in Chapter 8) plays a key role in guiding overall treatment goals of the SOS clinicians. The Emotion Regulation Guide, the central day-to-day tool for SOS clinicians, is introduced here and further described in Chapter 14.

Emotion Regulation Guide

 What it is: An individualized worksheet that identifies triggers, cues that the child is escalating, and appropriate interventions for various stages of escalation and traumatic states.

When to use it: At the beginning of each SOS session and throughout the SOS module.

Target goals: Child and parent learn to identify triggers and patterns of escalation and are able to intervene early in cycle of dysregulation. Also, to facilitate communication among providers.

The primary treatment tool used in SOS is the Emotion Regulation Guide (ER guide, for short). The ER guide is used in individual emotion regulation treatment as well as by the SOS clinicians. The ER guide is used to help clinicians, child, and family understand triggers, traumatic responses, and effective interventions, and it is also an important communication tool. It's a working document that gets filled out with the family during home visits.

 At the heart of the ER guide is a detailed analysis of what happens when the child becomes dysregulated—what happens right before, how the three A's change during, and what interventions or coping strategies helped to bring the child back to a regulating state afterward. Particularly in the beginning of treatment, families have a hard time observing all of these steps. It seems like a child goes from calm to behaviorally dysregulated with no steps in between. Office-based clinicians can do their best to help families remember what happened, but this approach has its limits. SOS clinicians are uniquely poised to help families observe, in the moment, what is happening. If SOS clinicians are present for episodes of dysreg-

> At the heart of the ER guide is a detailed analysis of what happens when the child becomes dysregulated—what happens right before, how the three A's change during, and what interventions or coping strategies helped to bring the child back to a regulating state afterward.

ulation, they can use their own observations to help the family and child begin to fill out the ER guide. This also gives the SOS clinicians a great opportunity to assess the triggers and, with the family, come up with solutions to minimize them. In essence, the ER guide is to help children and families move from "survival-in-the-moment" responses, as detailed in Chapter 2.

The Halftime Huddle: Communication with Other Providers

Imagine, if you will, an entire football team working toward the common goal of getting the football over that touchdown line. Now imagine that one player is on a playing field in Cambridge, the other is in Dorchester, and a third is only available to play every second Tuesday. So much for the Super Bowl!

Not necessarily. The team just needs to get creative about communication. And so it goes with the TST team. In order to get the most out of all of the collective skills and effort of the team, you need to make sure you are communicating— and when you don't all live and work in the same place (and we hope you don't), you need to get creative about the halftime huddle. The ER guide and the treatment plan can help.

 The ER guide is one of the key day-to-day communication links among the providers. Every provider should always have an updated ER guide. This means that whenever a session is held with the child or family— whether it be an individual office session or home-based SOS clinician meeting—any changes and additions to the guide are immediately communicated to the other clinicians/providers. E-mail attachments (with names removed for confidentiality), saving computerized updates on a common drive, or good old-fashioned hard-copy or fax handoffs can all be used. In addition, the family should always be left with an updated version. For SOS clinicians doing visits in the home, this may mean coming with at least two printed versions of the ER guide (with room to add new information) and handwriting changes on both copies. The family keeps one, and the other is used to update the master computer version.

> Whenever a session is held with the child or family— whether it be an individual office session or home-based SOS clinician meeting—any changes and additions to the guide are immediately communicated to the other clinicians/providers.

Psychopharmacologists, teachers, school counselors, or Department of Social Services (DSS) workers may all find a copy useful (assuming the family consents to its dissemination). Depending on the particular child, it may be helpful to include some of these providers in creating the guide. For instance, a psychopharmacologist may wish to add a section about current medications. Teachers may wish to highlight triggers and/or interventions that are possible in school. The guide can be expanded or adapted in any way that helps consolidate information and streamline treatment.

Similarly, the TST treatment plan is used to keep everyone up to date on the big picture. What is the priority problem again? What was the proposed solution? And who is working on that, anyway? The treatment plan can be passed among providers as a way of keeping everyone updated on progress toward goals, new information or circumstances, and any subsequent changes in treatment planning. Just as with the ER guide, it's important to keep everyone in the loop, including the family, by regularly circulating updated versions.

> The treatment plan can be passed among providers as a way of keeping everyone updated on progress toward goals, new information or circumstances, and any subsequent changes in treatment planning.

In addition, face-to-face meetings are a key component of coordinating care under the TST model. The weekly TST team meeting is used to conference new or urgent cases and is a good place for SOS clinicians to update other team members about their work with a shared case. We also recommend quarterly FCMs. For more acute cases, team meetings may need to occur more frequently.

One additional tool for helping to weave together different systems of care and providers is the closing ritual. A child in early phases of TST may have three or four different appointments with as many providers during a given week: his/her individual clinician, the SOS clinicians, the psychopharmacologist, and so on. Even though treatment goals may be very well coordinated, all of those people still will have very different styles and relationships with the child. The closing ritual is one way of reminding the child that we're all on the same team, working toward the same goal. The closing ritual can be anything that is quick, easy to do, and consistent across all of the different sessions—a handshake, a special way of saying goodbye, a favorite game, a few minutes of listening to music the child brings in. Sometimes this closing ritual can be developed at the end of the FCM as a symbolic kickoff to treatment. Other times it might need to emerge in an individual appointment and then get communicated to the rest of the team.

Terminating SOS: Knowing When to Phase Out

Knowing when to end SOS can be difficult, particularly because SOS is designed to help the family reach a more stable place—but not to continue through to the end of treatment. Thus a family is likely to still be struggling with a child's dysregulation and may feel far from "finished" or ready to say goodbye to the support offered by home-based clinicians. Close coordination with all providers can help communicate to the family that support will continue to be available after SOS services end.

> Can this home environment sufficiently contain this child's emotion dysregulation so that the home placement is not threatened? If the answer is yes, then the child has most likely completed the stabilizing phase.

In assessing whether it is time to terminate this phase, SOS clinicians should consider the initial goals. Ultimately, the question to ask is: Can this home environment sufficiently contain this child's emotion dysregulation so that the home placement is not threatened? If the answer is yes, then the child has most likely completed the stabilizing phase and is ready to begin the enduring phase of treatment. In this case, termination of SOS is appropriate. Ideally, SOS clinicians gradually diminish their in-home work with the family. If things have stabilized, family members may begin to focus their energy elsewhere. Other times, however, the process of ending SOS treatment feels threatening to families who have really benefited from the support, and problems can escalate as clinicians move closer to saying goodbye. Close coordination and communication with the individual therapist is very important in this situation, so that family members continue to feel supported and know that they still have someone to turn to. Ideally, SOS can be presented as an option that can be reengaged down the road if a family needs it—that is, if new environmental instabilities or regulatory problems emerge, creating a more acute clinical situation.

Closing Thoughts on SOS

SOS plays a crucial role in a child's treatment. SOS clinicians typically are involved at the most acute moments of a family's distress, and they engage in intensive services. Ideally, SOS services function as a continuation and intensification of ongoing services—an extra support during the most difficult times. By being in the home, SOS providers gain the important vantage point of seeing the environment in which the child lives. Parents may be too immersed in their own home to step back and see how certain elements of the environment may serve as triggers for the child's traumatic stress symptoms.

Close communication between SOS clinicians and other providers helps embed the services in the ongoing care, so that adding or terminating SOS services is not overly disruptive to treatment. Using consistent language and therapeutic approaches also helps weave the different treatment elements together so that the family feels supported, rather than overwhelmed, by having multiple providers.

Systems Advocacy

Integrating Advocacy into Clinical Treatment

WITH PAMELA TAMES

LEARNING OBJECTIVES

- To consider how families' basic needs impact child health and family stability

---

- To learn how advocacy fits within TST

- To learn how to be an effective advocate

Advocacy is one of the most important tools in TST for addressing instability in the social environment. As described in Chapter 8, systems advocacy is primarily used in the surviving and stabilizing phases of treatment, although it can be used in any phase when it is needed to remediate a key problem in the social environment.

Advocacy can address a family's needs for basic rights and safety, the absence of which may be directly contributing to a child's emotion dysregulation. Not knowing when you will get your next full meal, being scared to sleep because the locks on the door don't work, or being taught a school lesson that you can't understand is bad for any child's development. For most traumatized children, who associate feelings of fear or uncertainty with their trauma, these environmental problems can be toxic to their health. When specific environmental factors contribute to traumatic stress, advocacy for services or benefits to which the

---

Pamela Tames, Esq, is Senior Staff Attorney and Director of Education and Training at the Medical–Legal Partnership for Children (MLPC) at Boston Medical Center.

We would also like to acknowledge the contributions of Ellen Lawton and Amanda Sonis at MLPC in the development and writing of this chapter.

child and family are legally entitled can serve as an effective component of the treatment plan.

We have included a module on systems advocacy in TST for two reasons:

1. Inadequate food, shelter, clothing, and education can specifically contribute to emotion dysregulation and impede recovery in a traumatized child.
2. Some environmental triggers that lead to emotion dysregulation will not change unless the clinical team assumes an advocacy role.

What Is Systems Advocacy?

Advocacy generally means to plead the cause of another. It can be conducted with, or on behalf of, an individual or a group, and can be directed toward a range of targets—for example, a person, organization, administrative agency, legislature—depending on the nature and scope of the goal. In our TST context, *advocacy* means providing assistance to an individual or family to gain access to needed services or benefits programs. Our advocacy goal is to foster the self-empowerment of clients and their families by educating them about their rights and enabling them to secure needed services and benefits. In essence, advocacy is about changing the *trauma system*—ensuring that a family's rights and benefits are in place so that the systems designed to help a child *do* help a child.

> Advocacy is about changing the *trauma system*—ensuring that a family's rights and benefits are in place so that the systems designed to help a child *do* help a child.

In reality, clinicians practice advocacy on behalf of their clients whenever they call a school, refer a patient to a community resource agency, or follow up a medical referral denied by an insurer. Some concrete examples of advocacy interventions in the clinical setting are included in Table 12.1.

TABLE 12.1. Examples of Advocacy Interventions

Basic need	Advocacy intervention
Inadequate food	Encouraging a family that regularly visits a food pantry to appeal a denial of food stamps
Unsanitary housing	Writing a letter to a landlord addressing the impact of abysmal housing conditions on the child's health
Lost income	Writing a letter to the Social Security Administration, in support of Supplemental Security Income eligibility, explaining the severity of a child's mental disorder, the impact it has on his/her functioning, and on the parents' ability to maintain employment

Sometimes clinicians are successful in their efforts to advocate for their patients; other times they are as stymied by complex and fragmented bureaucracies as their patients are. Although clinicians have long sought to identify social or political problems that impact their patients' health, traditional clinical training does not generally offer a thorough understanding of social, legal, and political systems. Nor does it teach how to navigate these respective systems to remedy problems and effect improvement in health.

Figure 12.1 shows 10 domains that affect families.

But that's not the half of it! Multiple agencies may be involved or responsible for providing services and benefits related to any one of the 10 domains. Each agency or entity is governed by a different set of laws, rules, and policies, and the sheer complexity of multiple sets of laws, rules, and policies can deter families from accessing needed benefits and services. The complexity and fragmentation of this public "safety net" is sometimes beyond the grasp of clinicians—let alone traumatized children and their families.

Under TST, these barriers are not seen as a reason for clinicians to abandon advocacy. Rather, the TST model seeks to educate clinicians about how to do advocacy and about how to collaborate closely with professional advocates to provide essential parts of clinical care.

> Under TST, these barriers are not seen as a reason for clinicians to abandon advocacy. Rather, the TST model seeks to educate clinicians about how to do advocacy and about how to collaborate closely with professional advocates to provide essential parts of clinical care.

Lawyers are educated and trained to navigate government bureaucracies, to oppose illegal denials of

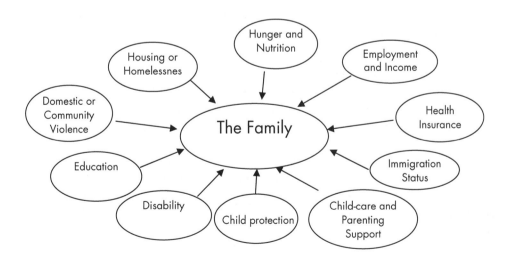

FIGURE 12.1. Domains that affect families.

government benefits and services, and to enforce families' rights to access basic needs. Although many clinicians are familiar with programs, services, and entitlements for which families may be eligible, lawyers are trained to understand the specific application of the law to particular family circumstances. Lawyers are also trained to take steps to recognize rights violations and to hold agencies accountable. Lawyers can serve as professional advocates! As we describe below, lawyers can be included in a TST treatment team at various levels. Depending on funding and availability, a lawyer can be hired to do the following:

1. Train the team on the specifics of families' rights to basic needs and relevant services and benefits and effective advocacy approaches to access these services and benefits.
2. Consult with the team on a given case.
3. Be a full member of the treatment team, providing ongoing consultation and advocacy expertise and helping identify when a referral to a lawyer is required.

 ## The Four-Step Advocacy Assessment and Plan

Under TST, the advocacy module is used when the following circumstances exist:

1. A social-environmental condition is determined to contribute to the child's difficulty in regulating emotional states, *and*
2. This social-environmental condition will not change unless services and/or benefits to which the child/family are entitled are put in place, *and*
3. These services and/or benefits are not in place and barriers exist that diminish the family's likelihood of accessing them, *so*
4. An advocacy plan is developed to maximize the family's likelihood of accessing needed services and benefits.

This four-step assessment and plan should always be used when the need is indicated. Advocacy interventions are most effective when there is specificity about the need that an advocacy approach is meant to address. This four-step advocacy assessment and plan gives clinicians and/or advocates this level of specificity.

The following case illustrates how this four-step assessment and plan can be used.

A grandmother, Sally, is the caregiver of a 12-year-old African American girl, Tanisha, who suffers extreme fear, withdrawal, and avoidance compounded by significant developmental delays, including selective mutism. Sometimes when Tanisha feels very frightened, she becomes severely aggressive. Tanisha endured severe neglect and was exposed to domestic violence while in the custody of her biological mother. After careening through the foster care system for years, at age 11 Tanisha was "temporarily" placed with Sally. Tanisha does not have any other relatives who are willing to care for her. Sally is an elderly but capable caregiver; however, there is some suspicion that she has allowed Tanisha unsupervised visits with her biological mother, possibly because she is unaware of whether she can prevent these visits. Often these visits are followed by increases in Tanisha's anxiety and aggression. Tanisha is enrolled in grade 5 of her local public school. Despite some specialized instruction, Tanisha consistently receives failing or near-failing grades. She was suspended several times for aggressive behavior and was recently put on permanent in-school suspension, such that she was told to simply report to the nurse's office each morning rather than her classroom. Sally does not recall when the school last reevaluated the appropriateness of Tanisha's education placement.

When viewed through an advocacy lens, several different social-environmental issues related to Tanisha's and her grandmother's basic needs and rights become apparent:

- Caregiver's "temporary" custody status
- Caregiver's understanding of her rights and obligations as guardian
- Ongoing exposure of child to an abusive/neglectful parent
- Adequacy and appropriateness of child's school and education
- Protections for child from inappropriate school discipline

Tanisha and her grandmother clearly have advocacy needs. In order to prioritize these issues and to advocacy effectiveness, the four-step advocacy assessment and plan was conducted below:

1. **What are the identified social-environmental issues that contribute to the child's difficulty regulating her emotional states?**

   Visits with biological mother and failure at school contribute to anxiety and aggression.

2. **Are services or benefits to which the family is entitled currently in place to help with these problems?**

   No.

3. **What barriers exist to putting in place appropriate services or benefits?**

   - Grandmother does not know that as a *guardian*, she has certain rights and obligations.

- Grandmother does not know whether or how she can diminish biological *mother's visits*.
- Grandmother does not know that Tanisha is entitled to certain *educational services* that may have a major impact on her functioning in school.

4. **What advocacy steps should be employed to address these barriers?**

   ✓ Educate grandmother about the impact of these environmental conditions on Tanisha's ability to heal.

   ✓ Understand grandmother's objectives regarding placement, educate her about her rights and obligations as guardian, and encourage her to seek permanent placement of Tanisha.

   ✓ Make clear recommendations to the Department of Social Services about permanency of placement.

   ✓ Encourage grandmother to seek supervised visits with mother.

   ✓ Make clear recommendations to the Department of Social Services about supervised visits by mother.

   ✓ Educate grandmother about Tanisha's right to an appropriate public education and protection from school discipline.

   ✓ Make clear recommendations to the school for the formulation of appropriate educational services and behavior plan.

   ✓ Work with grandmother on her own advocacy skills to empower her to be Tanisha's best advocate.

In the systems advocacy module, the clinician needs to be able to (1) recognize these issues, (2) help the family understand the importance of addressing them, and (3) work with the family to prioritize and resolve them. Advocacy can be conducted on many different levels, and it can be provided by different members of the TST team. The complexity of the advocacy issues, the acuity of the problems, the goals and strengths of the client and the family, and the resources of the team all must be weighed in deciding who should advocate, how, and for what reason. The four-step approach can be very helpful in making the advocacy intervention more effective.

Systems Advocacy Case Applications within TST

For families who are having trouble meeting their basic needs, there is good news and bad news. The good news first: To a certain extent, our government recognizes the importance of meeting the basic needs of a child's life and has put into place many federal and state programs to help families meet those needs. These include food stamps and nutrition supports, housing subsidies, homeless shelters and utilities assistance, income and employment supports, family and child protection programs, education, health care, and insurance. Laws governing the private sector—such as landlord–tenant, employment and consumer laws—also seek to prevent harm and protect families. Great! All we need is Uncle Sam on our treatment team, and we should be able to stabilize the environment for all of our families, right?

Now the bad news: it's not that simple. Despite all of these programs and protections, many families continue to live without adequate shelter, food, or safety and many children continue to be deprived of essential education or health care. In short, despite the fact that basic needs are often described as basic *rights* under our current laws and government programs, many obstacles prevent families from accessing these rights. A lack of awareness of programs and rights, intimidation or confusion in the face of bureaucratic barriers, literacy or linguistic impediments, or sheer exhaustion in the face of yet-another stack of forms can all deter families from accessing programs designed to help them. And as if that isn't bad enough, even when families navigate the complicated systems correctly, sometimes agencies or individuals incorrectly apply, or fail to comply with, the laws that are designed to protect families. As a result, families are often deprived of the benefits and services to which they are legally entitled.

> Despite all of these programs and protections, many families continue to live without adequate shelter, food, or safety and many children continue to be deprived of essential education or health care.

 Under TST, all of these barriers are viewed as parts of an environment that influence family stability and a child's ability to heal. They must be addressed as part of the treatment and recovery process. A clinician who works with family members to successfully advocate for changes in their environment empowers the family while helping the child recover.

> Under TST, all of these barriers are viewed as parts of an environment that influence family stability and a child's ability to heal.

In order to further illustrate how advocacy works in TST, we offer two more examples.

 Lara is a 14-year-old girl with a history of sexual abuse. She lives with her mother and eight extended family members in a substandard, three-bedroom apartment that is infested with rats. She reports that she lies awake at night terrified that someone will come into her room and hurt her. Sometimes when she hears the rats moving around, she thinks that it is someone coming after her. She is afraid to go to sleep because "something bad might happen." When she does sleep, she has terrible nightmares of sexual abuse. She is extremely tired during the day and has fallen asleep numerous times in class. Her school grades have dropped significantly.

Lara's housing conditions are creating problems on a number of levels. First, for *any* child, living in overcrowded housing with rats is a problem. For Lara, the rats in the house and the vulnerability of her sleeping situation are *traumatic reminders* that directly contribute to her symptoms. In order to provide effective treatment for Lara, the social environment—in this case, substandard housing—needs to be addressed. The four-step advocacy assessment and plan for Lara, described below, illustrates the case analysis and advocacy intervention.

1. **What is the identified social-environmental problem that contributes to the child's difficulty regulating her emotional states?**

   For Lara, who has been sexually abused, substandard housing and a rat infestation are strong trauma reminders and lead to sleep avoidance and nightmares.

2. **Are services or benefits to which the family is entitled currently in place to help with these problems?**

   No.

3. **What barriers exist to putting in place appropriate services or benefits?**
   - Mother does not know that housing laws prohibit unsanitary conditions.
   - Mother does not know how to advocate for better conditions, how to access alternate housing, or about the housing assistance programs for which her family may be eligible.
   - School does not understand how lack of sleep due to traumatic reminders is influencing daytime behavior and school performance.

4. **What advocacy steps should be employed to address these barriers?**
   - ✓ Educate parents about the impact of the housing conditions on Lara's ability to heal.
   - ✓ Educate mother about the family's housing rights and clarify her objectives regarding housing.
   - ✓ Educate mother about ways of approaching the landlord as well as seeking and financing alternate housing, and encourage her to seek improved conditions or alternative housing.
   - ✓ Work with mother and clinical team to present clear argument to landlord or to housing agency on how housing problem is specifically impacting Lara's health and education, and why improved conditions or alternate housing is essential.
   - ✓ Work with mother and school to address reasons for school difficulties and to discuss remedies for improvement.
   - ✓ Work with mother on her own advocacy skills to empower her to be Lara's best advocate.

Another example of how advocacy works is the case of Michael.

 Michael, an 8-year-old boy with a history of physical abuse by his father, is failing school. His parents are divorced and he lives with his mother. He states that when he is in the classroom, he has a hard time paying attention. There are 30 children in his "regular" classroom, and he often experiences an uncomfortable level of noise and disruption from other students. Michael says that sometimes he thinks he hears his dad yelling at him. Recently, he started refusing to go to school. The school, concerned that he was not passing, conducted psychological testing and found that Michael had normal intelligence and no specific learning disability. Based on these findings, the school stated that Michael could not receive special help at school.

Michael's symptoms of intrusive thoughts and possible auditory hallucinations are impeding his ability to learn in school. The school, not recognizing his mental health problems as a disability, is refusing to provide him with special services. As a result, Michael is missing out on his education—a basic right and need. In this case, helping the school to see the link between traumatic stress and school performance as well as how his current classroom is precipitating traumatic stress symptoms is extremely important. This specific information should be used to advocate for appropriate services. Advocacy could lead to the school's providing Michael with the support and structure he needs to help dampen his flood of traumatic memories and encourage his learning.

1. **What is the identified social-environmental problem that contributes to the child's difficulty regulating his emotional states?**

   Crowded classroom with high level of noise and disorganization. The noise and disruption frequently lead to intrusive memories and auditory hallucinations.

2. **Are services or benefits to which the family is entitled currently in place to help with the problem?**

   No. Michael is in a regular education classroom and is not receiving any special services.

3. **What barriers exist to putting in place appropriate services or benefits?**
   - Mother does not know her son's educational rights.
   - Mother does not know that she can, or how to, contest the school's decision regarding Michael's eligibility for special education or reasonable accommodations.
   - The school does not understand how classroom structure triggers traumatic stress symptoms and consequential poor school performance and has narrowly interpreted the protection of the education law to apply solely to students with disabilities.

4. **What advocacy steps should be employed to address these barriers?**

   ✓ Educate mother about the impact of these environmental conditions on Michael's ability to heal.

   ✓ Understand mother's objectives regarding Michael's schooling, educate her about the protections provided by the education laws to students such as Michael, and encourage her to contest the school's decision.

   ✓ Educate mother about ways of approaching the school and about the resources and information that will help the school reconsider its decision.

   ✓ Work with mother and the clinical team to present a clear argument to school on how the current classroom conditions are specifically impacting Michael's behavior and school performance.

   ✓ Work with school to understand reasons for school difficulties and make clear recommendations about appropriate supports and/or reasonable accommodations.

   ✓ Work with mother on her own advocacy skills to empower her to be Michael's best advocate.

In each of the above examples, barriers to services or benefits—whether with the landlord, government agencies, or the schools—significantly affected the child's mental health and recovery following trauma. In each case the social environment was fraught with traumatic reminders and therefore unable to contain the child's dysregulation. As we have described repeatedly, the effectiveness of individual psychotherapy and psychopharmacology is compromised unless the social environment is addressed. In these cases, an advocacy strategy is necessary to address the social-environmental problems.

How to Advocate under TST

As we have described, advocacy is a critical part of TST. We have defined advocacy and presented the four-step approach to assessing an advocacy problem. We now move to the practical aspects of integrating advocacy into clinical care.

Advocacy under TST can happen at any of several levels. Below we briefly describe these levels, starting with the least resource intensive and ending with the most resource intensive. In accordance with the principle to put scarce resources where they'll work, it is always preferable to use the least resource-heavy method of advocacy that can still be successful.

Support Families to Conduct Their Own Advocacy

Many times families do not advocate for themselves because (1) they don't know what their rights are, (2) they don't know how to advocate for what they need, or (3) they have not identified a particular problem as important enough to advocate for its change. All of these barriers can be addressed by providing the family with information and education about advocacy. Take the example of Lara, above. By providing her mother with information about her right to decent housing, helping her frame her argument to the landlord, and suggesting that she start by writing a letter, Lara's clinician can help the mother take the advocacy steps necessary to make an important change in her daughter's life. Helping parents advocate for themselves uses less TST team resources at the same time that it empowers parents with tools that allow them to continue to advocate for their family long after treatment has ended (remember Principle Ten from Chapter 6: Leave a better system).

Engage in Advocacy on Behalf of a Family

Although it is preferable to have families advocate for their own needs, sometimes it is not practical. Families may not succeed in advocating for themselves if (1) they don't have the necessary skills and can't learn them in time, or (2) they have tried advocating but an agency is just not responding to their efforts. In this case, the clinician will need to step up to the advocacy plate. Sometimes clinicians and a family can advocate simultaneously, making a stronger case for something. Take the example of Michael, above. The clinician helped the family frame its argument about a new classroom placement—but what if the school doesn't respond? A letter by a professional, on professional letterhead, sometimes attracts a little more attention. Parents can be experts on their own child, but as a clinician you can write a letter as an expert about child mental health. This kind of advocacy can be very powerful and is necessary at times to make a system move.

> Families may not succeed in advocating for themselves if (1) they don't have the necessary skills and can't learn them in time, or (2) they have tried advocating but an agency is just not responding to their efforts.

Provide a Referral to a Lawyer

The idea of sorting through immigration laws or arguing with a landlord about tenant rights may seem foreign or intimidating for many clinicians. And, in truth, some advocacy is beyond what a clinician can do—the family needs a lawyer. Knowing what a family's rights are, what you can do as a clinician, and when to refer a family to an expert is essential. If you have identified a central problem in the social environment that is directly contributing to a child's emotion dysregulation and that you don't have the expertise to fix, then a referral needs to be made. In these situations, the client actually

> The clinician's role here is to be very clear with the family and the lawyer about just which issue or problem should be the focus of advocacy. Close communication between clinician, lawyer, and family can help keep boundaries clear and treatment focused.

becomes a client of the lawyer, and the lawyer directly addresses the specific advocacy need of the family. The clinician's role here is to be very clear with the family and the lawyer about just which issue or problem should be the focus of advocacy. Close communication between clinician, lawyer, and family can help keep boundaries clear and treatment focused.

Immigration is a good example of an advocacy need that requires a referral. Take the case of a young boy from Haiti who experienced significant violence in his home country and fled to the United States on a boat. He wakes at night with nightmares and is constantly afraid that he will be sent back to Haiti. Indeed, the whole family is afraid of this and struggling to make it in the United States, as they don't have legal status and can't work. In this situation, the only real way to address the very significant threat in the social environment (being returned to a dangerous country) is to help the family file an asylum petition. Only a lawyer with expertise in this area can do this. Your job, as the child's clinician, is to help the family understand the need for a lawyer and to connect them with resources in the community. Learning about existing advocacy resources in your community and reaching out to appropriate resources are all parts of TST and are conducted as part of this services advocacy module.

Immigration is not the only legal need for which families would benefit from direct legal representation; however, a TST team needs to decide when a referral to a lawyer is both needed and prudent. Principle Eight from Chapter 5 must be considered: Put scarce resources where they'll work. Typically, communities have limited free legal resources. Whatever your arrangement with legal clinics or pro-bono time donations, you will need to carefully consider which cases (1) require a lawyer in order to remediate the social-environmental problem, (2) whether the social-environmental problem is contributing to a child's dysregulation, and (3) whether family members are ready to do their part in working with the lawyer on this particular problem. The third point is what we call "advocacy readiness." Families need to agree on the problem, agree on the solution (the treatment alliance), and be able to do what is required of them to work with the lawyer.

What to Do When Your Clinicians Don't Have Law Degrees

As we have discussed earlier, mental health clinicians rarely receive training in advocacy as part of their preparation to do their work. Yet we feel that advocacy-related is essential knowledge. How do we build that knowledge on a TST team?

There are several ways to go about training a TST team in basic advocacy skills. If you can do all of them, great; if you can do some of them, that will get you started. Every team's access to legal resources is different, so you will need to configure your advocacy training and consultation to reflect your resources. Ultimately, the goals are for team members to be able to the following:

1. Identify when advocacy could help remediate a social-environmental problem.
2. Have a repertoire of basic advocacy techniques.
3. Know when a referral to a lawyer is needed and how to make that referral.

How can these goals be achieved?

Advocacy Training

The clinicians on a TST team should have a working understanding of the basic rights of families protected by law, such as those relating to housing, immigration, food, income, education, child protection, and custody. Clinicians also should be trained in advocacy strategies for helping families ensure that their basic rights are met. Furthermore, clinicians should be aware of community resources and local advocacy organizations, with which they can consult, work, or refer families. Training of the staff in substantive rights, advocacy techniques, and existing resources is important to develop their advocacy skills.

> The clinicians on a TST team should have a working understanding of the basic rights of families protected by law, such as those relating to housing, immigration, food, income, education, child protection, and custody.

A lawyer who specializes in advocacy can provide trainings to TST team members about families' rights to services and about effective approaches to advocacy. By knowing a little bit about these areas, a clinician is better positioned to notice when the family is missing an opportunity to exercise its rights or meet a basic need. Clinicians can then provide advocacy education directly to families, thus empowering them to know, and advocate for, their own rights.

Take the example of a mother who brings her 9-year-old son in for help with his aggression, which has become a problem since he was sexually abused 2 years ago. As the mother is talking, she mentions that her son has been "permanently suspended" and has to stay home because the school says staff is unable to handle his behavior. If the clinician listening to this story has some familiarity with education laws, he/she would most likely hone in on the essential problem in this story: A child with a disability has a right to an education! All students with disabilities are entitled to a free and appropriate public education. Schools are prohibited from excluding students because of their disability. A first step in treatment should be to figure out how to help the family exercise this right. If

All students with disabilities are entitled to a free and appropriate public education. Schools are prohibited from excluding students because of their disability.

the clinician misses this problem and jumps into other elements of treatment with the child, an important chance to set the child on a positive educational trajectory would be missed. And, more than that, even if the specific issue *is* addressed, the larger picture of the child's mental health would be bleak: lost education, social isolation, and a self-esteem blow related to being "kicked out" of school. With appropriate training, a clinician will be able to detect the advocacy opportunity in any parent's story.

Being able to identify a basic need or right in a family's story and providing education about this right is an essential beginning, but knowing *what to do* in the situation demands a step up in knowledge. Let's say you are the clinician in the previous example, and the light bulb has gone on in your head—this child has a right to an education! What now?

Advocacy Consultation

Sometimes simply training the staff is not sufficient for complex service needs. In such cases, recognizing the need to get direct advice from a professional legal advocate can be very helpful in solving the problem.

With case consultation, a lawyer can provide the clinician with a menu of options or a sequence of next steps to address the specific problem at hand. These suggestions may be focused on how the clinician can educate and empower family members to advocate for themselves. For instance, a clinician might be able to suggest to the mother described above that she request an Individualized Education Program from the school by going to such-and-such office and saying such-and-such words. (Often just knowing the terminology can make an enormous difference in families being able to get their needs met!) At other times, a lawyer may suggest actions that the clinician can take—such as writing a letter to so and so, with (again) such-and-such phrasing. Either way, case consultation is a format that is appropriate for service needs that haven't yet been met because of lack of awareness or because of complex, confusing, or intimidating bureaucracy. Often all that is needed to get advocacy on track are a few well-targeted suggestions from a lawyer. Then the next time a clinician faces a similar situation, he/she will be armed with the knowledge of how best to approach the school. By conferencing the case at a team meeting, the knowledge can be transferred to the rest of the team as well.

Advocacy on the Team

If you are able to have a lawyer join TST team meetings, much of the learning about how to do advocacy can be accomplished in your meetings. The attorney becomes an integral part of the TST team. He/she plays a crucial role as an edu-cator of the clinicians and as a member of the TST team. Lawyers can listen to cases with an ear toward whether advocacy can make a difference, they can dis-cuss the best options in constructing the four-step advocacy plan, and they can troubleshoot stalled advocacy efforts and give tips for more successful strategies. The value of the lawyer pointing out these areas to the team is two-fold: Needed services and benefits for clients are identified, and the whole team learns about opportunities and strategies for advocacy intervention. We believe that having a professional legal advocate on the team is important. As will be detailed below, the standard we recommend is the advocate devote 2 hours a week to the team—one hour to be part of the team meeting and the other hour to be avail-able for any consultation calls.

Systems Advocacy Tools

Advocacy Screener

 Clinicians often have so many areas to cover in an intake that asking about basic needs—such as whether a family has enough to eat—gets lost in the shuffle. Families may not mention problems such as poor housing or hunger to the child's therapist because they don't think that the therapist can help or because they are ashamed to bring it up. Yet imagine what it must be like to spend an hour talking with a clinician about how to help your child while thinking the whole time, "Being able to give him dinner would help more than anything else."

The systems advocacy screener in Figure 12.2 (and in the Appendix) is our simple solution to these problems—a basic questionnaire that covers the 10 domains that systems advocacy addresses. We recommend that TST clinicians introduce the advocacy screener in the first session. Discuss the premise that the social environment affects a child's mental health and destigmatize poverty and related issues. Something as simple as "Before we finish up today, I'd like to spend a little time asking some questions about needs your family may have. We do this with all the families who come to our clinic, because we find that often a lot of the problems of daily life—such as just trying to make ends meet—can really affect everyone in the family. So part of my job in trying to help with Lola's behavior is to think about how we might be able to help with some of the problems of daily life."

TST Treatment Planning Form

 The TST Treatment Planning Form, introduced in Chapter 8, can help families and clinicians discuss and prioritize areas of intervention in the social environment. Legal advocacy should be done in the service

Systems Advocacy Screener	
Economic and income support	Do you ever have problems making ends meet?
Housing	Are you concerned about conditions, safety, or overcrowding at home?
Hunger	Do you ever have difficulty getting food for your family?
Child-care vouchers	Do you need, or are you eligible for, assistance paying for child care?
Education	Do you have any concerns about your child's learning or education?
Family law	Do you have questions about paternity, custody, or visitation? Have you ever had to file a restraining order?
Disability	Does your child have a disability that interferes with school performance or your work, home, or family life?
Immigration	Were you or your children born in a foreign country?

FIGURE 12.2. Systems Advocacy Screener.

of addressing a *priority problem.* Determining which priority problems require advocacy can be done by walking through the four-step advocacy plan. Once it has been determined that, indeed . . .

1. A social-environmental condition is contributing to the child's difficulty in regulating emotional states, *and*
2. This social-environmental condition will not change unless services and/ or benefits to which the child/family is entitled are put in place, *and*
3. These services and/or benefits are not in place and barriers exist that diminish the family's likelihood of accessing them, then . . .

A systems advocacy plan is developed to maximize the family's likelihood of accessing needed services and benefits. This advocacy plan is included as part of the TST Treatment Planning Form. It should specify (1) the priority problem to be addressed, (2) the advocacy solution to address it, and (3) what is expected of which treatment team members.

Tips . . . Tips . . . Tips

1. **Be specific!** To help a family receive what they need, and are entitled to, an explicit request to a specific agency or organization must be made. Your statement should expressly link the service or benefit need to the identified traumatic stress problem. Be methodical and data driven. Lay out the facts, as you have assessed them, and

explain the prognosis of the child should he/she receive, or not receive, the needed service.

2. **Don't give up.** If you are convinced that a family is entitled to a service or benefit that is essential to its recovery from traumatic stress, do not take "no" for an answer. Go to the supervisor of the person who said "no," and the supervisor's supervisor. Use your supervisor (and your supervisor's supervisor). Don't be afraid to be persistent. A negative answer may be wrong. You must persist if it is to be corrected.

3. **Clinicians and lawyers must be viewed as teammates.** Each brings critical skills to the table. Teach each other. Learn from each other. In order to advocate well, you *must* work together.

4. **Make sure that you know your stuff.** If you put your advocacy hat on and engage a service system to provide for your client, make sure that you truly do know the laws and entitlements. Speak the language of the agency or organization that you are calling. If you are not sure, ask your lawyer colleague.

5. **Always consider the policy implications of the work.** If you are advocating for a child, it is quite possible that you are working on a service need experienced by many similar children. Be aware of patterns of advocacy needs and advocate more broadly for change if you find the same problem emerge on the team again and again.

Developing Advocacy Resources for Your Clinic

If you work in a community mental health clinic (or just about any type of mental health clinic), right about now you are probably saying to yourself "Yeah, right, sounds nice—but just where are we supposed to find the money to hire a lawyer?"

Unfortunately, at present our systems of care do not recognize the role of lawyers in providing mental health treatment to traumatized children and their families. Until that happens, we need to be creative about how to fund advocacy.

Following are a few suggestions of ways to develop advocacy resources in your clinic. Each of them has its pluses and minuses, and we offer them as examples of ways to build on existing systems of care in providing the services that traumatized children and their families need and deserve. Again, the standard we recommend is 2 hours a week—one for the team meeting and one for as-needed phone calls.

Collaboration with Legal Service Programs

Legal services programs are federally and locally funded nonprofit organizations that provide free civil legal assistance to low-income individuals and families. Some legal services programs provide primarily advice and other limited forms of assistance so that they can serve large numbers of people who need their help. Other programs provide more extensive assistance to smaller numbers of clients. At least one program serves virtually every town, county, or city in the United States. The following link to a website lists legal services organization by county and state:

www.rin.lsc.gov/rinboard/rguide/pdir1.htm

Legal services provide much needed assistance to poor families but have a number of significant limitations in their practice. Many programs must now turn away approximately three out of five cases due to limited resources. Often, their offices are not located within the community served. Due to limited resources, agencies are frequently unable to provide linguistically appropriate services. For families with young children, gaining access to legal services can be extremely challenging.

Collaboration with Law School Clinics and Lawyers-in-Training

Many law schools have training opportunities in which students provide legal services to low-income families. Law schools are often open to participating in innovative programs. Most cities have a law school that can be approached for this type of collaboration.

Developing an On-Site Program through Grant Funding

Private foundations can be an excellent source of funding for innovative programs that serve traumatized children and families. Grant funding is often very flexible and allows you to tailor the advocacy program to your needs. The main drawbacks of grant funding are the effort and energy involved in applying for grants and the time-limited nature of the funding.

Developing Partnerships with Law Firms or Individual Lawyers

Many law firms routinely donate some time to pro-bono work. In addition, individual lawyers (practicing or retired) may be interested in volunteering to be a part of a TST team. It is always worth asking around at the law firms in town to see if someone with the appropriate skills would like to be a part of an innovative model of caring for traumatized children.

Plain Old Referrals

And finally, the local bar association maintains a list of referral attorneys who provide full-fee services and sliding-fee-scale services to families of low and moderate means.

Regardless of how you develop a partnership, it is important to keep in mind that not all lawyers were created equal. Not just any lawyer is equipped to advocate for patients; as in other disciplines, lawyers are trained as generalist advocates up to a point—then they become specialists. Lawyers who specialize in securing basic benefits and services for families are known as "legal services or legal aid attorneys." A lawyer joining a TST team will need extra guidance and education to understand the role of trauma and mental health in a child's development. To be effective, legal advocates must have an understanding of the health-related problems toward which their work is aimed.

> Lawyers who specialize in securing basic benefits and services for families are known as "legal services or legal aid attorneys."

Finally, remember that as with all other parts of TST, communication and teamwork are essential. Collaboration with a lawyer or legal organization is further complicated by the two different cultures (and, sometimes, ethical guidelines) of law and mental health. Several key principles have emerged from our ongoing collaboration with lawyers:

- ✓ Set advocacy priorities consistent with the overall treatment plan and communicate these priorities clearly to the lawyer if a referral is made.
- ✓ Respect ethical and professional responsibilities of different disciplines.
- ✓ Help make sure that families are "advocacy read" before making a referral to a lawyer—families need to agree on the plan and to follow through with what will be asked of them in the course of legal proceedings.

Closing Thoughts on Systems Advocacy

In some ways, advocacy requires pushing the boundaries of the clinician's job to be a little bit bigger. But looked at from another angle, advocacy is about finally having the tools to *do* our job. For clinicians, learning how to do advocacy can mean realizing that we don't just have to "accept the status quo" and tear out our hair over wishing things were different. For families, advocacy can make a powerful and lasting change in their children's lives. For everyone, advocacy can help to leave a better system.

Psychopharmacology

How Psychopharmacology Is Integrated within TST

LEARNING OBJECTIVES

- To detail principles of psychopharmacology within TST
- To describe the practice of psychopharmacology within TST
- To outline the psychiatric consultant's role within TST

There is no magic pill. TST is about focused services integration. Psychopharmacology can be a very useful service, but it must be integrated into care thoughtfully and clearly. Although we review various medications that can be useful for traumatized children, our main focus is about how the *principles and practice* of psychopharmacology fit within TST.

There is no magic pill.

This chapter also discusses the psychiatric consultant's role within TST and should be read carefully by all members of the TST treatment team. Psychiatric consultants should read the chapter to understand how their practice can and should be altered to fit within TST. Other clinicians should read this chapter to understand how to best use these services.

The first principle of TST is "Fix a broken system." This principle means that TST interventions are directed to the trauma system:

- A traumatized child who is not able to regulate emotional states.
- A social environment and/or system of care that is not able to sufficiently help the child to regulate these emotional states.

 Psychopharmacology, like all TST interventions, works toward this goal and is closely integrated with other interventions. The advantage of considering psychopharmacology within the TST framework is that the wider context of interventions are *built into* the framework. In other types of psychopharmacology practice, the psychopharmacologist often practices in isolation and either has to weave other interventions around the psychopharmacology interventions or must spend a great deal of time communicating with other providers in order to understand what services are being provided and how these services fit with the psychopharmacological interventions. Psychopharmacology within TST can be much more efficient than in other types of practice because this type of communication is, again, built into the framework.

The Role of the Psychiatric Consultant

There are a number of specific functions for a psychiatric consultant on a TST team. These include:

1. Directs psychopharmacological intervention.
2. Provides consultation on when a child needs a medical or neurological evaluation.
3. Provides consultation on diagnoses and differential diagnoses.
4. Provides oversight of the team's management of psychiatric emergencies.
5. Communicates with other medical providers and with psychiatric inpatient units.

In practice, a number of different medical professionals have the training to offer direct psychopharmacological services. These include psychiatrists, neurologists, behavioral and developmental pediatricians, and clinical nurse specialists. Whoever fills this role should have the breadth and depth of expertise necessary to perform the specific functions listed above. If it is not possible to have a psychopharmacologist with the knowledge base to provide such expertise, pairing a practitioner with a psychiatric consultant for additional consultation or supervision can work. For example, on our team a child and adolescent psychiatrist provides consultation in team meetings and supervision to a clinical nurse specialist. The clinical nurse specialist provides the bulk of the direct psychopharmacology services.

Psychopharmacology and the Survival Circuits

 As we reviewed in Chapter 2, psychopharmacology and psychotherapy work together on the brain pathways to diminish the amygdala's "hostile takeover of consciousness by emotion" (LeDoux, 2002, p. 226). These pathways, which we call the *survival circuits*, have evolved to help the individual survive in the face of threat and are central to the psychopathology of traumatic stress. In particular, when an individual with traumatic stress is presented with a stimulus that reminds him/her of the trauma, the response is immediate and extreme. This response, as detailed in Chapter 3, involves dramatic fluctuations in affect (or emotion), action (or behavior), and awareness (or consciousness), the three A's. It is these repeated changes in states of emotion when confronted by a stressor, mediated by the *survival circuits*, that define traumatic stress. During these emotional states the child is, to some

> These fluctuations are ultimately maladaptive because, in current reality, survival is not at stake.

degree, responding to the traumatic event in the present. The fluctuations in the three A's are expressions of a psychobiological system fighting to survive. These fluctuations are ultimately maladaptive because, in current reality, survival is not at stake. The child has not properly discerned that he/she is no longer under immediate life-threatening conditions.

Interventions help the child recognize that a stressor or traumatic reminder is not, in reality, a matter of survival. How can interventions help the child to change his/her way of responding when the brain has become predisposed to respond to stressful stimuli as if survival were at stake? Within TST, interventions are meant to work in the following way:

1. Social-environmental interventions work to diminish the stimuli.
2. Skill-based interventions (emotion regulation, cognitive processing, meaning making) engage and enhance contextual processing systems (hippocampus and cortex, LeDoux's "high road," Chapter 2) to more adaptively respond to stressful stimuli and, accordingly, to inhibit emergency response systems led by the amygdala (LeDoux's "low road").
3. Psychopharmacological agents work with skill-based interventions to inhibit this emergency response system.

> The psychiatric consultant stands arm-in-arm with the rest of the treatment team to work toward diminishing the stimulation and to give the child increasing emotion regulation skills.

The psychiatric consultant stands arm-in-arm with the rest of the treatment team to work toward diminishing the stimulation and to give the child increasing emotion regulation skills. In TST, all interventions fit together to fix a broken system (Principle One).

A number of specific psychopharmacological agents are known to diminish the reaction of this emergency response system or survival circuit. In essence, medications that diminish the activity of the amygdala will help shift the balance of the survival circuits to allow the child to use the brain's "high road" to stop, think, and plan instead of just reacting.

Medications known to inhibit (directly or indirectly) the amygdala, which has been implicated in a wide range of psychiatric disorders, include selective serotonin reuptake inhibitors (SSRIs), tricyclic antidepressants, benzodiazepines, mood stabilizers, and antipsychotics.

What about PTSD?

We reviewed PTSD in Chapter 3. In summary, we believe the disparate groupings of PTSD symptoms are a good start but are only the surface markers (symptoms) of the underlying processes that we describe in Chapters 2 and 3. Accordingly, PTSD misses a range of other surface markers that are at least as relevant.

 The targets of psychopharmacological treatment are the traumatized child's dramatic fluctuations in affect, action, and awareness when confronted by a stressor or traumatic reminder.

This definition of treatment target covers a wider range of symptoms than the PTSD diagnosis but more narrowly constrains the focus of intervention to one of *processes* (i.e., how specific stimuli lead to specific responses). Again: These processes are mediated by the dysfunction of the survival circuits.

Think Things and Not Words (Differential Diagnosis)

It is not entirely clear that the words used to describe different clinical problems truly describe different processes in nature or are, in fact, different words for the same thing. Justice Oliver Wendell Holmes's famous admonition to "think things and not words" is very relevant here. Is it PTSD or ADHD? Is it PTSD or depression? Is it PTSD or rapid-cycling juvenile bipolar disorder? Is it both? Is it all?! Is differential diagnosis different than comorbidity? Is there a more useful way of thinking about all this? Again: *Think things and not words!*

> It is not entirely clear that the words used to describe different clinical problems truly describe different processes in nature or are, in fact, different words for the same thing.

The brain can only unravel in certain ways. The brain is built of systems: attentional systems, mood systems, reality appraisal systems, motivational systems, and fear systems. If traumatic events influence these systems, then the types of problems expressed by the traumatized child would look similar to other conditions that are called by other names but influence the same systems. Our ways of arguing about whether these children are *really* ADHD or bipolar or psychotic or depressed may, again, reflect our preference to "think things and not words." If the brain processes underlying other conditions are the same or similar to brain processes related to traumatic events, it would be expected that medications helpful to other conditions would also be helpful for traumatic stress. Consider how traumatic stress likely shares processes important for other conditions.

Traumatic Stress and ADHD

The traumatized child may be processing internal information (e.g., traumatic memories, anxiety) at the expense of processing external information (such as school lessons). Furthermore, when the child is confronted with a reminder, there may be impulsive behavior and increased locomotor activity.

Traumatic Stress and Bipolar Disorder

In situations of high threat or stress, the child may experience rapidly changing affective states. These rapidly changing states may be accompanied by impulsive behavior.

Traumatic Stress and Depression

Traumatized children may experience a dramatic shutting down of their emotional responses such that they appear, and feel, numb and have difficulty feeling pleasure. In addition, they may have difficulty with attention, sleep, and appetite.

Traumatic Stress and Psychosis

Traumatized children may have trouble with their appraisal of sensation and reality.

Traumatized children may have trouble with their appraisal of sensation and reality. The sexually abused child, for example, sometimes hears the voice of the perpetrator. The Vietnam veteran sometimes hears the blades of the helicopters coming. Are these hallucinations, illusions, or perceptual distortions of some sort? If a hallucination is an internally driven perception of external stimulation that does not correspond to external reality, then it is hard to argue that these two examples are not hallucinations. Similarly, the abused child who scans the environment for signs that others might hurt him/her and misinterprets benign signals as threatening could be called delusional. If a delusion is a fixed, false idea, it is hard to argue that this problem is not a delusion.

Our overall approach to psychopharmacology is to make a clinical decision about whether a given target symptom is related to the traumatized child's dramatic fluctuations in affect, action, and awareness when confronted by a stressor or traumatic reminder. If this target symptom is consistent with the above definition, then we start by trying to diminish the amygdala's response. This approach is supplemented by psychopharmacological treatments that are known to be helpful to conditions that are more typically thought of as depression, psychosis, etc.

Adaptation

 Before we get specific about different medications, we must consider the crucial problem of *adaptation*. Our discussion of the survival circuits depends on the understanding that the life threat is in the past and the traumatized child is not fully able to discern that he/she is in a safer context. In the survival phase of treatment, however, there are genuine threats of harm. Therefore, the traumatized child's symptoms may be important adaptations to help with literal survival, and, if so, must never be treated. Consider the following examples:

> The traumatized child's symptoms may be important adaptations to help with literal survival, and, if so, must never be treated.

- The child who does not want to go to sleep because he/she is afraid of being abused in the night hours.
- The child who lives in a neighborhood where there is a gang war and who spends a lot of time scanning the environment for sources of threat.
- The child who avoids going to school because someone has threatened to kill him/her.
- The adolescent who is aggressive with his mother's boyfriend to protect her from getting beaten up.

These examples may seem obvious, but in busy psychopharmacological practice, particularly when it is disconnected from other therapeutic interventions, the adaptive nature of a child's response can easily be missed and treated like a symptom. From our point of view, this is a significant clinical and ethical problem. Treatment efforts in this situation must be aimed at decreasing the real threat in the environment.

What to Choose?

 The TST psychiatric consultant must choose a medication or medications to help the child's survival circuits return to baseline. Which ones?

We do not believe that our approach is the only approach. As we reviewed, many different medications can work to diminish the amygdala's threat response. Based on our understanding of safety, side effects, and effectiveness, we recommend a first-line approach to help stabilize the survival circuits and then other approaches for special cases.

First-Line Approach

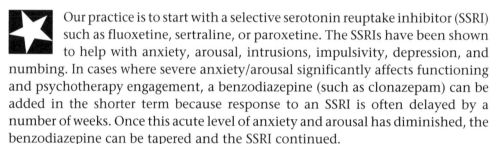 Our practice is to start with a selective serotonin reuptake inhibitor (SSRI) such as fluoxetine, sertraline, or paroxetine. The SSRIs have been shown to help with anxiety, arousal, intrusions, impulsivity, depression, and numbing. In cases where severe anxiety/arousal significantly affects functioning and psychotherapy engagement, a benzodiazepine (such as clonazepam) can be added in the shorter term because response to an SSRI is often delayed by a number of weeks. Once this acute level of anxiety and arousal has diminished, the benzodiazepine can be tapered and the SSRI continued.

Second-Line Approach

Other medication approaches include:

- Benzodiazepines alone
- Tricyclic antidepressants, such as imipramine or desipramine
- Atypical antipsychotic medications, such as risperidone or olanzapine. These medications should be reserved for severe anxiety that does not respond to other medications, particularly when the anxiety/arousal leads to disorganized thinking.

Special Cases

The following variations to our usual first-line practice occur when a specific problem is prominent:

Insomnia

- Making sure the child is not consuming products that are known to interfere with sleep (e.g., cigarettes, coffee, sodas, and, of course, illicit drugs).

- Sedating antidepressants such as trazodone and doxepine
- Benzodiazepines (not short acting)
- Alpha$_2$-adrenergic inhibitors such as clonidine or guanfacine

Impulsivity

We discuss behavioral dysregulation in Chapter 3. Posttraumatic emotional states sometimes become expressed in aggressive, risky, or self-destructive behaviors. Because these types of behaviors are typically part of the survival circuit response (behaviors used to survive, even though survival is not currently at stake), the usual first-line interventions should be tried initially. There are two cautions with this recommendation, however:

1. There is currently controversy about whether the SSRIs lead to increased impulsive and risky behavior. In our experience, these medications are more likely to help than hurt. However, because increases in risky behavior are possible with SSRIs, this should be monitored closely, particularly in the weeks after this medication is initiated.

2. Benzodiazepines can lead to disinhibition. It is our experience that, similar to the SSRIs, benzodiazepines are more likely to help than hurt. Nevertheless, because disinhibition is well documented following benzodiazepine treatment, these medications should be chosen as third- or fourth-line treatments for impulsivity and monitored carefully.

Medications that can also be helpful for impulsivity and should be considered second line, following a trial with an SSRI (and sometimes in addition to it, depending on the clinical circumstances), are:

- Mood stabilizers such as lithium, valproic acid, and carbamezepine
- Alpha$_2$-adrenergic inhibitors, such as clonidine or guanfacine
- Atypical antipsychotic medications, such as risperidone or olanzapine

Beware that impulsive behavior can sometimes be a first sign of alcohol or drug abuse. It is important, therefore, to keep a high index of suspicion about drug abuse in an impulsive adolescent or preadolescent.

Depression and Numbing

Traumatized children may experience dramatic shutting down of emotional responses that can significantly interfere with functioning and responsivness to skill-building interventions. In short, sometimes traumatized children get depressed.

Medications that can help with this shutting down of emotional responses, including major depression, include:

- SSRIs
- Tricyclic antidepressants
- Other antidepressants such as bupropion and venlafaxine

Disorganized/Idiosyncratic Thinking/Perceptual Distortions

- Start with the first-line approach because problems related to the appraisal of reality may be driven by survival-laden affect.
- As a second line, or occasionally as adjunct to this first line, use an atypical antipsychotic agent such as riperidone or olanzapine.
- If high levels of anxiety and disorganized/distorted perceptions and thinking are present, *and* risky behavior is present, we recommend starting with an atypical antipsychotic agent such as riperidone or olanzapine.

Inattention

- Start with the first-line approach because problems related to inattention may be related to survival-laden affect.
- As an adjunct to this first line, use a stimulant such as methylphenidate or dextroamphetamine.
- If the above approach does not work, consider bupropion or a tricyclic antidepressant.

Practice of Psychopharmacology in TST

 The psychiatric consultant should be familiar with the 10 treatment principles described in Chapter 6 for TST interventions. These principles guide all TST interventions, including psychopharmacology, and should be considered an overarching guide to psychopharmacology practice. We list these 10 principles again here (details about their use are given in Chapter 6):

1. Fix a broken system.
2. Put safety first.
3. Create clear, focused plans that are based on facts.
4. Don't "go" before you are "ready."

5. Put scarce resources where they'll work.

6. Insist on accountability, particularly your own.

7. Align with reality.

8. Take care of yourself and your team.

9. Build from strength.

10. Leave a better system.

Psychopharmacology fits closely with other treatment modalities in TST. In the earlier phases of treatment, the main use of psychopharmacology is to avert crisis. During these phases, when the social environment is unstable and the child is at high risk of engaging in dangerous behavior, psychopharmacology can be used to help prevent psychiatric emergencies, psychiatric hospitalizations, and out-of-home placements. Once the child transitions to the more advanced phases of treatment, the main goal of psychopharmacology is to enhance skill-building interventions.

An important part of TST is helping the child acquire the skills to (1) manage emotion, (2) process the trauma(s), and (3) create meaning out of the experience. This idea assumes that it is the building of these skills that will be most instrumental in helping the child to function better over the course of his/her life. Accordingly, the primary goal of psychopharmacology within TST, when crisis is not a salient part of the clinical picture, is to support these skill-building interventions. This goal is accomplished within TST via the very high degree of communication that is "built in" for all providers, the full integration of psychopharmacology within the larger TST treatment plan, and the phase-dependent clinical decisions that are integral to psychopharmacology within TST.

> The primary goal of psychopharmacology within TST, when crisis is not a salient part of the clinical picture, is to support skill-building interventions.

In this way, psychopharmacology is explicitly an adjunct or supportive intervention within TST. When the survival circuit is triggered, the child is often too aroused or disorganized to engage in skill-building interventions. Psychopharmacology is meant to diminish the responsivity of the survival circuit so that skill-building interventions can occur.

 Whenever psychopharmacology is used within TST, it is highly integrated with other interventions and providers. Psychopharmacology decisions are influenced by information from the team, are supported by the team, and affect decisions by other team members. Indeed, TST psychopharmacology is best characterized as a team intervention.

	Phase				
		Surviving	Stabilizing	Enduring	Understanding	Transcending
Module	Stabilization on Site (SOS)	***	***	–	–	–
	Services advocacy	***	**	*	*	*
	Psychopharmacology	**	**	**	*	*
	Emotion regulation	*	**	***	–	–
	Cognitive processing	–	–	–	***	–
	Meaning making	–	–	–	–	***

FIGURE 13.1. TST treatment modules used across treatment phases. *Note.* *** = essential; ** = often helpful; * = occasionally helpful; – = not used or contraindicated.

In order to see where psychopharmacology fits within the phases and modules of TST, we reproduce Figure 8.2 here (from Chapter 8) as Figure 13.1: As Figure 13.1 indicates, psychopharmacology is "often helpful" in the surviving, stabilizing, and enduring phases and is "occasionally helpful" in the understanding and transcending phases of treatment. It is never contraindicated nor is it ever considered "essential" within a given phase.

Day-to-Day Psychopharmacology Practice

 Referral to psychopharmacology intervention works like referral to any of the interventions. It fits within the overall assessment and treatment plan reviewed in the TST team. The psychiatric consultant is a part of this team meeting and can offer valued input to team discussion. All decisions about an intervention modality are team decisions and are based on a TST assessment and treatment plan. In this way the psychiatric consultant is never confused about the "referral question."

The Initial Meeting

When the psychiatric consultant has his/her first meeting with the family, he/she should have a copy of the TST Treatment Planning Form (discussed in Chapter 8 and reproduced in the Appendix), which fully outlines the results of the assessment and preliminary plans for treatment. At this meeting the psychiatric consultant should do the following:

- **Confirm the child and family's understanding of why they were referred and how psychopharmacology can fit within the rest of the family's care.** At this initial meeting it is extremely important that the child and family understand that the psychiatric consultant is part of the team and works very closely with the rest of the team and that medications, if they are recommended, are only a *part* of the overall treatment plan.

- **Detect the family's concerns about psychopharmacological interventions as early as possible and dispel any misunderstandings.** Families frequently have negative reactions to the possible use of medications, and addressing these concerns up-front can go a long way toward building the alliance.

- **Reassess the initial evaluation of emotional and behavioral dysregulation and psychiatric diagnoses.** The psychiatric consultant has particular expertise in these assessments and should confirm their initial formulations.

- **Assess the usual domains covered in a psychopharmacological evaluation (e.g., prior treatment history, medical history).**

- **Communicate to the family the results of the evaluation.** Make sure that the family understands that these results are preliminary and will be discussed with the team. Explain that the evaluation recommendations will be communicated to the family at the FCM, in which the psychiatric consultant will be present.

The Family Collaborative Meeting

The FCM, reviewed in Chapter 10, is the meeting in which all members of the team meet with the family to discuss the results of the evaluation and the preliminary treatment plan. The reason this treatment plan is considered preliminary is that it must be presented to the family as a first step in building an alliance around a treatment plan. The team must be clear on their overall plan and recommendations, including those involving psychopharmacology, and be open to the family's perspective. The goal of this meeting is to craft a plan that reflects what the team believes is needed and integrates the family's ideas about the problem and its solution. The psychiatric consultant should be thoroughly familiar with the ready–set–go module and address the treatment alliance regarding psychopharmacological issues from this perspective. Because treatment compliance can be a difficult problem in psychopharmacological practice, building the alliance within an overall agreement that includes all elements of treatment can be a powerful means of maximizing the chances of compliance. The plan, once agreed to by the family, is supported by all members of the treatment team. Family members' compliance with the psychopharmacology interventions are therefore considered by the team to be part of their overall adherence to the TST treatment plan. (The Treatment Planning Form is included in the Appendix and described in Chapter 8.)

Ongoing psychopharmacological practice, within TST, shares many elements with usual psychopharmacological practice. Follow-up meetings are usually held every 1–2 weeks until an effective dose of medication is found. Once the child is more stable, follow-up appointments are usually held every month. The psychiatric consultant's confidence in the treatment is enhanced by the unusually high degree of communication and treatment integration in TST. The following section describes how psychopharmacology is used in the different phases of TST treatment.

Psychopharmacology across the Phases of Treatment

As illustrated in Figure 13.1, psychopharmacology has a changing role in TST depending on the phase of treatment.

Surviving Phase

Psychopharmacology during the surviving phase is "often helpful." During this phase, the child exhibits significant behavioral dysregulation (i.e., is usually self-destructive or violent), and the social environment is threatening. Accordingly, the team is often in communication with the Department of Social Services, the police, psychiatric inpatient units, and hospital emergency rooms. Often the referral for psychopharmacology, in this context, is urgently needed to help regulate the child so that a psychiatric hospitalization can be prevented. The social environment may, however, be so unstable that the psychiatric consultant is not confident that parents or guardians can give consent to, or will use, the medications appropriately. In this case, it may be difficult to avoid psychiatric hospitalization. Social services agencies are frequently involved in the surviving phase and can at times either facilitate obtaining this consent from parents or give consent themselves. The psychiatric consultant's expertise in risk assessment can be invaluable to the team during this time. The psychiatric consultant should give his/her opinion on the level of risk and, if the team is still unsure, assess risk directly with the child and family. The psychiatric consultant can also be helpful to the team via his/her communication with medical/psychiatric staff on inpatient units and emergency rooms.

The psychiatric consultant must assess whether the presentation of a given symptom is really a needed "adaptation," as described above. In the survival phase of treatment there are significant threats of harm to the child. Such behaviors as aggression, vigilance, lack of sleep, and avoidance may be ways of *staying alive* and, if so, should never be medicated.

Stabilizing Phase

Psychopharmacology during the stabilizing phase is also "often helpful." During this phase, the child may be exhibiting significant emotional or behavioral dysregulation, and the social environment is distressed or threatening. The clinical picture, however, is not as urgent as in the surviving phase. During the stabilizing phase, the team is in the home conducting SOS interventions. These interventions are meant to diminish the sources of stimulation that repeatedly lead to dysregulation and to begin to introduce emotion regulation skill training. Receiving the information about what is occurring in the home is critical for psychopharmacology practice. The psychiatric consultant may have initiated a medication, for example, to help with the child's ability to regulate emotion. The child may initially not improve or even get worse. In this context, the psychiatric consultant is often inclined to increase the dose or change medications. However, if the SOS team provides information that there are increased stressors in the home, then the psychiatric consultant can avoid erroneously "chasing" symptoms with medication. Home-based care during this phase can also be very helpful in terms of assessing the family's compliance with medications and any barriers to compliance. This information can then be integrated into the psychopharmacological treatment plan.

> Home-based care during this phase can also be very helpful in terms of assessing the family's compliance with medications and any barriers to compliance. This information can then be integrated into the psychopharmacological treatment plan.

Enduring Phase

In the enduring phase, the child is more regulated and the environment more stable than in prior phases of treatment. This phase is largely defined by office-based emotion regulation skills training. In this phase, TST most resembles "typical" psychopharmacological practice. The therapist is trying to help the child regulate emotion, and the child may need medication to make the best use of this psychotherapeutic intervention. As described, the goal of psychopharmacology in the enduring phase is to help the child acquire the emotion regulation skills that are a central component of TST.

Accordingly, communication between the psychiatric consultant and the child's therapist is essential for the psychiatric consultant to determine if the child's emotional states are interfering with treatment. Children with mood disorders, ADHD, or disorganized thinking will need medication if these problems interfere with psychotherapy.

Understanding Phase

During the understanding phase of treatment, the environment is more stable and the child has sufficient emotion regulation skills to process the trauma cognitively. These cognitive-processing skills are the defining feature of the understanding phase of TST. Many children will not need medication during this phase of treatment, and some children will be tapered off their medications. As in the enduring phase, psychopharmacological decisions concern how to help the child best take advantage of cognitive-processing skills training. Learning occurs with an optimum level of arousal. Cognitive processing of the trauma requires an increase in arousal so that there can be some extinction of the trauma response. It is important, therefore, to *not* medicate this increased arousal unless it interferes with the child's functioning. Close consultation with the child's therapist will be important so that the psychiatric consultant will know . . .

> Cognitive processing of the trauma requires an increase in arousal so that there can be some extinction of the trauma response.

1. When to expect this increase of arousal related to trauma processing, *and*
2. Whether this increase in arousal is interfering with functioning.

The therapist can be very helpful in providing information about whether the level of arousal during the cognitive processing should be treated with medication.

Transcending Phase

The transcending phase is the last phase of TST and is devoted to helping the child gain a perspective about the trauma that will help create meaning for him/her. This phase also includes termination of TST treatment. Many children are sufficiently stable during the transcending phase to be tapered off medication. Some children, of course, need medications for a longer period of time. If no attempt has been made to taper medications, doing so should be tried during this final phase. If the child experiences an increase in emotion dysregulation during the taper, than the therapist should consider trying to improve emotion regulation skills to maximize the child's chance of not needing medications. If this enhancement of skills does not work, the child may need to take medications for longer periods of time. Ideally, children should be taken off medications before treatment ends. Integrating the psychotherapy with the medication taper can maximize the likelihood of this possibility. In practice, however, a taper does not work for all children.

Closing Thoughts on Psychopharmacology

Psychopharmacology can be a very useful intervention for children with traumatic stress. Psychopharmacology used within TST must be highly integrated with other TST interventions. Broadly speaking, the goal is to avert crises in the earlier phases of treatment and to enhance skill-building interventions in the later phase of treatment. The psychiatric consultant is a full member of the team and should always conduct care consistent with the principles of TST.

Emotion Regulation Skills

*How to Help Children
Regulate Emotional States*

LEARNING OBJECTIVES

- To help children acquire emotion regulation skills
- To help children learn how to label and talk about feelings
- To help children learn coping skills for when they feel upset
- To help family members learn when and how they can help their child regulate emotional states

---

Emotion regulation is a cornerstone of a child's recovery within TST. As described in previous chapters, child traumatic stress is related to (1) a child's difficulty in regulating emotional states, and (2) the incapacity of the child's social environment to help him/her regulate emotion. So, interventions should help a child regulate his/her emotions. That's half the pie—and what this chapter is all about. The emotion regulation (ER) module is a semistructured, office-based therapeutic approach that helps both parents and their children gain greater awareness of emotions and specific skills and strategies for regulation. This chapter presents the overall treatment goals for the ER module, suggested session structure, and key tools for implementing the treatment. Please be familiar with Chapter 2 and especially Chapter 3 for background that will help in implementing the ER module.

We would like to acknowledge the contributions of David Barlow and Liza Suarez in the development and writing of this chapter.

When to Use the ER Module

The ER module should be used once the child has been assessed with the TST Assessment Grid and it is determined that the child is in the enduring, stabilizing, or surviving phase. In general, the ER module is the primary treatment approach in the enduring phase. It may also be used in earlier phases under certain conditions. The emotion regulation module is appropriate for children who can't yet talk about, or be reminded of, their trauma without becoming numb, having overwhelming emotions, or engaging in inappropriate (or even dangerous) behaviors. The use of the ER module is somewhat different in the earlier phases (surviving or stabilizing phase) than in the enduring phase. We describe these differences next.

> The emotion regulation module is appropriate for children who can't yet talk about, or be reminded of, their trauma without becoming numb, having overwhelming emotions, or engaging in inappropriate (or even dangerous) behaviors.

ER Module in the Surviving and Stabilizing Phases

Children in the most acute phase of treatment need a lot of services, and ER treatment is a key part of the menu. ER treatment is conducted in coordination with SOS to help stabilize the child and give him/her basic coping skills. The "reacting" and "reexperiencing" sections of the ER guide (described below) are crucial. ER interventions are delivered in close coordination with SOS interventions and with other providers to extend this component into the home and across the different areas of treatment.

 Although kids in the surviving phase probably need a lot of help with emotion regulation, an outpatient setting might not be the right setting. If the child is suicidal or likely to hurt someone else, a higher level of care may be required, such as hospitalization. If—and only if—the child can remain in outpatient treatment safely (along with additional supports) can ER treatment begin.

ER Module in the Enduring Phase

Once the child has transitioned from the earlier surviving and stabilizing phases of treatment, ER therapy becomes much more office-based. Presumably the child's environment is stabler and the child's home placement is not at risk. During the enduring phase the therapist can focus on emotion regulation without needing to put out so many fires. The ER work done during the earlier phases is continued and enriched during the enduring phase. Children whose environment is relatively stable will start TST in the enduring phase. In this phase, the ER module is used to build a skill base to handle any new waves of crisis and to lay the groundwork for cognitive processing. ER treatment is designed to help the child gain the skills to experience emotions without being overwhelmed, and to label and talk about feelings. The skill-building activities and "maintenance" sections of the ER guide are especially important. Once children have these skills, they are ready to move on to cognitive processing (see Chapter 15).

 A note on the involvement of parents: Some caregivers may come equipped with good self-regulatory skills and a well-developed understanding of their child's needs and emotions. Other parents may require assistance in developing these skills before they are able to adequately assist their child with regulation. Although ideally every parent would be able to help his/her child in times of emotional distress, this, unfortunately, is not always possible. Personal emotional distress, cognitive limitations, or an unwillingness to engage in treatment may interfere with a parent's ability to attend to the child's emotions. In this case, the balance of treatment will focus on helping the child develop his/her own skills, as well as helping him/her identify adults in his/her life who are safe and effective resources. Remember, *build from strength* (Principle Nine). Meanwhile, getting the parent into his/her own treatment may be indicated.

> Personal emotional distress, cognitive limitations, or an unwillingness to engage in treatment may interfere with a parent's ability to attend to the child's emotions. In this case, the balance of treatment will focus on helping the child develop his/her own skills, as well as helping him/her identify adults in his/her life who are safe and effective resources.

Treatment Planning and the ER Module

Chapter 8 describes in detail how treatment planning works in TST. Whether you are moving between treatment phases or initiating treatment, you will want to make sure that the Treatment Planning Form accurately reflects the specific goals on which you are working within the ER module. As described above, the specific focus of ER work may change depending on whether a child is in the surviving, stabilizing, or enduring phase of treatment. Keeping the treatment plan current with the child's progress is essential to make sure that the team is acknowledging progress and focusing skills training at the right level of the child.

"Solutions" to priority problems are identified on page 311 of the Treatment Planning Form. Remember, priority problems specifically address patterns around a child's emotion dysregulation; emotion regulation skills directly address this area and should be included under "solutions." The TST team's presentation of initial ideas about treatment planning in the Family Collaborative

Meeting provides a perfect opportunity to educate the family about the ER module's importance and to enlist family members' support.

As is described later in this chapter, the ER module is built around a shared "working document" called the Emotion Regulation Guide (ER guide, for short). This guide is meant to be used by all the relevant TST team players. The ER guide is most effective if it is used consistently by the different team members—especially the family, the individual clinician, and (if involved) the SOS team. Treatment planning and the FCM are largely concerned with helping the different team players learn what is expected of them and then holding themselves and each other accountable to

> The ER guide is most effective if it is used consistently by the different team members—especially the family, the individual clinician, and (if involved) the SOS team.

these expectations. Thus, this is the time and place to introduce the idea that ER treatment will involve everyone agreeing to use the ER guide, in and out of treatment.

Domains of Treatment

The ER module is comprised of three domains of treatment (ACE, for short):

1. Assessment
2. Coping skills
3. Emotion identification

- **Assessment** runs throughout the course of treatment and helps identify which of the other two areas of treatment should be the central focus at any given time. The ER guide is the central tool for ongoing assessment.

- **Coping skills** provide concrete ways to regulate emotions and respond adaptively in times of stress.

- **Emotion identification** provides the skills children need to be able to apply some of the coping strategies. Children also learn how to talk about, show, and share their feelings. Parents are involved in each of these areas of treatment. We discuss these domains in more detail later in the chapter.

Treatment Structure

The ER module sessions are scheduled on a 1-hour per week basis for approximately 12–16 weeks. Typically, both the caregiver and child attend the first half of the session (**check-in** and **ER guide update**). The remainder of the session is devoted to working with the child to help him/her develop skills. The skills section of the session is typically one-on-one, although in some situations the parent can be involved as well.

Within-session structure includes:

1. **Check-in.** This is a 10-minute initial check-in with the parent and child together. During this time, try to learn the following information about the last week: Did the child experience any emotional or behavioral dysregulation? Did the child try any coping skills? Did the child have any experiences of staying calm even though there was a trigger in the environment? If the answer to any of these questions is "yes," then that answer guides the next phase of the session: updating the ER guide.

2. **ER guide update.** The next step is to review and update the ER guide based on the check-in report. Did the child escalate when triggered? Did he/she use coping skills to get back to a calm, regulated state, or did the child enter a reexperiencing state? If any episodes of reexperiencing occurred during the week, start here; if not, you can pick and choose whether you want to talk about when a child stayed calm despite a trigger (regulated), or when he/she got a little dysregulated (revved). Either way, the ER guide directs the conversation. Find out about precipitants to the emotion/behavior, internal and external cues, and any attempts the child made to use coping skills. The latter provides an opportunity to reinforce the child's efforts and to figure out if a particular coping strategy is a good one—or not—for this child. As you talk about all of these things, fill in the ER guide. If you have trouble filling out a part (e.g., the child can't tell you what he/she was feeling), that's a clue that you might want to work on that skill in the next part of the session.

3. **ER skill building.** The second half of session—about 20 minutes' worth—is devoted to a little more fun. Conveniently, it also is about building skills. Skills are divided into two main groups: coping and emotions. Coping skills activities provide the child with specific skills to use when upset and include relaxation skills, anger management, and social skills training. Emotions activities focus on helping the child *observe*, *name*, and *express* (ONE) emotions. The specific sets of skills will reflect the child's age, interests, and abilities.

4. **Closing ritual.** The last 5 minutes of the session are focused on a closing ritual that can help define the end of session, bring the child down if he/she got kind of excited during the session, and give a sense of predictability to an otherwise somewhat unpredictable world.

OK, now that you've got the structure down, don't forget that for some kids you may need to throw it out the window. How often you meet, and for how long, depends on the developmental level of the child. Younger children or older children with particular difficulties in tolerating a full 1-hour session may benefit from meeting twice weekly for 30 minutes. The session structure above is a general guideline; the big advantage of individual therapy is just that—it can be individualized.

The Emotion Regulation Guide

What it is: An individualized worksheet that identifies triggers, cues that the child is escalating, and appropriate interventions for various stages of escalation and traumatic states.

When to use it: At beginning of each ER session throughout ER module, and in conjunction with SOS or other providers.

Target goals: Child and parent will learn to identify triggers and patterns of escalation and be able to intervene early in cycle of dysregulation.

What It Is

The ER guide is a tool that is used in dialogue between parent, child, and therapist. Practically speaking, it is a document that is filled out collaboratively by the parent, child, therapist, and (if applicable) SOS team. The document remains a "work in progress" throughout therapy and is continually revised and updated as the family and providers become more aware of the child's strengths and needs, and as the strengths and needs change.

The ER guide is composed of four sections that follow a similar format. The four sections correspond to four different emotional states (discussed in Chapter 3) that may be seen in a traumatized child: *regulating* (being in control and feeling OK), reacting or *revving* (getting upset), *reexperiencing* (feeling and being out of control), and *reconstituting* (getting back in control). Within each section of the guide, two kinds of information are gathered:

1. Cues to identify that particular emotional state.
2. Interventions/maintenance activities to change or maintain that state.

Basically, we want to know:

1. How does the child, and how do other people, know that the child is in that emotional state?
2. What can the child and others do to change it (if it's a dysregulated state) or keep it going (if it's a regulated state)?

In addition, the reacting and reexperiencing sections include a list of traumatic reminders that lead to a child entering these emotional states.

As we described in Chapter 3, the four emotional states that traumatized children enter when triggered require different intervention approaches. The ER guide offers a framework for intervening depending on the emotional state the child is experiencing.

We now describe the details of the ER guide.

When to Use It

The ER guide should be introduced in the first ER session and used as an assessment of both the child's functioning and the child's and parent's current levels of understanding of the child's responses and emotions. The guide can then be used at the beginning of every session; information from the previous week regarding traumatic reminders, child behaviors, and effective interventions are used to update the guide.

 Similar to behavioral assessments used in dialectical behavioral therapy (DBT), the ER guide can be used to carefully assess precipitants and consequences of incidents that occurred during the week. The guide goes one step further, however, by incorporating a discussion of interventions. This conversation can lead to a selection of new coping strategies to learn during the latter part of session. New skills learned during the session can then be added to that week's ER guide.

 At the conclusion of each session the parent and child should be given an updated ER guide. If there are other providers involved, such as the SOS team or a psychiatrist, you may want to give them copies as well. By keeping everyone's ER guide up to date, you help team members use the same language, reinforce the same skills, and stay aware of any recent problems or successes. A blank ER guide is included in the Appendix.

The ER Guide, Step by Step

Following is a detailed description of the purpose of each section of the guide and how to use it. The description addresses each section of the guide in order.

Don't expect to get to the whole guide in one session! For the first few sessions, you might try taking one page (starting with page 1) and working on it. Then, after you have a few points on each page, you can elaborate and update it each week, based on the child's new experiences.

Page 1. Regulating or Being in Control and Feeling OK

The first step in addressing emotion dysregulation is understanding what a regulated state looks like. Many times parents focus on the moments when things go wrong and have a harder time identifying what contributes to a their child feeling in control and OK. By starting with talking about regulated states, you help to focus attention on what the child is doing *well*.

Cues of a Regulated State

Let's say you're driving down the highway and you notice that the temperature gauge on your car engine reads 72 degrees. If you know as much about cars as we do, you might be wondering whether this is good or bad. What is the car engine temperature usually? Is it heating up? Or is it normally this way? To have that number mean anything, you need to have paid attention to what your car temp is on a typical, no-problem day. The same point applies to kids who have emotion regulation problems. An awareness of the child's *normal* state is essential to be able to identify changes in that state.

> An awareness of the child's *normal* state is essential to be able to identify changes in that state.

 The concept of mindfulness (Hahn, 1976) describes the process of tuning into one's internal experience and simply noticing what one's current state is. The goal of this section of the ER module is to make the client more aware of emotions, physiology, thoughts, and behaviors during normally regulated moments.

The idea of paying attention to "normal" states of being may be new to both parent and child. You may spend a good portion of the first session just focusing on this first page of the guide and helping the family get the idea of how it works. A possible dialogue might sound like this:

THERAPIST: OK, so I've heard a little bit about how Janice sometimes has a hard time. What I'd like to do now is hear a little bit about what things are like when she's not having a hard time—when things seem to be going along OK. Janice, why don't we start with a time when you were feeling really in control of what you were doing—even if you felt scared or upset. Tell me about a time when that was true.

JANICE: Well, I've been pretty OK today. Like even right now. I was a little scared to come here, now I feel OK.

THERAPIST: OK, great, let's take right now as an example. So you were feeling a little scared, and now you feel OK. Let's start with the feeling. How do you know you're feeling OK? (*Silence.*) That's kind of a hard question, I know. But feelings can have a lot of different parts to them—sometimes we feel them in our body, like when we have butterflies in our stomach. So how our bodies feel is one way we know how we're feeling something. And sometimes when we have a feeling we do things—such as jumping around when we're excited or making a face when we're grossed out by something. So the things we are doing also tell us something about our feelings. Let's start with that. So you're here, in my office, and you say you're feeling OK. What are you doing right now that helps us know that you're feeling OK?

JANICE: Well, I'm just sitting and talking . . .

THERAPIST: Great! Yes. You're able to sit and have a conversation with me and listen really carefully and pay attention. So those might be clues that you're feeling OK. In fact, I remember from when we were talking earlier that when you're really angry, you do *not* sit and have a conversation—your Mom said you shut yourself in your room and won't talk to anyone. So let's put "sitting and talking" under things you do when you're feeling OK, right here in this box of the guide. OK, now Mom, I'm curious, have you noticed some things that Janice does when she's feeling OK?

MOM: Sometimes I'll hear her singing to herself . . .

In this way the family is introduced to the idea of the ER guide in the context of the child's strengths and successes in regulation.

Importantly, successful emotion regulation does not mean experiencing just positive emotions. A child might be sad or frustrated but experience those emotions within a range that allows him/her to remain in control. If a parent identifies only positive emotions in this list, talk to him/her about the fact that negative emotions are a normal part of life and that it's OK for the child to feel them. Another misperception that may need to be addressed is that *not* feeling is a form of emotion regulation. In reality, emotion regulation means being able to experience all emotions without being overwhelmed—so clamping down on emotions and not feeling them is actually another form of emotion *dys*regulation. Try and help the child think of times he/she has had unpleasant feelings that were tolerable and maybe even helpful (such as feeling some worry about a test, leading to studying).

Note on filling out the guide: You will see that cues are noted in two columns, one labeled "Ask Others" and the other "Ask Myself." The "Ask Others" column is for external cues (e.g., a smile), that can be identified by an observer. The "Ask Myself" column is for internal cues that only the child can identify in him/herself (e.g., feeling happy). Initially, the external cue list is likely to be much more fully developed. Over time, however, children may be able to take greater responsibility for identifying their own internal cues and letting others know what they are experiencing.

Maintenance Activities: How to Keep Feeling OK and Being in Control

Once everyone can identify when the child is in a regulated state, the question becomes *how can you keep him/her there*? This section of the guide encourages activities that help build the child's esteem, promote positive relationships with family and friends, and generally bolster his/her sense of well-being. Skills are categorized as either "Things an adult can help me with" (mutual regulation) or "Things I can do on my own" (self-regulation). Fill out this part of the guide by doing the following:

- Brainstorm with the child and parent about **things the child is good at doing**. If you do not know the child well yet, this part may take some exploration. Does the child dance? Play some music and find out. Does he/she enjoy drawing? Can he/she identify every character by name on his/her favorite TV show? Place this list in the column of ""Things I can do on my own," under maintenance activities on the first page of the guide.
- Think about **activities that help promote positive interactions** between the child and others. When you have identified a list of things the parent and child can do to build their positive interactions, place this list under "Things an adult can help me with," under maintenance activities.

Make sure you periodically check in with the parent and child to see if they are doing the activities they've listed.

Page 2. Reacting or "Revving": Getting Upset

The section on escalation begins on page 2 of the ER guide. This section describes the early stage of distress following exposure to a traumatic reminder or stressor, the revving stage. There may be changes in the child's three A's: affect, awareness, and action. In the ER guide, this stage is conceptualized as early in the dysregulation pattern; although there may be changes in each of these domains, typically they are not very extreme yet. Without immediate intervention, however, they may escalate to more difficult or even dangerous feelings and behaviors—which is what happens when a child enters a re-experiencing emotional state. During the course of a traumatized child's day, there may be many revving episodes. These episodes may either terminate due to the child's having sufficient coping skills to regulate emotion and therefore

The goal during the revving
state is to facilitate the transition
back to the regulated state
and to prevent the
reexperiencing state.

to transition back to the regulated state, or they may lead to the reexperiencing state. The goal during the revving state is to facilitate the transition back to the regulated state and to prevent the reexperiencing state.

Sometimes the change of affect that takes place in response to a stressor is to feel *less*, not more. Emotional numbing is a core symptom of PTSD, and for some children, a traumatic reminder quickly leads them to exert rigid control over their whole emotional experience. They may control these feelings by avoiding situations that elicit strong feelings, or they may avoid thinking about things that lead to these feelings. Although these strategies may seem to help in the short term, in the long run they can prevent a child from having necessary and normal life experiences and emotions. As discussed earlier, not experiencing emotions is as much a part of dysregulation as is being overwhelmed by emotions. If a child struggles with experiencing feelings, this numbness, or the avoidance of things and thoughts that lead to emotions, can be noted in this part of the ER guide and specifically addressed.

Often, checking in about problems in the past week will elicit specific examples of times when children became revved. By "walking through" the incident, step by step, with parent and child, information on triggers, internal and external cues, and even ways of effectively coping, can be identified. This section describes how to use the ER guide to walk through an incident.

Traumatic Reminders/Stressors

On top of page 2 you'll see a section labeled "Reminders/Stressors." Parent, child, and clinician work together to identify what factors (internally or in the environment) can shift the child from his/her regulated state and into a revving state.

As the triggers are identified, the clinician works with the parent to reduce or eliminate those that are within the parent's control and are unnecessary for the child to learn to tolerate (e.g., certain TV programs or trips to overstimulating places). Particularly when the child is in an early phase of treatment (surviving or stabilizing phases), one of the most potent interventions may be to help the parent decrease the traumatic reminders in the child's environment. Over time, as the child gains greater regulatory capacities, some triggers may cease to be problematic and can be removed from the list (and returned to the environment).

It is important for the parent to understand that it may be neither possible nor desirable to eliminate all triggers from the child's environment. Indeed, if a child is triggered by essential activities of life, such as being around other people or going out of the house, then removing these triggers would reinforce avoidance strategies and hinder the child's development. Sometimes a child will purposefully avoid certain settings or situations that lead to distress. Sometimes this avoidance itself becomes the first problem to treat. Unless a child begins to have the experience of facing a feared (but necessary for full life) stressor and successfully managing the distress, it will be impossible to help him/her practice building regulatory skills. The clinician can remind the parent that it is the process of helping the child to learn to regulate his/her emotions (rather than just avoiding dysregulation) that leads to recovery.

> If a child is triggered by essential activities of life, such as being around other people or going out of the house, then removing these triggers would reinforce avoidance strategies and hinder the child's development.

Following is a child's hypothetical list of triggers and a commentary on whether or not these should be removed from the child's environment:

- "When my teacher tells me I need to sit down": Learning to be a part of a classroom is essential in life—assuming the classroom is appropriate for this child, this is a trigger that should not be eliminated. Instead, the child needs to work on skills for regulating in that moment.

- "On the bus, when all the kids are throwing things": Being able to be with other kids is essential—tolerating a rowdy bus is not. If this context consistently triggers the child, consider advocating to have a bus monitor put on the bus.

- "At home when my big brother and his friends watch sexy movies": Watching movies is not only nonessential, in this case, it also seems age-inappropriate. The therapist should work with the parent to provide better monitoring or work with the whole family to help everyone understand why these movies can't be watched at home right now.

- "Going to school": Unless there are extraordinary circumstances, a child needs to go to school. A child who refuses to go to school may be avoiding the resulting feelings of distress. In this situation, gradually helping the child introduce more and more aspects of the school day into his/her life again may help him/her learn that he/she can manage attending without being overwhelmed by his/her feelings.

Cues of the Revving State

This part of the guide should look familiar from page 1. Just as you did when you helped the child identify cues for knowing he/she was in a regulated state, try to find out what changes occur when the child begins to rev. This is usually best done with a specific example or two of times when the child began to get dysregulated. It is not necessary to have every category filled in to begin with—in fact, discovering which categories are hard to fill in can help provide information about which skills need to be the focus of skill building later in session. For example, if a child cannot identify how he/she feels, activities that focus on emotion identification skills are in order. A sample follows.

Ask Others	Ask Myself
Affect: What expression does my face show? How do I say I feel? *My mouth gets tight, I stop smiling, I make fists. I tell people I'm mad.*	**Affect:** How do I feel? What does my body feel like? *Angry. Really mad.*
Awareness: Do I seem spaced out or in my own world? How well am I paying attention to things? *Mom says I don't answer her, don't seem to notice her. I sometimes get in trouble for not paying attention at school.*	**Awareness:** What's going on around me? What am I thinking about? *Don't know.*
Action: What do I do? What do I say? *I say, "Get out of my face, leave me alone."*	**Action:** What do I feel like doing? *I feel like punching someone, or yelling.*

Based on this cue chart, the therapist can identify that the child needs help developing strategies for regulating when he/she is angry, as well as help identifying internal body signals. He/she may also benefit eventually from activities that help him/her ground (if, in fact, he/she is not answering his mom because he/she is dissociating or otherwise overwhelmed with internal stimuli).

Interventions for the Child in a Revving Emotional State

It's not enough just to know when the child is getting out of control; the family needs some concrete things to *do* when this happens. This section contains a list of emotion regulation techniques that are individualized to the child. This list can grow and change over time. Some techniques that initially the child needs someone else to help him/her with, over time, may become internalized, and the child may be able to do them alone. Talking about what's bothering him/her or getting a hug are strategies that clearly involve another person. Drawing pictures together, going on a walk, or doing relaxation exercises are all techniques that might eventually be employed by the child alone but may initially need to be initiated and modeled by a parent.

The child may not have many things to put on this list when you start. That's where you come in. Section 2 of this chapter, "Emotion Regulation Skill Building," provides specific activities that help children develop coping skills. Each time a child learns a new coping skill, such as a new relaxation technique, he/she can list that skill in the intervention box. What is most important is that the child develop these skills so that once he/she (or a caregiver) recognizes that a revving state is occurring, he/she can apply these skills to transition back to the regulated state.

Things an *adult can help me with:*	Things I can *do on my own:*
Have someone joke around with me.	*Take deep breaths.*
Play basketball.	*"Connect to the universe" activity.*
Mom: Give a time out.	*Favorite room visualization.*

Page 3. Reexperiencing: Feeling and Being Out of Control

You will notice that this page looks a lot like page 2 of the guide. The format is the same; what has changed is the child's state. If a child continues to escalate until he/she reexperiences the prior traumatic event, the whole playing field changes. Suddenly the same things that might have calmed a child earlier (e.g., joking around with him/her) become a trigger. Interventions that might have worked 10 minutes ago (e.g., suggesting he/she put on music) are irrelevant, and meanwhile the danger is escalating—the child is about to throw something or is curled up in a ball in a dissociated state. What now? In essence, this page of the guide becomes a crisis management plan.

 As children become increasingly dysregulated, they may engage in more crisis-oriented behaviors. In this stage their ability to choose how they respond is narrowed; they may feel, in fact, that they have no choice in, or control over, their behavior. This state was described in detail in Chapter 3. As children transition into a reexperiencing state, their affect, awareness, and action change dramatically. They are experiencing themselves back at the time of the traumatic event or events or reexperiencing emotions and arousal and a sense of loss of control much like when the trauma happened. Accordingly, their capacity to feel, think, and behave is radically altered. As described in Chapter 7, when a child experiences changes in the three A's and is engag-

> They are experiencing themselves back at the time of the traumatic event or events or reexperiencing emotions and arousal and a sense of loss of control much like when the trauma happened.

ing in potentially dangerous behaviors, we say that he/she is behaviorally dysregulated. When the child is not engaging in potentially dangerous behaviors, we say that he/she is emotionally dysregulated.

Initially it may seem that a child moves immediately from a traumatic reminder to the reexperiencing state. One of the therapeutic goals is to lengthen the time between the traumatic reminder and the entrance into crisis behaviors; efforts to identify and intervene earlier are part of this process. Once a child reaches the reexperiencing state, there may be fewer options for intervention; the focus of the interventions shifts to maintaining the safety of the child and others.

Traumatic Reminders and Stressors

The first step in helping a child who is in a reexperiencing state is to figure out if there is anything in the environment that is perpetuating this reaction. Previously benign elements of the environment may suddenly be perceived as threatening and thereby contribute to the dysregulation. For instance, for a child who has entered a reexperiencing state a noisy environment may be overwhelming. The list of traumatic reminders and stressors generated here are not likely to be removed from the child's environment during most times; however, if a crisis is brewing, these triggers should be minimized immediately. Removal of these stressors is temporary, and once the child has returned to a regulated state they can be reintroduced. Examples:

- Noisy environment
- Presence of peers/siblings
- Verbal threats of consequences (consequences may appear later)
- Some kinds of music
- The person with whom the child is currently in conflict

Cues of a Reexperiencing State

Knowing when a child is entering a reexperiencing state is critical to helping the child and, particularly, preventing dangerous behaviors. Differences between cues for revving and reexperiencing states may be subtle, but they are very important. Again, talking about specific examples of times the child reexperienced a trauma will be helpful in filling out this information.

Ask Others	Ask Myself
Affect: What expression does my face show? How do I say I feel?	**Affect:** How do I feel? What does my body feel like?
I breathe hard.	*Angry. A 9 on 1–10 scale. I feel really strong.*
Awareness: Do I seem spaced out or in my own world? How well am I paying attention to things?	**Awareness:** What's going on around me? What am I thinking about?
Can't remember—Mom says she does things and tells me thing, but I never remember it.	*My body feels all hot.*

Action: What do I do? What do I say?	**Action:** What do I feel like doing?
I say swear words, a lot of things about the other person. Sometimes I hit my little sister or hit my head against the wall.	I feel like killing someone.

Interventions for Reexperiencing

At this point, interventions are focused on the maintenance of safety and the containment of the child's behavior. Mutual regulation techniques often include reducing or eliminating the new set of traumatic reminders. For example, a child who cannot tolerate loud noise and high levels of stimulation when he/she is in a reexperiencing state could be taken to a quieter room, or other family members might be asked to leave the room. Consequences, which might be highly effective with a child during most times, may seem threatening and further escalate the child's behavior during these times. For instance, a time-out is not an appropriate strategy when a child is physically out of control. Instead, an intervention that focuses on calmly redirecting the behavior might be more helpful. This intervention section can also be used as an emergency/crisis plan, so that parents have a list of numbers to call in an emergency

Things an *adult can help me with:*	Things I can *do on my own:*
Make sister leave the room.	Try "walking and breathing" technique.
Don't yell, just talk normally.	Draw a really big picture on the butcher paper on the ground.
Put the big glass vase and other breakable things where they can't be reached.	Cheerlead self: "I can stay in control, I can stay in control, I can stay in control."
If hitting head on wall, hold me in big hug.	
Call SOS team at 867-5309.	
If I can't calm down and you are worried about my safety or someone else's, call 911.	

Page 4. Reconstitution: "Getting Back in Control Again"

Equally important as knowing when a child is entering a reexperiencing state is knowing when he/she has returned to feeling in more control. How does a child communicate when he/she is feeling in control again? How does he/she feel about him/herself once the crisis is over? This is the focus of page 4 of the guide: reconstitution. During this time, children are particularly vulnerable to new triggers.

Page 4 is also important for the session *process*. Walking step by step through a crisis event that took place over the week may leave the child feeling ashamed or feeling other emotions that led to the event. Thus, within session, it is important to end the discussion by focusing on the eventual success of regulating.

Maybe he/she didn't calm down until he/she reached the hospital, or maybe he/she calmed down fairly quickly at home; either way, spend some time talking with parent and child about how everyone knew the crisis had passed, and what helped get everyone to that place.

Sometimes what the child did during a reexperiencing state has lasting effects or has caused other people to feel hurt or angry. Part of reconstitution is coming up with a plan for what the child can do to repair some of the damage—literal or metaphorical. This aspect is important not only to help diminish other people's feelings of anger, but also to help the child manage his/her own feelings of shame. Can a child put his/her allowance toward replacing a broken object? Can he/she write a letter of apology? Can he/she help clean up the mess? These "repair" items can be listed under the intervention section at the bottom of the page.

> Part of reconstitution is coming up with a plan for what the child can do to repair some of the damage—literal or metaphorical.

Follow the same format of filling out the cue chart and include repair activities in the "maintenance and repair activities" section.

Ask Others	Ask Myself
Affect: What expression does my face show? How do I say I feel?	**Affect:** How do I feel? What does my body feel like?
I look calm, kind of relaxed.	*Tired. I feel like I'm bad because I hurt my sister.*
Awareness: Do I seem spaced out or in my own world? How well am I paying attention to things?	**Awareness:** What's going on around me? What am I thinking about?
I can pay attention again. I notice a lot of things, like how upset Mom is.	*My body feels like a noodle. I don't know what I'm thinking, nothing.*
Action: What do I do? What do I say?	**Action:** What do I feel like doing?
I say I'm sorry, that I won't do it again, sometimes I help clean up.	*Nothing.*

Maintenance and repair activities: things I can do to keep myself in control and to fix the problems I contributed to.

Things an *adult can help me with:*	Things I can *do on my own:*
Go to the store and buy new toy to replace the one of my sister's that broke.	*Use my allowance to buy the toy.*
	Pick up the stuff I threw.
	Tell my sister and mom I'm sorry, and that I love them.

Emotion Regulation Skill Building

Once the ER guide has been used to check in about the past week and to guide the first half of session, the focus then shifts to introducing or practicing specific skills. The activities or skills can be tailored to the child's developmental level, personal interests, and needs. There are two primary types of skills that need to be built:

1. Emotion coping skills
2. Emotion identification skills

The next two sections detail the goals of each of these skill areas and provide examples of activities that encourage skill development.

Emotion Coping Skills

Emotion coping skills are practical ways of handling difficult feelings and situations. Specifically, they involve *relaxation* skills and *affect management* strategies. Coping skills are often introduced very early in the ER module, thus giving the child concrete, practical skills to try out in times of distress. The specific goals of each type of coping skill (relaxation and affect management) are discussed below, followed by a toolbox of activities that encourage the development of that specific skill.

> Emotion coping skills are practical ways of handling difficult feelings and situations. Specifically, they involve *relaxation* skills and *affect management* strategies.

What skills: Relaxation and affect management (RA)

When to use them: Emphasized early in ER module to provide immediate set of skills to use in response to emotion dysregulation

Target goals: Child and parent have repertoire of coping skills and knowledge of when to employ them to prevent further dysregulation.

Relaxation

Relaxation skills are critical to help the child calm down, counteract physiological arousal, take a mental and behavioral "pause," and create an opportunity to shift an escalating trajectory. Learning to relax can also help a child gain a greater awareness of changes in his/her body and to become more attuned to when his/her body is reacting to a stressor. Relaxation skills can encompass body movement, breathing, and visualization.

Not all of the activities listed here are going to work with every child. Make sure you consider the child's developmental level and natural interests when selecting an activity. For instance, visualization techniques may be too quiet, demanding of the imagination, or difficult to focus on for some (particularly younger) children. If this is they case, try making the exercises shorter and more concrete. Some clients may not be comfortable closing their eyes. Younger clients may be able to engage in drawings that follow themes similar to the visualizations suggested below.

 RELAXATION TOOLBOX: BODY MOVEMENT, BREATHING, AND VISUALIZATION ACTIVITIES

Activity: Mirroring

Skills: Body awareness, sense of control over body, mindfulness, physiological calming

Stand facing the client. Tell him/her you are each looking into a magical mirror, where each person is the other's reflection. Start by having the child make slow movements and mirror his/her body movements with your own body. After a few minutes, switch, so that the child follows yours. Then change again, with neither person identified as the lead—this time either person can make movements, and you both take turns without verbally telling the other when you are changing. Try making different emotional expressions and moving very slowly. Rules: Do not touch the mirror (the other person), use slow-motion movements only, and make no sound.

Activity: Hand drawing

Skills: Body awareness, visualization

Place a blank piece of paper in front of both you and your client. Explain that you are each going to draw a picture of your hand, but that you have to place your hand on the table in such a way that you can't see the paper while you draw. You may need to tape the paper down so that it doesn't move. Encourage your client to draw lots of details on the hand, such as fingernails and knuckle wrinkles. When both of you have finished, look at the drawings you made. This is an important activity to participate in with your client, because usually the drawings are very silly looking. Rules: Do not peek at the paper, keep your eyes on the hand you are drawing the entire time.

Activity: Strike a pose

Skills: Body awareness, sense of body control

Take turns having you or the client strike a pose. The other person has to mimic that pose. The initiator then has to comment on three things he/she notices about the pose (e.g., "All your weight is on your left foot," "It's hard to balance," "The world looks upside down!") before you can shift and have the other person strike a pose. Try some poses that are more inward focused (e.g., hugging your knees or placing your arms tight across your chest) and some positions that are very open (e.g., on tiptoes, arms flung up and out or stretched toward the sky). Talk about the different feelings you have in each of the poses. Rules: The position has to be physically possible for both therapist and client.

Activity: Statue

Skills: Body awareness, collaboration, trust

Explain to the child that one of you is a great artist who is going to make a statue out of magical putty. The putty is magical because it will move where you want it to move—without being touched! All the sculptor has to do is describe to the putty what to do. Unfortunately, the putty doesn't understand things unless the statements are very specific; for instance, it won't respond to "Sit down"—you have to say "Bend the left knee, now lower your bottom toward the floor, put the left foot on the floor. . . . " Take turns being the "sculptor" and the "putty," and talk each other into sculpture positions. The sculptor needs to tell the putty as specifically as possible how to move (e.g., "Take your left arm and move it up; now take your thumb and make it stick up, curl your other fingers into a fist"). The putty needs to listen carefully and respond very literally to the commands. Rules: No touching or inappropriate positions.

Activity: Being a noodle

Skills: Body awareness, muscle relaxation, visualization

Ask the child if he/she has ever seen a spaghetti noodle before and after it's been cooked. Talk about how stiff and rigid it is before, and how floppy and flexible it becomes. Then have the child act like an uncooked noodle (guide him/her verbally to tighten different muscles, stand stiff, and be as tight and rigid as possible). Talk the child through the cooking process, relaxing him/her as you go: "OK, the noodle is being put in a big pot of hot water! It's in there, and OH! It's starting to get sort of soft in the middle! It's bending a little bit at the middle . . . now up top it's getting a little floppy, relax your neck a little bit . . . now the arms are beginning to wiggle around a little bit. . . . Uh-oh, the legs are getting so soft I'm not sure they'll be able to hold the noodle straight anymore!" Continue in this fashion until the child is totally relaxed. Then let the child take a turn "cooking" you.

Activity: Connect to the universe

Skills: Body awareness, body control, sense of groundedness

Start by talking about how, thanks to gravity, it is virtually impossible not to be connected to the earth. Explain that today we're going to see just HOW connected we can get. Start by observing how many different points of the body are touching the earth just then (e.g., two feet on the ground, one bottom on the chair, an arm on the arm rest makes four points). Then ask the child if he/she can make zero points touch the ground (e.g., by jumping). Ask him/her to place one point down (e.g., one foot or one bottom). Keep increasing the number of points, until he/she can't put any more points down. Talk about how different it feels when you have one point versus eight (or whatever limit he/she reached).

Activity: Walking and breathing (adapted from Linehan, 1993)

Skills: Control over body, physiological calming, breathing awareness

Begin by walking slowly around the room in pace with your client. Have your client count how many steps he/she is taking with each breath. After about five steps ask the child to slow his/her breathing so that he/she takes three steps per breath. Continue gradually increasing the number of breaths per step until the breaths are long and slow (but not to the point of being forced).

Activity: Deep breathing

Skills: Physiological calming, breathing awareness, control over body

Have your client sit in a comfortable position or lie on the floor on his/her back. Tell the client to breathe normally, then verbally draw his/her attention to the way the stomach and chest move as he/she breathes. Start by commenting "Breathe in . . . breathe out" in time with the client's natural breathing. Gradually slow him/her down so that he/she is pausing a moment at the top of the breath before slowly exhaling. Do this for about 10 breaths. For young children, put a stuffed animal on their abdomen and have them watch it move up and down with their breathing.

Addendum: Particularly for the child who finds deep breathing boring, it can be helpful to include a before and after "pulse test." Have the child find his/her pulse while he/she is breathing normally, and count the beats for 10 seconds. Multiply this number by 6 to get his/her pulse rate. Then complete the deep breathing and retake the pulse. Compare the numbers and see if he/she was able to bring his/her heart rate down.

Activity: Favorite room

Skills: Distraction, self-soothing, mindfulness

Help your client visualize a room that feels safe and comfortable. Ask questions about what furniture and toys he/she would put in the room. Who would he/she let visit in his/her room? What kinds of games would they play or what would they talk about in the room? Are there windows? What is the view from the window? Are there pictures on the wall? What is in the pictures? Is there music playing? Let the child be queen or king of the room, totally in control of the imaginary space.

Activity: Four-seasons mountain meditation

Skills: Self-soothing, mindfulness, focus

Have the client sit comfortably, preferably in a cross-legged position (like a mountain). Ask him/her to think of a mountain, a beautiful mountain, real or imagined. Provide the child with a series of elaborations, such as "There is a stream on the mountain that falls over some rocks. What does the stream sound like? Imagine an animal drinking from the stream. What kind of animal do you see?" Include trees, the sky, and the ground. Ask about details that appeal to different senses, such as temperature, bird, or wind sounds, or the feel of the ground under his/her feet. After the child has a sufficiently elaborate mountain in mind, tell him/her that fall is coming and ask him/her to imagine changes. Then bring in a winter storm and snowfall and ask the child to imagine how things change. Do this again for spring and summer, ending on an image that is full of life.

Affect Management

As another key area of coping skills, affect management provides children with skills by which they can calm themselves when they are upset. These skills are focused on in-the-moment activities that help to calm a child and prevent him/her from acting impulsively. Affect management skills include refocusing and self-coaching.

 AFFECT MANAGEMENT TOOLBOX:
REFOCUSING AND SELF-COACHING

Activity: My list of things I do

Skills: Refocusing

Work with parent and child to generate a list of things the child likes to do. Try to get the child to really stretch beyond the usual (e.g., "I like to draw and watch TV"), and come up with an exhaustive list. Does he/she like to skip down the hall? Sit on the top stair and watch the light coming in the window? Eat apples with the skin peeled off? Wash his/her hands in hot water? Take a bubble bath? Try to come up with sensory activities. Have the child decorate the list or turn it into a poster so that it can go up at home in a visible place. When he/she's feeling upset, have him/her pick something off the list and do it, whether he/she feels like it or not. If the child is scientifically minded, you can have him/her create a rating column next to the activities so that he/she can rate how well they worked (or do a rating of how distressed he/she is on a 1–10 scale before he/she tries it and then after).

Activity: Affirmations

Skills: Inserting a "wedge" of cognition, refocusing, positive self-talk

Collaborate with the child to find an affirmation, slogan, word, or phrase that he/she can repeat to him/herself or visualize when he/she is having a hard time. For instance, "I am lovable," "I am here to learn, I don't have to get it right the first time—just try," "I know people who believe in me." When a booster message has been selected, you can reinforce it by making banners, using puffy-paint on a T-shirt, or making a poster. Have the child practice saying it aloud as well as to him/herself. When the child begins to get upset, encourage him/her to visualize the poster or repeat the slogan in his/her mind 10 times.

Activity: Imaginary school bus

Skills: Internalizing positive self-image, idea generation

Work with the child to generate a list of people who are supportive of the child or who the child thinks would support him/her (e.g., superheroes or celebrity figures). Feel free to put yourself on the list, teachers, or anyone else the child might not think of, whom you suspect could be a supportive person. Then ask the child to visualize getting on a school bus and seeing each of those people in a seat. Help the child visualize this in a way that is easiest for him/her—drawing a picture of the bus, putting names of people on seats (who would sit next to whom?), or closing his/her eyes and having you describe all the people in the bus. Have the child imagine which seat each would pick— who would each sit near? Have the child imagine that everyone on the bus wants the child to sit next to him/her. If the child is having a specific problem (e.g., friends at school teasing him/her), ask the child to imagine the whole bus of hand-picked people generating ideas of what he/she could do. What would Mom say? What would J-Lo say?

Activity: Coach the therapist

Skills: Idea generation, self-talk

Talk with the child about a sports coach (he/she may have one he/she admires, or you can talk about a hypothetical team coach). Talk about how a coach's job is both to encourage and support team members as well as challenge them to do their best. Have the child imagine how a coach stands at the side of the basketball court, calling out encouragement and ideas. Now suggest that the child be the coach and you will be the player. Pick a recent incident when the child was having a little trouble regulating emotions (e.g., having trouble staying in his/her seat at school). Do a role play, with you acting like the child (and verbalizing out loud your thoughts and reactions). Ask the child to play the coach and to stand on the sideline yelling support and encouragement and providing suggestions and tips. If the child is having trouble, switch roles and you be the coach, then switch back so the child has practice verbalizing the coaching role. Suggest that the child can visualize his/her coach when he/she is next in school. You can refer back to this image later, asking things such as "What would the coach say?" when the child comes in with a new problem.

Activity: Bigger than a breadbox: The emotion continuum

Skills: Emotion identification, self-confidence, emotion regulation

This exercise works best when the child has had trouble regulating emotions in the past week and comes in with a specific incident to talk about (e.g., he/she got in a fight at school when someone teased him/her). Ask the child to pick up a handful of rocks (or crayons, jelly beans, paper clips, or whatever small object you have on hand in large quantity) and make a pile to represent how angry he/she felt during that time. Then ask the child to think of another time he/she was angry—but a little less angry (place a smaller pile of rocks in front of him/her). Ask how he/she coped with the anger that time. Keep going down in size, until the child finally reaches a point where he/she tells a story about a time he/she was angry but successfully coped with it. Compare the two piles of rocks—one that represents how much anger he/she felt when he/she successfully regulated the anger, and one that represents how much anger he/she felt when he/she was dysregulated. Point out that he/she really *does* know how to regulate and only needs to work on coping with more and more rocks (angry feelings) in successful ways.

Emotion Identification Skills

Being able to experience, identify, and express emotions forms the foundation for successful emotion regulation. These abilities are also essential for cognitive processing. Part of the goal of the ER module is to make sure the child has the skills to experience, identify, and express feelings. If the child has trouble identifying his/her feelings when you do the ER guide, that's a good clue that you need to spend some time on these skills. You can do emotion identification skills interchangeably with emotion coping skills during the second half of the session; both types of activities reinforce the other.

> If the child has trouble identifying his/her feelings when you do the ER guide, that's a good clue that you need to spend some time on these skills.

We've divided emotion identification skills into two sections: (1) Observing and naming skills focuses on helping the child become aware of his/her emotions and put words to the feeling. (2) Expression, on the other hand, focuses on ways of allowing that feeling to be shared with another person, or even fully experienced by oneself. For children who experience numbing or avoidance of feelings, these skills may form the central portion of the ER work.

What skills: Observe, name, and express feelings (ONE)

When to use them: Emphasized in the more advanced phases of the ER module to provide skill building in times of regulation or early on, if a child is unable to experience feelings. Prerequisite for cognitive-processing module.

Target goals: Child can experience a range of emotions, can identify emotions in self and others, has vocabulary to label specific feelings, understands concepts of *mixed feelings* and *different intensities* of feelings, has repertoire of safe ways to express feelings.

Observing and Naming Feelings

Observing and naming feelings are critical underlying skills for all emotion regulation work. In the course of using the ER guide, children become more familiar with observing their internal and external responses and learning to put words to that emotion. The process of playing and talking in session frequently gives rise to opportunities to explore how the child is feeling in the moment. Pausing in your activities to discuss physiological changes, action urges, and emotions provides the child with immediate feedback and practice in labeling feelings in the moment.

> Pausing in your activities to discuss physiological changes, action urges, and emotions provides the child with immediate feedback and practice in labeling feelings in the moment.

The therapist's own emotional responses provide another opportunity for modeling the process of observing and naming. Particularly if a child appears to be attempting to elicit a certain emotion (e.g., anger), it can be helpful to pause and identify for the child the fact that you are feeling that emotion, as well as how you plan to handle it. Using your own responses in session allows you to model the crucial learning that emotions are controllable and that the child's actions have an effect on the environment.

In-session process work can be augmented by skill-building activities that help the child develop a vocabulary for, and understanding of, a wide range of emotions.

Expressing Feelings

Skills for expressing feelings can be divided into two groups: (1) skills that allow a child to experience feelings (e.g., expressing them to him/herself), and (2) skills that help a child communicate these feelings to others. Expressive feeling skills can involve art, dance, music, writing, or any medium that resonates with a particular child. For some children who are especially numb to feelings or who actively avoid anything that leads to certain physical sensations, activities that elicit different emotions and give them the chance to experience the physical sensations associated with feelings may be necessary.

Activities that help children experience emotions are most important for those children who avoid experiencing emotions, avoid situations that might lead to such emotions, or are numb to some or all emotions. They may not be appropriate for children who have difficulty controlling their anger. Skills involving communicating with others may also help increase a child's social skills: How do you express your anger to someone through words, rather than fists? How can you communicate to others the different feelings you have about something?

 EMOTION IDENTIFICATION TOOLBOX: OBSERVING, NAMING, AND EXPRESSING (ONE)

Activity: Emotion portfolio

Skills: Emotion identification, self-awareness, emotion vocabulary

Part 1: Emotion faces. On a piece of paper trace or draw a large circle. Ask the child to name an emotion and draw a corresponding face. Have the child write the emotion name on top. Do this for as many emotions as the child can think of (or until you have a range of basic emotions), each on a different sheet of paper. If there are any critical emotions missing (e.g., anger, fear), prompt the child by thinking about scenarios in which that feeling is likely to occur. If the child is having difficulty thinking of what the facial expression looks like for a particular emotion, take turns trying to act out that feeling and showing it on your face. You can also take this time to talk about how different people show emotions in different ways.

Part 2: "I feel X when . . . " On the bottom of each emotion face page, write "I feel [whichever emotion] when. . . . " Help the child brainstorm different activities or events that make him/her feel a certain way, and write these on the bottom of the face page. Some items may show up on more than one emotion face page. Point this out and talk about how you can have more than one feeling about the same thing.

Part 3: Emotion words. On the back of each emotion face page, brainstorm a list of related emotion words. By taking turns with the child, thinking of other related emotions, you can introduce the child to words that he/she may not know. Spend some time thinking together about how the different words might provide different information (e.g., *glad* vs. *joyful* vs. *content*) and making up scenarios in which you (or a puppet or a friend) might feel the different ways.

The emotion portfolio can be worked on and developed over time. New experiences or words can be added to the face sheets as you go. Ultimately, the different emotion face sheets can be collected and made into a book.

The emotion portfolio can also be adapted for different ages. Older children, for instance, may choose to do more abstract representations of feelings within the circle on the page. Younger children may need to see predrawn faces and then can participate by trying to guess the feeling depicted.

Activity: Emotional drama

Skills: Emotion identification, emotion vocabulary

Write a variety of emotion words on different slips of paper and put them in a hat. Hand a copy of the "boring script" (see Appendix) to both you and the child. (The boring script can be the one provided in this book, something you have made up beforehand, or something that you write together. The idea is to have a script of a brief, neutral dialogue that the two of you can enact). Read through the script together once, with each of you taking a role. Now each of you draws an emotion from the hat, without showing the other. Reread the script, but this time each person enacts his/her role as if he/she were experiencing the emotion that he/she drew from the hat. Try to guess each other's emotion and give feedback about why you guessed that emotion.

Continue drawing emotions and reenacting the script until all of the emotions have been drawn.

Activity: The feelings interview

Skills: Emotion identification, physiological awareness, normalizing

Provide the child with a set of about 10 sheets of paper that have the following format:

WHAT PEOPLE'S BODIES DO WHEN THEY ARE MAD			
Reaction	Yes	No	What Helps?
SHAKING			
GET HOT			
CRY			
FEEL SICK TO STOMACH			
GET TIGHT/TENSE			
OTHER _____			

Together, fill out the left column (the list of possible reactions when someone is angry). Then ask the child to interview 10 people in the next week, about times when they were mad and if they have ever had their body react a certain way (e.g., shaking). Also have the child ask what that person does to feel better. When the child brings the forms back, discuss how bodies respond to anger. You can do a similar activity for different feelings.

Activity: Basket of feelings

Skills: Identify feelings, understand mixed emotions, communicate feelings

Have the child come up with a list of feelings and write each one in large letters (or draw a face showing it) on a different piece of paper. Spread the paper out in front of you. Then show the child a basket with a bunch of things in it—a bunch of crayons, lots of little stones, jelly bellies, whatever comes in many little pieces. Model for the child, bringing up a time when you had a strong feeling (e.g., when you had to give a talk in front of a bunch of people). For each feeling you had during that experience, place a handful of the objects—a big handful if you had a lot of those feelings, a little handful if you had a little. You might have lots of jelly beans on nervous and scared, and a few on excited, and one or two on confident. Then have the child do the same thing, either with his/her own emotional experience or a specific event that you are helping him/her talk about. This activity can be done over and over during the course of treatment, to talk about how feelings change. It can also be used to help communicate to parents how a child feels about something.

Activity: Color your life

Skills: Communicating emotions, identifying feelings

Have the child make a list of feelings, each in a different color. Then draw a large circle on a piece of paper, telling the child that the circle represents him/her right now, and have the child fill in the circle with colors that represent his/her different feelings. Then do this with other events in their lives or for other people so that the child can see how he/she felt about different things. You can have family members, and yourself, do this as well and compare with the child the different perspectives on how people felt.

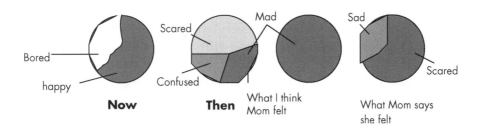

An alternative is to have the child color a timeline of his/her life, going from left (birth) to right (present). Then go back and have the child explain which events are represented by the different colors.

Activity: Name that feeling/name that tune

Skills: Identifying feelings, experiencing emotions

Bring in a selection of music (the child can as well). Take turns playing the music and being the "feeling actor." The feeling actor needs to decide what feeling that particular piece of music evokes and then act it out (with facial expressions and body language). The other person needs to guess the feeling. Talk about whether listening to different types of music actually makes you feel different.

Activity: Stop everything and feel!

Skills: Identifying feelings, generating coping strategies

Write a story together, alternating lines or having the child dictate it (if he/she can generate it on his/her own). Periodically ring a bell (clap, bang a drum, etc.). Whenever the bell rings, the story stops and you answer the following questions: How is the character feeling? How can you tell he/she feels that way? What can he/she do next to let people know he/she feels that way? Does he/she want to keep feeling this way? If not, what could he/she do to change his/her feelings? When you've had a sufficient discussion about the character's feelings, ring the bell and let the story continue. The character does not have to take the advice you might have come up with during the discussion (e.g., does not have to express his/her feelings to someone or change the way he/she feels).

Activities: The last straw, sit and spin, and hearts up! (adapted from Barlow, Allen, & Choate, 2005)

Skills: Experiencing emotions (each of these activities is for children who avoid different physical sensations because they associate them with feeling upset. "The last straw" is for children who avoid feeling lightheaded or hyperventilated, "sit and spin" is for children who avoid feeling dizzy, and "hearts up!" is for children who avoid rapid heart beats).

This exercise is for children who are very avoidant of emotions. Tell them you want to help them get used to feeling different sensations in their body and learning that it's OK, that nothing bad happens. Talk about how everyone has different feelings all the time—like an itch, for instance—that are pretty normal. But if you get too focused on that feeling or too scared that that feeling "means something" or is the beginning of something bigger and worse, then simply having that little itch can throw off your whole day. For some kids that "itch" might be their heart speeding up a little or their head feeling a little light or getting a little dizzy on the tire swing. Talk about how these are normal daily feelings that come and go, and that if they are really avoiding one of them, or scared by one, it's good to get used to having them. Ultimately, you want the children to understand that the feeling itself isn't a problem and that sometimes that feeling is very manageable. The following activities can help children experience whichever feeling they are avoiding in a safe, controlled way.

Sit and spin. Have the child sit in an office chair that can spin. Ask the child to list any sensations he/she notices in his/her body and any thoughts he/she has. Can the child feel his/her heart beat? Does he/she notice the speed of his/her breath? Then tell the child that you are going to spin him/her around very fast in the chair, and you want the child to pay attention to see if there are any changes to the feelings, sensations, and thoughts he/she just identified. Spin the chair long enough for the child's physiology to react—usually between 30 seconds and 2 minutes. Then stop the chair and ask the same questions you asked prior to spinning. "What has changed? Does the feeling in your body remind you of an emotion? Have you felt that way before? Have you ever done something to *avoid* feeling that way?" Help the child track how the feelings keep changing over time, gradually becoming less intense. Talk about "riding the wave" of emotion, and how there is a moment of peak intensity that is typically followed by a drop-off. Once the child has "ridden the wave" back down, try another exercise to start another wave. If the child is reticent to do this, remind him/her that this is different from other emotional experiences he/she may have had because he/she is literally in the "drivers' seat": He/she is choosing to start the wave.

The last straw. Have on hand two drinking straws. Tell the child that you are both going to breathe through the straw for a while. First have the child note all the physical sensations, thoughts, and feelings he/she can identify. Do this again after breathing through the straw long enough to feel your own internal sensations change. Did the internal sensations remind the child of a feeling he/she has had before? Did the child notice his/her emotions change, or did emotions appear? Talk about "riding the wave," as described in the exercise above. Now try a coffee straw. . . .

Hearts up! For this exercise, follow the basic outline described above (having the child note his/her physical sensations, thoughts, feelings, etc.). Then pick a cardiovascular exercise—say, running in place or running up the stairwell. As described above, have the child note changes in his/her feelings and emotions and talk about "riding the wave."

Activity: Feelings . . . are they really worth it?

Skills: Experiencing emotions

If a child is very resistant to the idea of experiencing emotions, you may need to start by helping him/her (and sometimes the parents) understand the value of emotions. Here are three situations you can pose to the child. In each case, see if the child can think of any important results that can be linked to having that emotion or physical sensation.

- You put your hand on the burner on the stove and discover it is hot. What if you couldn't feel any pain? What might happen then? What does pain lead you to do?
- You have a test at school at the end of the week and you haven't read the chapter yet. What if you don't feel anxious at all? What might you do? What might you do differently if you did feel anxious? How might reading the chapter change what you feel? How might reading the chapter change how you do in on the test?
- You borrow a friend's new shirt and get a big stain on it. What are some emotions you might feel? What might those feelings motivate you to do? Let's say you didn't have *any* feelings. Would that change what you did? Let's say you returned the shirt to the friend with the stain (even though you have enough money to buy the friend a new one, or even though you could have tried spot remover on it). How might that action affect your friend and your friendship?

Can the child think of other examples that show how emotions can be helpful? Can he/she think of times when he/she had emotions that were helpful, or when having a certain emotion would have helped?

Activity: Picture this (adapted from Barlow, Allen, & Choate, 2005)

Skills: Experiencing emotions

Have a selection of photographs or magazine pictures on hand that evoke different emotions. Look at them with the child and ask questions to get him/her thinking about the image. What is happening in the picture? What might the people in the picture be feeling? What is the child feeling, looking at the picture? If the child identifies a feeling, spend some time helping him/her describe that feeling as well as any associated thoughts or fears he/she might be having related to that feeling. After the feeling has been explored, move to the next picture. At the end, reflect back on how feelings were transient, how they could be changed, and how the child was able to tolerate all of those different feelings without anything bad happening. Pay attention to whether the child is trying to avoid experiencing emotions during this time by looking away from the pictures or trying to distract him/herself. The child may need some encouragement to go ahead and really let him/herself feel—you can remind him or her about how sometimes feelings end up being helpful.

Activity: Avoiding avoidance (adapted from Barlow, Allen, & Choate, 2005)

Skills: Experiencing emotions

This activity is designed for children who are avoiding some essential part of life in an effort to avoid becoming distressed. First identify the activity or setting that is being avoided and talk about why that is an essential part of life. Examples include going to school (essential for learning, making friends, and achieving independence), riding in a car (essential for getting around), being in public (essential for being a part of a community, maintaining daily life needs). Once you've picked an avoided activity on which to work, help the child construct a list of ways he/she could start chipping away at that avoidance. For instance, if a child is avoiding getting in the car because he/she was in a car accident, the list might include:

1. Look at the car.
2. Look at a picture of a car.
3. Watch someone else drive around in a car.
4. Sit in the car with it turned off, then on.
5. Drive in the car for a short distance.
6. Drive in the car for a long distance.

With the child, put the list in order from easiest to hardest (e.g., looking at a picture of a car might come before going outside and looking at a real car). Working from the list, start by doing the easiest activity. While the child is doing that, have him/her report on his/her emotions and physical sensations. How is he/she feeling? What is he/she thinking? The key to this exercise is that the child has to stick with it until any wave of emotion has subsided. You may need to do the activity several times (show several pictures or the same picture again and again) until the child's emotions get less intense and dissipate faster. Then move to step 2 of the list. Moving through the whole list may take several sessions.

Terminating the ER Module:
Knowing When to Transition

Refining emotion regulation techniques is a lifelong process. Within the TST approach, however, the goal is to transfer the knowledge and skills necessary to refine and practice emotion regulation to the parent and child; ultimately, the most important work in emotion regulation will take place outside of the therapy office. Thus termination of the ER module depends on achievement of three goals:

1. The child is able to regulate his/her emotions effectively in response to a normal range of stressors.
2. The child and parent have a working knowledge of the child's traumatic reminders, changes that signal a shift in state, and appropriate interventions to help the child regulate.
3. The child has developed the necessary emotion coping and emotion identification skills to move on to cognitive processing.

Each of these goals can be monitored through use of the ER guide. Over time, the guide will provide an assessment of the child's increasing capacity to regulate emotion in the face of upsetting events. In addition, as the parent and child gain a greater understanding of when and how to implement emotion regulation techniques, they can gradually assume responsibility for filling out the guide.

As the client achieves his/her ER goals, the therapist gradually transitions from the ER module to the cognitive-processing (CP) module. Although the therapist will continue to monitor the child's emotion regulation progress, the focus of the sessions will shift to cognitive processing. The therapist should encourage the child to continue using the emotion regulation guide, and they may wish to review and update the guide together periodically. Because it is likely that the child will occasionally return to experiencing difficulties with emotion regulation (e.g., due to external events or developmental transitions), it is helpful to maintain some fluidity in moving between the ER and CP modules.

At times, the boundary between CP and ER modules may seem unclear. Some clients want to talk about what happened, and it is important not to send a message that they "shouldn't" talk yet or that the trauma is so big and bad that it can't be handled. On the other hand, sometimes children want to talk about the trauma but really are not ready to process what happened and could place themselves at risk of engaging in dangerous behavior. The best approach to take is one that allows the child to bring up whatever is on his/her mind (including the trauma), but use that topic to engage in skill building rather than cognitive processing. As an example, you might choose to work on emotion identification regarding the trauma (e.g., the basket of feelings exercise), which allows for some discussion of the trauma without yet working on the trauma narrative (cognitive processing). Finally, there are times when a child needs to tell his/her

> The best approach to take is one that allows the child to bring up whatever is on his/her mind (including the trauma), but use that topic to engage in skill building rather than cognitive processing.

story—because he/she wants to; because there is no one else to tell it and you want to understand what happened, so you ask her to; or because she is flooded with intrusive thoughts. CP techniques might come in earlier than usual in these cases, but the actual work of cognitive processing occurs in depth later, when the child has the requisite skills. Regardless of whether or not the child is talking about the trauma, basic emotion and coping skills should be taught as part of the overall intervention. The ER module should never be skipped unless the child comes in with a full set of skills and the ability to stay regulated.

Closing Thoughts on Emotion Regulation

The activities in this chapter are by no means exhaustive. Rather, they are suggestions to fuel your own thoughts on what might help develop these skills in the child with whom you are working.

As you begin to transition into CP, it can be helpful to review the progress made. If you have collected a copy of the ER guide each week, then the copies can be reviewed as a record of progress. Comparing early and more recent copies will hopefully show a progression of the child's ability to identify internal and external cues. It may also show a growing repertoire of self-regulating skills. Finally, things that were listed as triggers early on may no longer be identified as such. Remembering where the child began and how far he/she has come can be a moment of important validation for everyone involved—parent, child, and therapist.

When you believe a child is ready to move on to CP, it can be helpful to call another Family Collaborative Meeting to review the treatment plan. By now the child has sufficient regulation skills and a sufficiently stable environment so that he/she can move to the understanding phase.

APPENDIX 14.1. The Boring Script

Following is a very boring script for use in the emotional drama exercise.

Scene: A donut shop.

Customer: Hello, I'd like to have a coffee, with milk, and a donut.

Sales clerk: We're out of coffee.

Customer: Oh. Out of coffee? I'll just have tea then.

Sales clerk: We're out of tea.

Customer: Oh. Well, could I just have the milk then?

Sales clerk: Nope, no milk either.

Customer: What? No milk?

Sales clerk: No milk. None at all.

Customer: Well, I guess I will just have the frosted donut.

Sales clerk: We're out of donuts.

Customer: You are out of donuts?

Sales clerk: Yup. Out.

Customer: Well, OK, I guess I'll have to go somewhere else. Is there anywhere else I can go around here for a cup of coffee and some donuts?

Sales clerk: Out the door and to the left. Third door down.

Customer: Thanks. Goodbye.

Sales clerk: Have a nice day.

(We *told* you it was boring!)

Cognitive Processing Skills

*How to Help Children Think and Talk
about Their Traumatic Experiences*

LEARNING OBJECTIVES

- To help children acquire cognitive coping skills
- To help children increase their tolerance for discussions about the trauma
- To help children decrease the intensity of emotion associated with the trauma
- To help improve communication about the trauma among family members

---

We know that a child has reached a critical milestone when he/she is able to begin discussing thoughts and feelings about the trauma. This important transition is the focus of the cognitive processing skills (CPS) module. This module is comprised of exercises and activities that help the child minimize negative reactions to reminders of the trauma and learn how to communicate about the trauma with family members. Specifically, this module helps the child to . . .

1. Build upon his/her ER skills to incorporate cognitive coping skills.
2. Increase his/her ability to tolerate talking about the traumatic event.
3. Decrease the intensity of emotions associated with thoughts of the trauma.
4. Facilitate communication about the trauma among family members.

How to Know If a Child Is Ready for Cognitive Processing

Cognitive processing is appropriate for children in the understanding phase of treatment. Because many of the exercises in the CPS module require the child to remember the trauma in detail and talk about his/

her feelings, it is necessary for the child to have acquired sufficient ER skills before beginning this module. The clinician can feel comfortable beginning this module if:

1. The child can regulate his/her emotions effectively in response to a normal range of stressors.
2. The child and caregiver have a working knowledge of the child's traumatic reminders, changes that signal a shift in mental state, and tools to help the child regulate emotions.
3. The caregiver is able to help the child with his/her emotion regulation.
4. Developmentally, the child is ready to talk and think about his/her emotional reactions to the trauma. (Generally, the exercises in this module were designed for children age 6 years and above.)
5. The social environment is not threatening.

It is important to remember that the CPS module requires some flexibility on the therapist's part to be able to shift from CP exercises to ER exercises during the session, particularly in the early stages of the module. The child is likely to show some initial resistance to processing the traumatic material, which may manifest as emotion dysregulation (such as crying) or overt avoidance (such as changing the subject or trying to leave room). During these situations, the therapist can help the child remember the ER skills that he/she learned previously in treatment and make use of the ER guide when necessary (see Chapter 14).

As children transition into the Understanding phase and begin cognitive processing, the treatment plan needs to be revisited. The primary work of individual therapy will now focus on the four domains of cognitive processing. As always, meeting to review the treatment plan is also an opportunity to review expectations about (1) what the CP module is, (2) why families should expect it to help, and (3) what is expected from the different team members (including the family). Particularly in the CP module, children and families have difficult work to do; the treatment alliance needs to be strong and accountability clear.

Domains of Treatment

The CPS module is comprised of four domains of treatment (COPE, for short):

1. Cognitive coping skills
2. Observation of thoughts, feelings, and behaviors
3. Processing the trauma
4. Exchanging stories with caregivers

The child is taught cognitive coping skills in the beginning of the CPS module in order to help counter the negative, and often overwhelming, feelings that may be associated with memories of the trauma. Next, the child is taught to notice how thoughts and feelings affect behavior and how to generate more adaptive thoughts. Creative techniques are then used to help the child process thoughts, feelings, and behaviors associated with the trauma. Finally, bringing the child and family together to discuss the child's trauma narrative can be important both to ensure that parents and children understand the events of the past and also to facilitate open dialogue within the family. Each of these treatment domains is explained in greater detail later in this chapter.

Treatment Structure

Therapy sessions in the CPS module are scheduled on a 1-hour per week basis for up to 3 months. Within-session structure includes:

1. **Check-in.** A 10-minute initial check-in with the parent and child together. During this time, the therapist reviews the child's emotions and behaviors throughout the past week. In addition, the Cognitive Coping Log (discussed later in this chapter) is reviewed.
2. **CP skills.** Approximately 35 minutes, during which time one of the four COPE treatment domains is addressed.
3. **Review and closing ritual.** At the end of the session, 10 minutes are spent alone with the caregiver, reviewing the child's work for the day and processing the caregiver's own reactions. Finally, the last 5 minutes of the session are focused on a closing ritual, during which both the child and caregiver jointly participate (see Chapter 11 for a description of the closing ritual).

The next section describes each of the treatment domains found within the CPS module, as well as accompanying exercises and tools used to help the child process thoughts and feelings associated with the trauma.

Cognitive Coping Skills

We start with the first domain of treatment, cognitive coping skills. One of the main skills addressed in this domain is how to control one's own thoughts. Many children who have been traumatized have intrusive thoughts about the traumatic event and feel as though these intrusive thoughts are totally out of their control. Other children may not identify thoughts specifically related to a trauma, but they do report generally "unhelpful" thoughts—negative thoughts about their own self-worth or generalized fears about bad things happening.

In their manualized treatments for sexually abused and traumatically bereaved children, Cohen and her colleagues (Cohen et al., 2001; Cole, Mannarino, & Deblinger, 2003) describe the use of **thought-stopping techniques** to help children gain more control over their cognitions. Thought stopping is accomplished by helping the child to move his/her attention away from a traumatic or unhelpful thought. Both verbal (e.g., saying *stop*) and/or physical (e.g., snapping a rubber band on one's wrist) techniques can be used to interrupt an intrusive thought. The following case illustrates the use of thought stopping with a traumatized child.

> Kelly is a 12-year-old girl who was sexually abused by her stepfather. She has recurring, intrusive thoughts about her perpetrator. She states, "Sometimes I can't get his words out of my head. He told me that if I told anyone what he did to me, then I would never see my mom again. When I think about it, I feel sick to my stomach."

Although a critical step in Kelly's treatment will later involve in-depth processing of these intrusive thoughts and images, the initial goal in the cognitive coping skills domain is to help her put a stop to thoughts that are distracting and upsetting. The therapist might help Kelly to combat these intrusive thoughts by saying, "As soon as you realize that you are hearing his voice in your head, I want you to picture a large stop sign, and I want you to yell to yourself, *Stop!* You can even yell *stop* out loud if you are by yourself."

 It is important for the therapist to be able to help the child see the difference between *controlling* intrusive thoughts when necessary and *avoiding* all thoughts of the trauma all of the time. Although the cognitive coping skills domain is focused on techniques that distract children from negative and intrusive thoughts, this is not meant to discourage children from having any thoughts of the trauma whatsoever. This domain should be used to help children learn how to identify thoughts that are limiting their ability to function (e.g., difficulty concentrating in school) and then distract themselves from those thoughts so that they are better able to handle the tasks of daily life.

> Although the cognitive coping skills domain is focused on techniques that distract children from negative and intrusive thoughts, this is not meant to discourage children from having any thoughts of the trauma whatsoever.

 Once the child has mastered thought stopping, a useful accompanying skill is **positive self-talk**, a concept also described by Cohen and colleagues (2001, 2003), during which the child focuses on positive and optimistic thoughts about him/herself or coping with the trauma. As the child learns to interrupt intrusive thoughts using thought-stopping techniques, he/she can also learn to focus on alternative, more adaptive thoughts through the use of positive self-talk. Using the previous case illustration, the therapist can help Kelly generate a list of alternative thoughts and focus on these thoughts instead of the threats that her abusive stepfather made. These more adaptive thoughts might include: "It's over now"; "I know my mom is safe"; "He can't hurt any of us anymore"; "There are lots of people protecting me." The therapist should initially have the child attempt to generate alternative thoughts on his/ her own, and if the child has difficulty, the therapist can help. It is a good idea to have the child take the list home to revisit whenever necessary.

 Make sure that the alternative thoughts you help the child generate are real—that is, don't encourage a child to think "I won't be mugged again in my neighborhood" if it might, in fact, happen. If the social environment is still distressed and the child is accurately perceiving this threat, focus instead on things the child can control. For instance, the statement "I know I can knock on a neighbors' door or call for help if I'm feeling scared in the neighborhood" acknowledges the potential threat while giving the child a greater sense of control.

Observation of Thoughts, Feelings, and Behaviors

Now, let's turn to the second domain of treatment, **observation of thoughts, feelings, and behaviors.** This domain is used to help the child understand how and why thoughts influence feelings and behaviors. By actively changing his/her thoughts, the child can see firsthand how feelings and behaviors can change as a result. This is important because traumatized children often have difficulty identifying the ways in which traumatic thoughts or reminders are influencing their feelings, and in turn, their behavior. It is often helpful to provide the child with an example. The therapist might state:

> By actively changing his/her thoughts, the child can see firsthand how feelings and behaviors can change as a result.

> "Let's say you are walking down the street during the middle of the day, and you hear someone running behind you. You glance behind you and see a boy from your class running toward you, and it looks like he is holding something. He's yelling at you to stop. You think to yourself, "That guy from my class is chasing me, and it looks like he might try to hurt me." You then feel panicked and start to run as fast as you can. You later realize that you must have dropped your wallet earlier when you were walking down the street. You feel disappointed because you have no idea where it is at this point.

"Now let's change the scenario a little bit. You are walking down the street and you hear someone running behind you. You glance behind you and see a boy from your class running toward you, and it looks like he's holding something. You think to yourself, 'That guy from my class is trying to get my attention. I wonder what he wants.' You feel calm and comfortable and walk toward him. Sure enough, you had dropped your wallet, and he was trying to give it back to you. You feel relieved and happy. Do you see how your thoughts affected the way you felt and behaved in each scenario? That's why it's so important to pay attention to your thoughts and attempt to change them if they are making you feel bad or making you act in ways that are not helpful."

 Clinicians can use the **Cognitive Coping Log** (CCL) (in the Appendix) to help demonstrate the ways in which thoughts can influence feelings and behavior.

>   **What it is:** An individualized worksheet that identifies thoughts, feelings, and behaviors associated with dysregulated states as well as adaptive, alternative thoughts.
>   **When to use it:** At the beginning of each CPS session as well as during episodes of dysregulation at home and/or at school.
>   **Target goals:** Child and caregiver will learn to identify links between the child's thoughts, feelings, and behaviors as well as adaptive ways of countering automatic thoughts.

The CCL is a therapeutic tool that serves a variety of purposes. The CCL is:

1. A means of helping children become aware of thoughts and feelings that lead to unhealthy behaviors.
2. A guide for generating alternative, adaptive responses to intrusive thoughts and traumatic triggers.
3. A record of progress.
4. An assessment of areas that need more attention.
5. A way to structure the session.

Similar to the ER guide, the CCL is a tool that should be used collaboratively between the caregiver, child, and therapist. The worksheet is used after the child has had an episode of dysregulation, whether at home or at school. The caregiver and child are asked to fill out the worksheet together at home. The child then brings the CCL to the next treatment session for review. The child is asked to complete one CCL per week for the duration of the CPS module.

The CCL comprises four sections, including a description of the incident, "What happened to make me feel or act upset," and the three R's: recounting, reflecting, and rewarding. In the first section, the child is asked to describe a situation during which he/she felt or acted "upset." The following CCL was completed by Kelly, the case example presented previously.

What happened to make me feel or act upset:

Someone at school told me that they heard my stepfather was getting out of jail, and I got really scared and ran out of the class and hid in the bathroom.

In the next section, recounting, the child is asked to describe in greater detail what he/she was thinking, feeling, and doing during the incident. It may be difficult for some children to reflect on their upsetting experience and provide details about how they were feeling at the time. This may require some coaching from the therapist as well as returning to the ER guide to help the child remember the types of external and internal cues that are indicative of certain emotions.

Recounting: What I was thinking, feeling, and doing at the time

What I Was Thinking	What I Was Feeling	What I Was Doing
What if he really is getting out of jail? Is he going to come to school to look for me? What if he tries to hurt me or my mom?	*Scared and worried.*	*Ran out of class and hid in the bathroom in case he was really getting out of jail.*

The next section, reflecting, asks the child to use his/her newly developed cognitive coping skills to replace the recounting thought with a more adaptive, helpful thought. As with the previous section, the reflecting section may require the therapist to help the child reflect on positive self-statements that he/she had generated in previous sessions. This section can be extremely beneficial in helping the child visualize positive outcomes stemming from his/her ability to change thought patterns at the time of an upsetting event.

Reflecting: What I could have thought, felt, and done instead

What I Could Have Thought	What I Would Have Felt	What I Would Have Done
I know my mom would have told me if he's getting out of jail. And even if he does get out of jail, I know that I'm safe right now.	*I probably would have felt calmer and not as scared.*	*I would have stayed at my desk and finished my assignment.*

The final section of the CCL, rewarding, is used as a means of encouraging the child to complete the CCL at home and/or at school. It is also a useful way of helping children learn how to reward themselves and engage in self-soothing behaviors. Finally, it sends an important message that completing the CCL is hard work and the child deserves to feel proud of this accomplishment. The child may wish to reflect on the self-regulation techniques that he/she recorded in the ER guide in order to generate ideas for rewards.

Rewarding: How can I reward myself after completing this worksheet?

I could reward myself by listening to my favorite CD and making bracelets with my bead set.

As the child continues to complete each CCL, he/she will find that attempts to change thoughts in the moment will become easier and easier. Whereas caregivers may need to play a large role in the initial completion of the CCL, by the end of the CPS module, the child should be able to complete the CCL independently.

Processing the Trauma

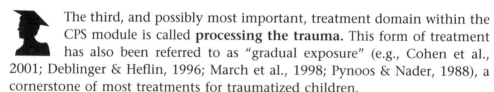 The third, and possibly most important, treatment domain within the CPS module is called **processing the trauma.** This form of treatment has also been referred to as "gradual exposure" (e.g., Cohen et al., 2001; Deblinger & Heflin, 1996; March et al., 1998; Pynoos & Nader, 1988), a cornerstone of most treatments for traumatized children.

Often, caregivers believe that their children will "only feel worse" after talking about the trauma, so they avoid any discussion of it in an effort to prevent their children from getting upset. These caregivers will need psychoeducation regarding the benefits of openly discussing their children's thoughts and feelings surrounding the traumatic event. In addition, some caregivers have difficulty hearing about their child's experience due to their own unresolved traumatic reactions or feelings of guilt that they did not protect their child. A continuing assessment of the caregiver's ability to *help* the child regulate during this time is important. It may become necessary to refer a caregiver to an individual therapist during this phase of treatment in order to address the caregiver's own symptoms.

In order to help children and caregivers understand why talking about the traumatic event is helpful, Cohen and colleagues (2001, 2003) provide a very effective metaphor for therapists to use in treating traumatized children and their caregivers. The therapist might say:

"Let's pretend that a little girl your age is riding her bike along a bumpy road, falls off of the bike, and scrapes her knee. In order to make sure that the girl's knee does not become infected, it will be important to clean out the wound, right? So even though cleaning the cut may hurt at first, it helps the wound to heal much faster and it will stop hurting over time. If the girl were to leave the cut and not wash it out, it would end up hurting more and more over time because it is likely to get infected. It's kind of the same thing when we begin to talk about the trauma because at first, it hurts. But the more we talk about it, the less it hurts, and the less likely it is to hurt over time."

The method of trauma processing that the therapist chooses to use should match the skills and interests of the child. For example, if a child enjoys singing or writing rap music, the trauma can be processed using song lyrics or raps. Other examples include making collages or drawings and writing poetry, play scripts, or books. Whatever the medium, the key is to help the child put a story together about what he/she experienced, including facts, feelings, and a sense of time that separates past, present, and future.

Using the Trauma Narrative

Much of the purpose of doing a trauma narrative is accomplished simply in the act of putting the story together. However, most children will need encouragement and coaching to help elaborate the story. The following paragraph is taken from Kelly's initial trauma narrative, which she wrote as part of making a book; it exemplifies the level of detail that can be expected after a child's first pass at a trauma narrative:

"My stepfather had sex with me. When he did it, I was crying. He told me to take my clothes off. I almost ran out of the room, but then he locked the door. When my mother came home, I told her what happened. She said to him, 'Why did you do that?' and he said, 'What did I do?' "

The next narrative illustrates the ways in which the therapist was able to help Kelly expand on her previous narrative and incorporate more detail, including her own feelings, observations of others' emotions and reactions, additional traumatic aspects, as well as rescripting. *Rescripting* refers to the child's attempts to rewrite the ending of his/her own trauma experience. It is a useful means of helping the child gain a sense of mastery or identifying potential maladaptive thoughts that may need to be addressed. It is also a powerful means of engaging the brain's contextual processing system, as detailed in Chapter 2.

Kelly writes:

> "My stepfather was mean. He had sex with me. When he did it I was crying, but
> he is not in my family now, so he can't hurt anyone in my family. I was mad
> when he did it to me. He called me to come to the room and then he told me
> to take my clothes off. I almost ran out of the room but he locked the door. I
> felt mad when he asked me to take my clothes off. I also felt like I must have
> done something wrong, like he was punishing me for something. The worst
> part was when I was trying to get up and he pinned me down and covered my
> mouth. When my mother came home from work I told her what happened
> . . . that he had sex with me, even though he told me not to tell anyone or he'd
> kill my mom. First I told my mom, 'Dad had sex with me.' My mom got mad.
> Her face looked really angry. When he came home from work, my mother
> said, 'Why did you do that?' and he said, 'What did I do?' I felt mad when I
> heard them arguing. I felt like I shouldn't have said anything because then
> they wouldn't be fighting. I was scared that he would hurt my mom. This is
> what I wish would have happened: I would get my brothers and sisters ready
> at the front door and when my stepfather started to call me into the room, I
> would run past him, run to the front door, and run to my aunt's house with all
> of my brothers and sisters."

There is obviously a great deal of material to work with in the previous trauma
narrative. As an example, Kelly's narrative contains elements of self-blame such
as, "I felt like I must have done something wrong, like he was punishing me for
something," and "I felt like I shouldn't have said anything because then they
wouldn't be fighting." Cohen and colleagues (2001, 2003) describe the use of
progressive logical questioning to address inaccurate or unhelpful thoughts. The
following example demonstrates how a therapist might use this technique with
Kelly to address her statements of self-blame:

THERAPIST: Can you help me find a sentence in this chapter that may be
  unhelpful or untrue?

KELLY: Maybe the sentence about how I must have done something wrong?

THERAPIST: When you say that you felt like you had done something wrong,
  that's really a thought. Can you tell me what the feeling is?

KELLY: Guilty. Like it was my fault that it was happening because he was
  trying to punish me for something.

THERAPIST: So when you think to yourself that you must have done something wrong, that makes you feel guilty. You also said that it felt like he
  was punishing you. What do you think he was punishing you for?

KELLY: Well . . . I did forget to clean my room that day.

THERAPIST: Now let's think about that for a minute. We may never know why your stepfather hurt you in the way that he did. But it sounds like he has a lot of problems and that his reasons for hurting you have absolutely nothing to do with anything that you did. But what if what you're saying is true? Everyone makes mistakes sometimes, right? What if you had forgotten to clean your room? Do you think that means that your stepfather has a right to punish you in that way . . . to rape you?

KELLY: No. I don't deserve that just because I didn't clean my room.

THERAPIST: That's right. Can you think of *anything* that you could have done that would have made it OK for your stepfather to rape you?

KELLY: No. It wasn't fair. I don't deserve to be treated like that, even if I do something wrong.

THERAPIST: You're absolutely right. Raping someone is a terrible thing to do and should NEVER be used as a form of punishment. It is also illegal, and that is why your stepfather is going to jail. So instead of thinking to yourself, "I felt like I must have done something wrong, like he was punishing me for something," what could you think to yourself that might be more helpful and accurate?

KELLY: I know that I didn't do anything wrong, and even if I made a mistake, he should never have raped me. I didn't deserve that. No one deserves that.

If left unaddressed, cognitive distortions can become extremely damaging in that they can develop into permanent, global statements related to the child's self-concept. Consequently, helping a child identify and change unhelpful and/ or inaccurate thoughts about the traumatic event is a critical step in ensuring his/her future psychological health. Because these thoughts can be so powerful, it may take several sessions to fully process their meaning and help the child generate more adaptive thoughts. The following dialogue provides another example of how to address an unhelpful thought:

THERAPIST: Can you find another sentence in there that may be unhelpful?

KELLY: I guess it's not helpful to think that I shouldn't have said anything because it made them fight.

THERAPIST: What makes this thought unhelpful? What does it make you feel when you think about it?

KELLY: It's unhelpful because I feel guilty again. Like it's my fault that they were fighting.

THERAPIST: What do you think would have happened if you hadn't said anything?

KELLY: They wouldn't have been fighting. He wouldn't have tried to hurt my mom.

THERAPIST: That might be true. But can you think of anything bad that might have happened if you hadn't said anything?

KELLY: He probably would have done it again . . . I mean, raped me. And maybe not just to me . . . maybe to my sister too.

THERAPIST: So by telling your mom, you were protecting yourself and also your sister. Those are two very important reasons for telling your mom, don't you think?

KELLY: Yeah. I guess if I hadn't told her, he could still be living with us . . . and still abusing me.

THERAPIST: It sounds like you made a very smart and also very brave decision to tell your mom what he did. And your sister is very lucky to have you looking out for her. So let's go back to the unhelpful sentence that we started with: "I felt like I shouldn't have said anything because then they wouldn't be fighting." What would be a more helpful thought to have?

KELLY: If I never said anything, my stepdad could still be abusing me and my sister. It was important to tell my mom so that she could help protect us.

It is important to note that the therapist should not begin to address cognitive distortions in the child's narrative until the entire narrative has been written by the child. If the therapist were to address unhelpful thoughts too early, it might make the child feel inhibited and reluctant to write about thoughts or feelings that may be considered inaccurate or unhelpful.

> The creation of a book is an ideal way of helping the child to process the trauma because there is evidence that the act of writing about the trauma can be healing in itself.

The creation of a book is an ideal way of helping the child to process the trauma because there is evidence that the act of writing about the trauma can be healing in itself (Donnelly & Murray, 1991; Esterling, L'Abate, & Murray, 1999). However, it is critical that the child also write about thoughts and feelings associated with the trauma, because research suggests that the integration of thoughts and feelings within the trauma narrative is essential for improving psychological health (Pennebaker & Francis, 1996). As suggested by Cohen and colleagues (2001), the therapist should have the child begin with "neutral" information, such as name, birthdate, grade in school, etc., in order to help the child begin to feel comfortable with the process. Next, the therapist should help the child move toward gathering "facts" about the trauma, such as what happened, where the trauma took place, who was there, etc. Finally, the therapist should help the child process thoughts and feelings associated with the traumatic incident(s) and address cognitive distortions that are likely to arise during the writing of the trauma narrative. This process is described in more detail below.

Toolbox for Trauma Processing

The following section provides detailed outlines of two books that can be used to help the child process a traumatic event. The child may wish to give the book his/her own title. The first outline is designed for use with single-event traumas, or in situations in which a child can identify a specific series of related events. The second outline can be used for children who have experienced chronic, systemic disruption to their social environment and who may have a hard time identifying a specific bad event; this narrative strives to help the child put order and structure to an otherwise chaotic life experience.

Every trauma narrative will look different, and the guide and prompts used with each child will need to be tailored by the therapist. For instance, children who experienced trauma when they were very young may not even have verbal memories of what happened—although the experience may have deeply affected them, telling the story about it may be different than for a child who remembers and can describe the traumatic event. The book outlines provided below are tools to help therapists think about the type of questions that would be helpful in getting a narrative started. These outlines can be adapted and changed depending on the developmental stage and the specific experiences of the child. The therapist and child will probably not have time to discuss each question, but by picking the questions that seem most applicable to a particular child's situation, the therapist can help guide the development of the child's narrative.

Narrative 1: Specific event

Chapter 1: All about Me	Goals of Chapter 1:
What does the child like about him- or herself?	Introduce the book, help the child become comfortable writing about him/herself through easy, familiar topics.
What is he/she good at? Have the child list some favorite things, such as a food, a color, or a TV show.	
Who is he/she close to? Does he/she have a best friend? Who is it?	
Chapter 2: My Family	**Goals of Chapter 2:**
Have the child list the people in his/her family.	Introduce key players and introduce discussion of both positive and negative aspects of a child's life.
Who does he/she live with? What does his/her home look like? Who takes care of him/her? Who else is especially important to him/her?	Depending on the child's situation, this chapter may already delve into difficult territory. In this case, adding questions about supportive people outside the family is important.
What does he/she like about his/her family? What does he/she not like?	

Chapter 3: Something Bad Happened to Me	Goals of Chapter 3:
For first two sessions: Facts about the traumatic event (who, what, when, where, why). Does child remember sights, sounds, smells? Does child remember what he/she said or did? Who else was involved? What did he/she say and do? **Next two sessions:** What was the child thinking and feeling during the traumatic event? What did the child's body feel like? Are there parts of the event that he/she can't remember? What does the child say other people were thinking and feeling during the event? What was the worst part? What does the child wish would have happened instead?	The goal of Chapter 3 is to help the child recall and begin to verbalize what happened during the traumatic event. The therapist should plan to spend at least four sessions working on this chapter with the child.
Chapter 4: Things Changed after the Bad Thing Happened The therapist should help the child describe things that may have changed immediately after the traumatic event as well as over time (e.g., removal of perpetrator from home, mother became depressed, moved to a new location).	**Goals of Chapter 4:** This chapter can help a child explore the many different ways in which the trauma may have affected his/her life—for better or worse. On the positive side, there may be people who stepped up to help or changes that led to greater safety. It's also possible that the traumatic event led to grieving, problems at school, or new difficulties at home. In writing this chapter, it may become evident that the child should write another book using other traumatic events.
Chapter 5: Some Things Stayed the Same after the Bad Thing Happened The therapist should help the child describe things that have remained consistent since the traumatic event. These can be both positive and negative (e.g., child still does well in school, child still enjoys playing basketball, child still argues with siblings).	**Goals of Chapter 5:** This chapter is useful in helping the child feel reassured that, amidst all of the changes that may have taken place since the trauma, he/she can count on a number of things to remain the same.

Chapter 6: People Who Care about Me	Goals of Chapters 6–8:
The therapist should help the child list as many people as possible on whom he/she can rely (the therapist should remember to add him/herself to the list if the child forgets). The list can include family, friends, teachers, guidance counselors, clergy, as well as religious/spiritual figures.	The next set of chapters helps the child identify supports and strengths in his/her life—both what other people bring to the child, as well as what the child has learned him/herself. The goal of these chapters is to help the child feel empowered, as well as to review the skills covered in earlier therapy sessions.
Chapter 7: What I Can Do to Protect Myself in the Future	
The therapist should help the child generate a list of possible safety measures that he/she could take in the event that something like the trauma were to happen again. It is obviously important to strike a balance between providing the child with an internal locus of control while not inadvertently sending a message that the child is to blame for what happened.	
Chapter 8: Skills I Have Learned to Use When My Bad Thoughts Get in the Way	
The therapist should help the child describe coping skills that he/she has learned in therapy, including thought stopping, positive self-statements, activities that he/she enjoys, and talking to a trusted adult/friend.	
Chapter 9: What I Learned from the Bad Thing	Goals of Chapters 9 and 10:
The therapist should help the child reflect on any positive life lessons that may have resulted from the traumatic event. If the child has trouble, the therapist can ask the child what he/she would say to someone who just experienced the same traumatic event. What advice or wisdom would he/she give to the person?	The final chapters are intended to empower the child and help him/her recognize that the traumatic event does not have to define the child's identity or future self. Chapters 9 and 10 also serve as the foundation for the next phase of treatment, meaning-making skills. As the child is working on his/her book, it will be important to share the child's progress with the caregiver. This is done to ensure that the caregiver is kept up to date with the child's trauma processing, to provide an opportunity for gradual exposure with the caregiver alone, and to assess the caregiver's thoughts and feelings with regard to the trauma. It also begins the final domain of treatment in the CPS module: exchanging stories with the caregiver.
Chapter 10: My Future Is Bright	
The therapist should have the child describe what he/she hopes to do in the future (e.g., career goals, family aspirations, travel).	
The therapist should help the child generate steps that he/she can take, beginning right now, to reach his/her goals.	

Narrative 2: Chronic trauma

Chapter 1: All about Me Same as above version. **Chapter 2: My Family** Same as above, with additional questions if the child is having trouble defining family: "There's no one definition for what a family is, so there's no right or wrong answers here. What do you think *family* means? What is the job of a family? Does anyone do that for you? Do you think families stay the same, or do they change? Can you think of families that look different from one another but are both still families? What makes each of them a family?"	**Goals of Chapters 1 and 2:** Same as above. Note that for children who have experienced many changes in who they live with, it may be hard to define *family*; sample questions to help the child decide who belongs in this chapter are provided.
Illustration 1: My Timeline The therapist can help the child draw a timeline with all of the important events of his/her life. It can help to start with a blank graphic with "My Birth" on the far left side of the page, and "Today" on the far right side of the page. Explain how a timeline works and ask the child to put important events on it. You may need to help younger children sequence things as they go; they can decide what is important. After the child has filled in all that he/she can think of, ask some probe questions. Has the child always lived with the same caregivers or in the same city? If not, make sure these changes are noted. Has the child lost anyone important to him/her? Did anything upsetting happen? Did anything really good happen? By this time, the therapist usually knows if certain events (e.g., death, divorce) were important parts of the child's history and can ask appropriate probes to help him/her acknowledge and sequence these things.	**Goals of Timeline:** The goal of this exercise is both to help the child begin the process of putting order to their life events, as well as to learn what life events are most salient to the child. If a child seems to be avoiding some important events (e.g. there is no mention of when child was taken from parents and placed in foster care) it will be important to introduce this and help the child acknowledge and place it on the timeline.
Chapter 3: When I Was a Baby Facts about the child when he/she was a baby: who took care of him/her, where he/she lived, important people in his/her life.	**Goals of Chapters 3–5** In this section, the therapist helps the child begin to verbally sequence events and to make his/her life story into a

Because the child will not remember what life was like when he/she was a baby, try to elicit what he/she may have heard from others about what life was like for him/her then.

What are some important things that happened to him/her when he/she was a baby?

Is there anything the child wishes he/she knew about his/her babyhood?

What are some questions he/she would like to ask his/her parent or caregiver about his/her babyhood?

narrative. Children who have had very inconsistent caregiving may have more questions than answers.

The time frame you pick to help the child build the chapters should be changed depending on how the child remembers events—for instance, instead of "When I First Went to School," you might choose to call the chapter "When I Moved to Grandma's House." Regardless of the timelines, an important thread to follow through the child's life is the presence or absence of important people—who is still there, who has gone.

Chapter 4: When I First Went to School

Facts about going to school (how old was the child, where did he/she live then, what school did he/she go to, who did he/she live with then).

What did he/she like about school? What did he/she not like about school?

What kinds of things did he/she like to do?

What was he/she really good at?

What was it like to come home after school? What kinds of stuff did he/she do at home? Who else lived at home? What kinds of stuff did they do?

What are some important things that happened when he/she was just starting school?

Who were the important people in the child's life back then? (Refer back to the list of important people from when the child was a baby—were those people still important?)

Chapter 5: My Life Today

Facts about the child's life today (age, current school, who is in the home, location of the child's home).

Help the child identify how life now may be different from when he/she was younger.

Think about how his/her family, home, or self may have changed.

Also help the child think about the ways in which his/her life is the same as it was when he/she was younger.	
Chapter 6: Best and Worse, Hopes and Fears Have the child look back over the last chapter and timeline and identify the best times. What made them the best? What were the worst times? What made them the worst? Ask the child to look ahead and say what he/she hopes will happen in his/her life. What would he/she like to see happen tomorrow? Next year? Five years from now? When he/she is grown up? Now ask the same questions regarding what the child worries will happen.	**Goals of Chapter 6:** This chapter asks the child to reflect on the life events in the timeline and identify the most difficult times and the best times. The second half of the chapter—on hopes and fears—orients the child toward the future.
Illustration 2: My Support Tree In this section the therapist helps the child draw a support tree, which is like a family tree, only in this tree all the different kinds of people who are supportive to the child are listed: Family he/she lives with, family he/she doesn't live with, friends, and mentors. Go through each category with the child and help him/her think of who is supportive and list them on the tree. If the child likes to draw, he/she can draw his/her own tree; a blank tree can also be filled in. During this time, the therapist can also ask about people who used to be important but are not on the support tree. **Chapter 7: People Who Care about Me** The therapist can help the child write about the people on the support tree. Who helps with what kinds of problems? Who does the child trust and talk to?	**Goals of Illustration 2 and Chapter 7:** The goals of these sections are to help the child identify supports in his/her life.
Chapter 8: What I Have Learned from the Tough Times Have the child identify skills he/she has. The therapist should help the child describe coping skills that he/she has learned in therapy, including thought stopping, positive self-statements, activities that he/she enjoys, and talking to a trusted adult/friend.	**Goals of Chapters 8–9:** The final chapters lay the groundwork for the next module, meaning making. Chapter 8 helps the child to become an expert on him/herself and his/her experiences, and reflect on what he/she has learned. Chapter 9 orients the child to the future; you can even add a "future" timeline, so that the child can

What would the child tell someone else who was having a tough time?	imagine events that he/she hopes will happen in his/her life.
Chapter 9: My Future Is Bright The therapist should have the child describe what he/she hopes to do in the future (e.g., career goals, family aspirations, travel). The therapist should help the child generate steps that he/she can take, beginning right now, to reach his/her goals.	

Narratives in Other Media

COLLAGES OR DRAWINGS

Provide three large pieces of paper labeled *PAST*, *PRESENT*, and *FUTURE*. Have the child complete collages for each of these, and then do an interview with the child. In the interview include questions about the facts of each time period, as well as emotions the child experienced.

POETRY

Use existing poems to provide inspiration or a starting structure for the child. For example, Wallace Stevens's "13 Ways of Looking at a Blackbird" could be read, and then the theme of "13 ways of looking at my life" could be used. Another good poem is Robert Frost's "The Road Not Taken": Read the poem, then have the child or adolescent write one poem about "the road behind me," one poem about "the road I'm on," and one poem about "the road I'm going to take." After the child is done writing, interview him/her about the poetry to generate elaboration of the facts, feelings, and chronology of his/her life.

Exchanging Stories with Caregivers

The final treatment domain within the CPS module is **exchanging stories with caregivers**. Before beginning this particular domain, it is important for the therapist to carefully assess the caregiver's progress with regard to processing the trauma. The key element of this domain is the joint sharing and open discussion of the trauma, so it is essential that the caregiver is able to offer support to the child during the joint sessions. The structure of these three to four sessions is slightly different from the others in that the majority of the time is spent with both the child and caregiver. The first 10 minutes of the session is still used as an opportunity to review the child's CCL and behavior and mood over the last week. However, the next 35 minutes are devoted to the joint processing of the traumatic event by sharing the child's narrative (or other means) as a guide. The next 10 minutes are spent with the caregiver alone in order to process what he/ she heard in session as well as to prepare for the next session. The last 5 minutes are again used for the closing ritual.

If using the child's book as a guide, the therapist should plan to review approximately three chapters per session with the caregiver and the child. It is useful for the child to read the chapters to the caregiver and then to have the caregiver offer his/her own thoughts and feelings after the child is done reading. The caregiver should also be able to praise the child.

The therapist may wish to prepare the caregiver regarding what kind of statements may be helpful or unhelpful in this situation. For example, after Kelly read her narrative to her mother, her mother stated, "I'm so sorry that happened to you. It makes me very sad to hear how upset you were, but I'm so proud of you for being able to talk about it." When Kelly's mother met with the therapist alone, she stated, "I completely blame myself for what happened. I should have kicked him out of the house way before that. I guess this just confirms that I'm a horrible mother." Clearly, this latter statement would not have been helpful for Kelly to hear, and thankfully, Kelly's mother was insightful enough to suppress these statements while in session with Kelly, instead discussing these thoughts later during her individual time with the therapist. If necessary, the therapist may find it useful to conduct a **role play** with the caregiver (e.g., parent pretends to be the child, and the therapist pretends to be the parent) if he/she appears to be having difficulty providing support to the child during the joint session.

 It is important for the child and the caregiver to discuss the "hardest parts" of the narrative to think about and/or talk about. Without this important component, it is likely that the child and/or caregiver will be at greater risk of future avoidance and possibly the resurgence of trauma symptoms. It is possible that the therapist will need to spend more than four sessions in this domain of treatment if it appears that there are a number of traumatic aspects of the event that have not been openly discussed yet.

Terminating the CPS Module: Knowing When to Transition

Termination of the CPS module depends on the achievement of three goals:

1. The child is able to effectively demonstrate cognitive coping skills, such as thought stopping and positive self-talk.

2. The child is able to think and talk about the trauma without experiencing overwhelming negative affect.

3. The caregiver and child feel comfortable openly discussing thoughts and emotions associated with the trauma.

When the child completes the CP module, he/she should be ready to graduate to the final phase of treatment: transcending. As the child transitions to the next phase of treatment and the corresponding meaning-making treatment module, the therapist should encourage him/her to continue using the CCL and may suggest reviewing it together periodically. The child's cognitive processing of the trauma is likely to continue as he/she develops and encounters new transitions in life. However, if the child has the appropriate cognitive coping skills and a supportive and receptive caregiver, he/she should be able to face these transitions with courage and hope, particularly as the child and caregiver begin to make meaning out of difficult times, with the help of their therapist.

Meaning-Making Skills

How to Help Children Make Meaning Out of Their Traumatic Experiences and Move On with Their Lives

---

LEARNING OBJECTIVES

- To help children recognize and articulate important lessons learned from the trauma
- To help children reinvent themselves and plan for the future
- To help children enact meaningful and sustaining experiences related to the trauma
- To come to a close in treatment and say goodbye

We must never forget that we may also find meaning in life even when confronted with a hopeless situation, when facing a fate that cannot be changed. For what then matters is to bear witness to the uniquely human potential at its best, which is to transform a personal tragedy into triumph, to turn one's predicament into a human achievement. (Frankl, 1963, p. 135)

Meaning making is the final module of TST. Meaning making is necessary for both the child and the clinician. After months or even years of working together, experiencing suffering or being witness to that suffering, it is essential to try to understand the meaning in what has come before—and what lies ahead.

In his book *Man's Search for Meaning* (1963), Viktor Frankl describes his horrific experiences in a concentration camp and his resulting creation of "logotherapy," a meaning-centered form of psychotherapy that focuses on "the meaning of human existence as well as on man's search for such a meaning."

Two of the central areas Frankl identifies as ways to discover meaning in life are (1) by creating something, and (2) by experiencing another human being in all of his/her uniqueness. These two ways of finding meaning form the foundations of this module, meaning making.

Why Meaning Making?

Current treatments for traumatized children often overlook the necessity of helping children make meaning out of their traumatic events. It is likely that the acquisition of meaning-making skills following a traumatic event can serve as a protective mechanism and buffer children from future symptom relapse. Meaning-making skills can provide children with hope for the future and allow them to focus on the positive aspects of their lives as opposed to dwelling on the tragedies that they were forced to endure. In essence, the activity of creating meaning out of a traumatic experience allows children and families to put the event in context so that they are no longer consumed by the past but can move into their future.

> In essence, the activity of creating meaning out of a traumatic experience allows children and families to put the event in context so that they are no longer consumed by the past but can move into their future.

The meaning-making module also provides an important time in treatment to explore the therapeutic relationship and to say goodbye. As we talked about in Chapter 5, the therapeutic relationship is central to successful treatment—particularly to the treatment of traumatized children. A child's relationship with his/her therapist may have been his/her first experience of a truly caring, consistent individual. Both therapist and child may have experienced another human being in all his/her uniqueness—an experience that Frankl calls central to finding meaning in life. Saying goodbye is no small task. Thus the meaning-making module is devoted to gradually transitioning to saying goodbye, while helping the child find meaning in both the challenges of the past and the hopes for the future.

 ... life is potentially meaningful under any conditions, even those which are most miserable.... This in turn presupposes the human capacity to creatively turn life's negative aspects into something positive or constructive. (Frankl, 1963, p. 162)

The meaning-making module is devoted to three overarching goals:

1. To create new ways of viewing the trauma and its consequences.
2. To instill hope and actively encourage the pursuit of a brighter future.
3. To say goodbye.

How to Know If a Child Is Ready for Meaning Making

 Because meaning making is the final module of treatment in TST, beginning this module signals that many of the goals of treatment have been accomplished. The social environment is no longer threatening or distressed. Ideally the caregiver is able to actively help and protect the child. The child must be able to regulate emotions well enough so that he/she can navigate the innate stressors of life. In addition, the child's trauma narrative must have been explored so that, although talking about the trauma may never be easy, it is neither avoided nor overwhelming to the child.

To summarize, the therapist can feel comfortable beginning the meaning-making module if . . .

1. The child is able to effectively demonstrate emotion regulation and cognitive coping skills.
2. The child is able to think and talk about the trauma without experiencing overwhelming negative affect.
3. The caregiver and child feel comfortable openly discussing thoughts and emotions associated with the trauma.
4. The social environment is stable.

As with every transition to a new phase of treatment, the TST Treatment Planning Form should be revisited. By this time, there may be significantly fewer treatment team members than there were in the beginning. Priority problems should be greatly diminished in number and intensity now. Revisiting the TST treatment plan can be a chance for family and therapist to consider what is left to do before treatment ends—in essence, before the therapist can *leave a better system* (TST Principle Ten, Chapter 6).

Domains of Treatment

The meaning-making module comprises four domains of treatment (LIFE, for short):

1. Lessons learned
2. Invention of a new self
3. Future goals
4. Enacting meaning

The therapist begins the module by helping the child generate important life lessons that may have resulted from the trauma. Next, the child identifies ways in which the traumatic experience has changed him/her in a positive way. The child is then encouraged to think carefully about future goals and use problem-solving skills to combat any obstacles that might stand in his/her way of achieving those goals. Finally, the child is engaged in thinking about activities that might create lasting meaning out of the experience of trauma and the process of recovery. The child and therapist work together to enact this meaningful activity; for example, helping others, serving as an example for children who experienced a similar trauma, finding creative expression through art, song, etc. Each of the treatment domains is explained in greater detail later in this chapter.

In addition to these four domains, throughout this module the therapist and child have an additional, and very important, task: saying goodbye to each other. At the end of the meaning-making module, most children will be ready to transition out of therapy. Throughout this module, the therapist and child work not only to help the child find meaning in the events of the past and goals for the future, but to understand the transformative meaning of the therapist–child relationship.

Treatment Structure

In the meaning-making module, therapy no longer occurs on a weekly basis. Part of getting ready to say goodbye involves tapering off the frequency of sessions. At the beginning of this module, sessions can be conducted every other week. By the end of the module, it may be best to move to a once-a-month check-in. Overall, this module typically involves about six to eight sessions, spread out over 3 months. Even after saying goodbye, we recommend scheduling a 6-month check-in; this leaves the door open for the family to reengage if they need to, and sends a message that the therapist continues to care about the child even after treatment officially ends. These sessions may be concluded with the parent and child together, or primarily with the child alone, depending on the pattern that has been established over the course of treatment. Regardless, be sure to reserve some time for talking about ending therapy with any family members who have been centrally involved in treatment. Within-session structure includes:

1. **Check-in.** A 10-minute initial check-in with the parent and child together. During this time, the therapist reviews the child's emotions and behaviors throughout the past week. This time is generally used to ensure that there are no major crises that need immediate attention.

2. **Meaning-making skills.** Each of the LIFE (lessons learned; invention of a new self; future goals; enacting meaning) treatment domains consists of approximately two sessions. Each session devotes 35 minutes to exploring one of the domains.

3. **Open ending.** At the end of the session, 10 minutes is provided for more open-ended discussion of saying goodbye. This can take many forms, including introducing the topic and simply playing together. Suggestions for ways to tie this conversation to the meaning-making skills are provided at the end of the discussion of each domain, below.

4. **Closing ritual.** Finally, the last 5 minutes of the session are focused on a closing ritual, during which both the child and caregiver jointly participate (see Chapter 11 for a description of the closing ritual).

The next section describes each of the four treatment domains within the meaning-making module.

It is important to note that these exercises can feel invalidating to children if they have not had sufficient time to express their negative emotions regarding the trauma.

It is important to note that these exercises can feel invalidating to children if they have not had sufficient time to express their negative emotions regarding the trauma. The last thing the therapist would want to do is make the child think that the trauma was actually "a good thing" and to feel that the therapist is suggesting to "just look on the bright side." However, if the child has been able to express, and gain perspective on, his/her thoughts and feelings about the upsetting consequences of the trauma throughout the CPS module, the exercises in this module should feel encouraging and hopeful as well as help the child recognize that it is possible to "turn life's negative aspects into something positive or constructive" (Frankl, 1963, p. 162).

Lessons Learned

We start with the first domain of treatment, lessons learned. If the child used the book/trauma narrative outline from the CPS module, then he/she will have already completed "Chapter 9: What I Learned from the Bad Thing." The lessons learned treatment domain can be thought of as an extension of this work. Generally, children are able to identify more and more "lessons" learned from their traumatic experiences as time passes. These lessons may take on many different forms. Some children's lessons pertain to things that they learned about themselves, about others, or about life in general.

Some of the lessons that a child identifies are likely to be negative (e.g., "You can't always trust the people in your family"), in such cases the therapist should help the child find a lesson that will have utility for him/her in the future. Using the previous example, instead of focusing on the very painful lesson that "you can't trust people in your family," the therapist can help the child identify ways in which the traumatic experience showed him/her whom he/she *can* trust (e.g., "You can trust certain people in your family") or how he/she can better discriminate people who are trustworthy from those who are not (e.g., "You are better able to protect yourself because you are better able to know who you can trust").

It may be very difficult for some children to find meaning in their traumatic experiences. Consequently, the therapist may need to be actively involved in helping the child generate ideas. It is often useful to have the child talk about what helped him/her to get through the traumatic experience. The following dialogue with Kelly, a 12-year-old child who was sexually abused, illustrates this concept:

THERAPIST: What do you think you may have learned about yourself since having this experience?

KELLY: I don't know.

THERAPIST: How about if we try a different question? What do you think helped you get through the experience itself? You mentioned that you "almost gave up" at times and even thought about hurting yourself. What was it that kept you from doing that?

KELLY: I just kept thinking about my little sister. I wanted to make sure that this [the abuse] didn't happen to her because I didn't think she'd be able to handle it.

THERAPIST: So it sounds like you wanted to be there to protect your sister.

KELLY: Yes. I'm the only one who would really look out for her.

THERAPIST: And it also sounds like you felt like you were stronger than your sister in some ways.

KELLY: Well, I'm older . . . and, yeah, I guess I'm stronger than her. I don't think I even knew how strong I was until this happened to me.

THERAPIST: Could that be one potentially positive thing that you take away from this experience? That you learned just how strong of a person you really are?

KELLY: Yeah. I definitely feel like what happened has made me stronger . . . more brave. I think I could pretty much handle anything now.

It is clear that initially Kelly has a difficult time identifying ways in which the traumatic experience may have taught her something about herself. But with some guidance, reflection, and further questioning by the therapist, she was finally able to see how the abuse led to a belief in her inner strength—a strength that she hadn't recognized until she had overcome tragedy.

It may also be helpful to have the child think about what he/she might say to another child who is going through a similar trauma. This approach can be beneficial in that it encourages children to discuss potential lessons learned in a more optimistic way. The following dialogue with Billy, a 10-year-old boy whose father was murdered, provides a good example of this. He had not seen his father for over a year at the time of the murder.

> THERAPIST: When kids go through really difficult times, it can be helpful to think about the things that they may have learned from their experiences. Can you think of anything that you may have learned from losing your dad?
>
> BILLY: I learned that I can miss my dad, but I'm still allowed to have fun. Like, I'm still a kid, and I don't have to be sad for the rest of my life.
>
> THERAPIST: That's a very important lesson—that you can miss your dad but also live a happy life at the same time.
>
> BILLY: Yeah. I felt bad at first because I think everyone expected me to be sad and crying all the time because everyone else was. But I didn't really know my dad that well.
>
> THERAPIST: It's hard when other people expect you to feel exactly how they feel. If one of your good friends lost his dad, what do you think you'd want to tell him to help him get through it?
>
> BILLY: I'd tell him to talk to someone about how he's feeling. And don't think that he has to feel the way everyone else does all the time. That no one else can tell you how to feel.
>
> THERAPIST: So it sounds like you may have learned a couple of important lessons from this experience: that it helps to talk about your feelings, and that only you can decide what you really feel.

It may be helpful to have the child add more "lessons learned" to Chapter 9 in his/her trauma narrative so that he/she can reflect on the information later. It is also important to help children understand that they will continue to learn things about themselves, others, and life in general as a result of the trauma, and that these lessons will accumulate as they transition into adulthood.

In addition, the ideas in this treatment domain can be applied to other difficult situations that the child may encounter. The ability to turn tragedy into something meaningful is an invaluable skill that will serve the child well in the future.

Identifying lessons learned can apply not only to the child's trauma but to both the child and therapist in the course of therapy. During this phase of meaning making, the idea of saying goodbye should be introduced. A conversation about what child and therapist have taught each other can help the child begin to think about the relationship with his/her therapist, and can help each articulate what it has meant to work together.

When a therapist shares with a child what he/she has learned from him/her, it communicates several points: (1) that the child has things of value to share with other people, (2) that what the child says and does influences those around him, and (3) that the therapist, also, has been changed by the therapy.

Invention of a New Self

 Man does not simply exist, but always decides what his existence will be, what he will become in the next moment. By the same token, every human being has the freedom to change at any instant. (Frankl, 1963, p. 154)

Inherent in the nature of therapy is the human capacity for change (or a system's capacity to change, for which we strive for in TST). To have graduated to the meaning-making module signals for many children that they have experienced and participated in tremendous change. But the changes will not end with therapy; rather, the foundation has been laid for the child's continued growth and development into his/her full potential. Part of meaning making is to make sure the building blocks are in place for a child to continue this healthy trajectory.

After a traumatic event, children's identities sometimes change for the worse. After being abandoned by a parent, for example, a child may see him/herself as "unwanted" or "lost." After being raped by her stepfather, a child may see herself as "damaged" or "worthless." These maladaptive identities may be even more difficult to change if the trauma has been chronic. Even after a child has processed his/her thoughts and feelings about the abuse, negative self-images may persist indefinitely unless they are directly addressed, challenged, and modified.

> Even after a child has processed his/her thoughts and feelings about the abuse, negative self-images may persist indefinitely unless they are directly addressed, challenged, and modified.

A goal of the first exercise in this treatment for children who hold falsely negative self-images is to elicit their self-perceptions and compare them to their "real" selves. Two exercises for younger children are also included below, which may be used to facilitate the conversation.

Happily, some children are able to maintain positive self-images despite having experienced traumatic events. For these children, the meaning-making module can be a time of exploring how they see themselves now and what they hope to be like in the future.

 The first exercise is called "Then and Now." This exercise is designed to help children identify negative self-images that they may have had since the trauma (or before) as well as positive self-images that they hope to maintain, starting now. For this exercise, the therapist will need to supply:

1. Two or three magazines
2. Scissors
3. Glue stick
4. Markers
5. One sheet of construction paper
6. One sheet of transparent paper

First, the child is asked to cut out words or images from the magazines that describe how the child felt about him/herself during the time of the trauma. The child should paste the cutouts on the sheet of construction paper and title it *Then*. Next, the child is asked to cut out words or images from the magazines that describe how the child feels about him/herself currently. He/she should paste these cutouts on the sheet of transparent paper and title it *Now*. Finally, the therapist should help the child staple the transparent paper on top of the construction paper. Through this exercise, the therapist can help the child visually understand that his/her negative self-images are now "behind" him/her and he/she has the opportunity to make his/her current self, his/her real self. In addition, viewing the negative self-images that the child once had can help him/her see just how much progress has been made.

A similar exercise that can be used with younger children is entitled "Old Me, New Me." For this exercise, the therapist will need to supply:

1. Two styrofoam cups, one larger than the other
2. Markers

First, the child is asked to draw a face on the smaller styrofoam cup that exemplifies how he/she felt about him/herself during the time of the trauma. Then the therapist should help the child generate words that would describe his/her self-image during this time and write them all over the paper cup (e.g., *abused, worthless, bad, unloved*). Next, the child is asked to draw a face on the larger cup that exemplifies how he/she feels about him/herself currently. If this current self-image appears to be negative, the therapist should ask the child to draw a face that shows how he/she *would like* to feel. Again, the therapist should help the child generate words that describe this self-image and write them all over the cup (e.g., *confident, lovable, good*). The child is then asked to place the larger cup over the smaller cup to visually demonstrate how those negative self-concepts can be overpowered by positive self-concepts. This also helps the child understand how his/her "old self" can be replaced by his/her "new self."

The therapist's job during this treatment domain is to help the child gain control over his/her self-image and actively construct the type of self-image that the child would like to have. Because so many traumatized children have learned to define themselves by what others have told them (e.g., "You're a bad kid"), this can be a very empowering and necessary experience for them.

Discussions about changes in self-perception lend themselves readily to a conversation about how the child has changed since the beginning of therapy. During this domain, encourage the child to reflect on how much has changed since you started working together—how well you've gotten to know each other, how much better you are at the high-five handshake, the way the child used to have trouble at school and recently received the spirit award . . . and so on. Help the child reflect on all of the hard work and positive changes, and also on how your own relationship with each other has grown. It often is important to include the parent in these conversations, so that the important changes are seen and acknowledged at home as well. Sometimes change is so gradual, it is easy to forget how far a child has come!

Future Goals

 . . . mental health is based on a certain degree of tension, the tension between what one has already achieved and what one still ought to accomplish, or the gap between what one is and what one should become. (Frankl, 1963, p. 127)

Imagine you are moving to a new city that you've never seen. How much harder it is to say goodbye to all of your old friends and your favorite cafés if you have no idea what you will find in the new place! As children begin to transition out of therapy, you are a part of what they know. Where they are headed is often unknown. Helping children prepare for the transition out of therapy means helping them to think about what lies ahead and what they can look forward to.

This future orientation can be particularly important for children who have been traumatized. Sometimes traumatized children have difficulty imagining themselves in the future. This difficulty may reflect an adaptive response for a child who is living a life in constant fear and is simply trying to make it through the day. However, at this point in the treatment, the child's environment should be stabilized, he/she should feel in control of his/her thoughts and feelings, and he/she should be ready to start thinking about the future and setting goals outside of the therapy.

Goal setting can serve as a powerful means of motivation for children and can help them see "a light at the end of the tunnel." In other words, goals are the building blocks for a brighter future.

Why is it important to set goals? Children who are able to set future goals for themselves are more likely to see meaning in their lives and are less likely to give up. Goal setting can serve as a powerful means of motivation for children and can help them see "a light at the end of the tunnel." In other words, goals are the building blocks for a brighter future.

 The Goal-Setting Guide (GSG) is designed to help children generate realistic goals for themselves and identify the steps they will need to take to get there.

> **What it is:** An individualized worksheet on which children identify their strengths, desires, future goals, and specific actions needed to accomplish these goals.
>
> **When to use it:** During the *future goals* treatment domain.
>
> **Target goals:** The child will identify his/her strengths, learn how to set goals, and develop a specific plan to achieve them.

The GSG comprises four sections: "What I Am Good At," "What I Like to Do," "What I Want to Do in the Future," and "What Steps I Need to Take to Get There." A copy of the GSG is included in the Appendix. The following GSG was completed by Kelly, age 12, with the help of her therapist. The therapist's questions are included to demonstrate the types of prompts that may be necessary to help the child generate responses to each section.

> THERAPIST: This worksheet is designed to help kids figure out the things that they're good at, how to set goals for the future, and how to accomplish those goals. So let's start with the things you are good at. Can you make a list of everything you can think of that you're good at?
>
> KELLY: (*Makes list.*)
>
> > *What I Am Good At:*
> > 1. *Making necklaces*
> > 2. *Braiding hair*
> > 3. *Making people laugh*
> > 4. *Taking care of my pets*
>
> THERAPIST: That's a great start. Can you think of anything else that you're good at? What do other people tell you that you're good at?

KELLY: Well, my friends tell me that I'm a good listener. And I'm pretty good at taking care of my sister.

THERAPIST: Great! Let's add those to the list.

KELLY: (*Adds to list.*)

> What I Am Good At:
>   1. Making necklaces
>   2. Braiding hair
>   3. Making people laugh
>   4. Taking care of my pets
>   5. Listening
>   6. Taking care of my sister

THERAPIST: Good job. Now, can you make a list of the things that you like to do? They can be the same or different from the things that you are good at.

KELLY: (*Makes list.*)

> What I Like to Do:
>   1. Make necklaces
>   2. Make people laugh
>   3. Take care of animals
>   4. Watch Animal Planet
>   5. Draw pictures of my pets

THERAPIST: That looks like a good list. When you read over the list, is there anything that stands out? Are there some things that you like to do that have a common theme?

KELLY: Animals . . . I love animals.

THERAPIST: It sure looks that way! And it looks like you not only enjoy animals, but you're good at taking care of them too. When you're thinking about your future goals, it's great to think about the things that you like to do, and it's even better if the things you like to do are also things that you're good at. So based on what you are good at and what you like to do, what is it that you'd like to do in the future more than anything else?

KELLY: (*Responds in writing.*)

> What I Want to Do in the Future:
>   Take care of animals

THERAPIST: Great. Now, when you say "take care of animals," what do you mean? Can you tell me more about that?

KELLY: Heal them when they are sick and help them to get better. Like a doctor for animals. A veteran.

THERAPIST: I think you mean a *veterinarian*, right? It sounds like you would make a great veterinarian.

KELLY: Can you help me spell it (*writing on GSG*)?

> *What I Want to Do in the Future:*
>> *Take care of animals, be a veterinarian*

THERAPIST: Now let's think about what you would need to do to become a veterinarian. I can help you with this part if you get stuck. But why don't you start by listing some of the steps that you think you would need to take.

KELLY: *(Makes list.)*

> *What Steps I Need to Take To Get There:*
>> 1. *Graduate from high school*
>> 2. *Go to college*
>> 3. *Graduate from college*
>> 4. *Go to school for veterinarians*
>> 5. *Graduate from school for veterinarians*

THERAPIST: Great start. Can you think of anything that you could be doing while you're in school to prepare yourself for becoming a veterinarian?

KELLY: I bet it would help to take some science classes . . . they talk about animals a lot. And I probably need good grades to get into a good college.

THERAPIST: Those are great steps to take. How about adding those in the order that you think they should happen?

KELLY: *(Adds to list.)*

> *What Steps I Need to Take to Get There:*
>> 1. *Get good grades*
>> 2. *Take some science classes*
>> 3. *Graduate from high school*
>> 4. *Go to college*
>> 5. *Graduate from college*
>> 6. *Go to school for veterinarians*
>> 7. *Graduate from school for veterinarians*

THERAPIST: It sounds like you're on your way! You know, another good thing to do when you're thinking about future goals is to find people who are doing what you want to be doing and ask them questions about how they were able to do it. So, for you, it might be a good idea to talk to a veterinarian about the things that you can do to prepare yourself for that job. Do you know any veterinarians?

KELLY: Yeah! I've taken my dog to see one a few times. I'm going to ask him the next time I go there.

THERAPIST: It might be a good idea to write down some questions ahead of time that you'd like to ask. Would you like to do that now?

KELLY: Sure!

As seen in this example, some children may need more coaching than others, but most children will be able to identify at least one future goal. This guide is useful in not only helping children recognize their own strengths, but also helping them to develop goal-setting skills, which will continue to be useful throughout their lives. The future goals treatment domain can help to instill hope in children who have had little, or no, reason to believe in themselves or a future filled with opportunities.

> This guide is useful in not only helping children recognize their own strengths, but also helping them to develop goal-setting skills, which will continue to be useful throughout their lives.

The ability to set, plan, and achieve realistic goals is critical for happiness and success in life. As discussed in Chapters 2 and 3, children with traumatic stress usually spend their lives *reacting* to events. Accordingly, they often have not developed the skills to approach life proactively through this ability to set, plan, and achieve realistic goals. The meaning-making module aims to provide children with these skills.

By this point in treatment, you are only a few sessions away from saying good-bye. You've talked a lot about the future in the above exercise—now it is time to talk about how your therapy relationship will be different in the future, too. How much longer will you be working together? Will you be around for any of the goals listed on the worksheet? If not, can you still be found in each other's hearts? Again, this discussion of the future related to the therapeutic relationship is an integral part of planning, anticipating, and goal setting.

Enacting Meaning

> . . . the true meaning of life is to be discovered in the world rather than within man or his own psyche, as though it were a closed system . . . being human always points, and is directed, to something or someone other than oneself—be it a meaning to fulfill or another human to encounter. (Frankl, 1963, p. 133)

In the above quotation, Frankl talks about the importance of being a part of the world, not just in the closed system of one's own psyche. Likewise, the ultimate goal of TST is to transition away from the *trauma system* and into the world. Frankl talks about two ways that this transition can be achieved: by creating something, or by truly coming to know another person. In this last section of treatment, the child is encouraged to leave behind the trauma system by engaging in an activity that will create lasting meaning out of the trauma experience and the recovery process.

This is a very individualized section of treatment that must come from the child's sense of him/herself and his/her place in the world. The therapist is only a guide and a witness to the child's creative process of enacting meaning.

The possibilities for enacting meaning are endless and may involve creative expression through art, music, writing, or altruistic expression through charity, teaching, or political action. Enacting meaning may involve changes in career path in order to acquire the skills to make meaning throughout the child's life.

The historical development of culture and religion can be seen as a natural and time-tested process for enacting meaning.

The child's culture or religion may contain powerful rituals for enacting meaning. These should be understood and used if the child believes they are meaningful. The historical development of culture and religion can be seen as a natural and time-tested process for enacting meaning.

For many children, the experience of tragedy ultimately brings about a strong need to live life to its fullest and to serve as a source of hope for others. As one child who lost her mother to a murder stated in session, "I want her to know, wherever she is, that I went on to do great things because she never got to do them. I want to use the gifts that she passed on to me. . . . I know that's what she would have wanted."

Following are a few real-life examples of how children were able to enact meaning from their traumatic experiences.

Victoria is a 16-year-old Sudanese girl with an extensive and complicated trauma history. While in the Sudan as a child, she was raped by militia and threatened with female genital cutting (FGC). In order to escape FGC, she ran away from her village and, ultimately, to the United States. When she arrived in the United States at age 16, she was experiencing major depression and PTSD. She had attempted suicide twice.

Victoria was an exceptionally talented artist. At the start of treatment, she drew several pictures that resonated with themes of emptiness, loss, and powerlessness. Her self-portrait showed a girl with a blank expression, and she explained that the girl did not have hope.

As treatment continued, Victoria's therapist encouraged her to explore new themes with her art. She painted a series of paintings about the process of FGC rituals, showing young girls being prepared for this procedure. She explained that she wanted the world to understand what was happening back in Africa. Toward the end of her treatment, she shifted her topic yet again and did a series of portraits of self and others. Each of these was of a young woman, beautiful and physically powerful looking. One she described as "finding love"; another she described as a self-portrait of herself crossing a bridge, leaving the horrors of the past behind her. Victoria continues to paint and hopes to pursue a career in art.

Kenny is an 8-year-old boy who lost his father in a gang-related shooting. Kenny was not witness to the shooting, but went to the hospital with his mother immediately afterward and observed the doctors attempting to resuscitate his father, who died in front of him.

When Kenny began individual therapy, he was experiencing significant symptoms of PTSD, including flashbacks of his father in the hospital, nightmares, and overt avoidance of anything that might remind him of the shooting. He was also experiencing separation anxiety and did not want to attend school.

As Kenny progressed in therapy, it was clear that there were many layers to his traumatic experience. It became evident that one of the most traumatic aspects of the event was standing alone outside of his father's hospital room with no one to comfort him as he watched his father die. In one particularly moving session, Kenny stated, "I would hate for other kids to feel that way—like they're the only person in the world, like they're all alone."

At the next session, Kenny drew a picture of two boys. The first boy looked very sad; underneath the boy, Kenny wrote, "I know how you feel." The second boy looked very happy, and underneath this boy, Kenny wrote, "Some day you will feel like this again." At the very bottom of the page Kenny wrote, in bold letters, "YOU ARE NOT ALONE." Kenny asked if he could give this to the hospital where his father died so that other kids could see it. This picture now hangs right next to the door of his late father's hospital room. According to one of the nurses, a child about Kenny's age has already asked if she could take it home with her.

 Michael is a 17-year-old boy who was in a serious car accident 1 year before treatment began. He had several broken bones but was able to heal rapidly. Unfortunately, his girlfriend of 1 year had been in the passenger seat and experienced severe injuries to her head and her neck. She is now completely paralyzed from the neck down.

When Michael began therapy, he was extremely guilt-ridden over his girlfriend's situation and was experiencing major depressive symptoms, including suicidal ideation. He also had symptoms of PTSD, such as frequent nightmares, flashbacks of the accident, and avoidance of the site of the car crash.

Throughout the course of therapy, Michael began to identify healthy ways of alleviating his feelings of guilt. He spent a great deal of time with his girlfriend, offering her emotional support and providing her with information about new technologies that may be able to assist in her recovery. Providing her with hope was healing for Michael as well. He also began fundraising efforts at his high school to raise money for his girlfriend so that she could afford the newest advances in medicine. At his high school homecoming dance, Michael was able to raise money, through ticket sales; $5 of each ticket was given to his girlfriend's fund.

These are just three examples of the ways in which children can make meaning out of their trauma and convey this meaning to others. The important point to remember is that it is up to the child to decide how he/she would like to use the lessons that he/she has learned from the traumatic experience.

By the end of this module, children should not only be able to think about the future but to see themselves as effective creators of a meaningful future. If the

By the end of this module, children should not only be able to think about the future but to see themselves as effective creators of a meaningful future.

child is able to shift his/her view in this way, he/she now has initiated a brand new journey with a different destination in mind—one that has the potential for reparative experiences and new ways of looking at the world.

Saying Goodbye

A child's journey through treatment can be long, full of joy and pain, at times uncertain, and ultimately life changing. A therapist is witness and partner in all of this. Ultimately treatment must end. The child, parents, and therapist must say goodbye, which can be difficult for everyone involved. Saying goodbye also has critical therapeutic value regarding everything this chapter is about: leading a meaningful life beyond the trauma of the past.

Premature or De Facto Goodbyes

Before talking about how we like to bring therapy to a close in TST, we need to acknowledge that you may not ever get here. Although in a perfect therapy world treatment ends when everyone involved is ready for it to end, that doesn't always happen. An intern finishes her rotation and has to transfer a family midstream, a child's symptoms improve and Mom doesn't see a need to bring him to therapy anymore, or sometimes a family just stops coming and you don't ever learn why. These can be difficult endings, because so much is left unfinished or unsaid. Although maybe we don't see the child again, we can guess that it is hard for him/her.

And it's hard for the therapist, too! Unplanned endings can leave a therapist wondering what he/she did wrong or that what he/she did wasn't enough. Maybe the child is still having a lot of trouble, and the therapist feels like a failure. It's hard for everyone not to have closure.

But it's also important not to despair just because you didn't make it all the way to the meaning-making module. Truthfully, healing rarely happens in a straight line.

But it's also important not to despair just because you didn't make it all the way to the meaning-making module. Truthfully, healing rarely happens in a straight line. Maybe the family has done all they can do for now—but you've given them a gift of opening the door to treatment, and they will come back when they are ready for the next step. Maybe you've expressed that one compliment that the child is going to hold in his/her heart during the hard times ahead. Maybe you'll never know that, but you can rest assured that there's meaning in the therapist–client relationship that is impossible to see on the surface.

Special Vulnerabilities of the Traumatized Child at the End of Treatment

Traumatized children often have long and painful histories of loss and abandonment. The notion of ending treatment may provoke memories and emotions related to these experiences. Sometimes these experiences occurred at a very young age, before the child was able to form and store declarative memories of them. In these cases, the child may still respond to stimuli signaling the end of treatment with emotion related to loss and abandonment, but not know why he/she is responding in such ways.

The therapist should expect some exacerbation of symptoms around the time of treatment termination. In a way, this phase is a good test of the child's new emotion regulation, cognitive processing, and meaning-making skills. The essence of the treatment approach during this increase in symptoms is to help the child use these new skills to manage emotion related to the end of treatment and to help the child and family see that they can use these new skills to manage stressors after treatment ends.

> The essence of the treatment approach during this increase in symptoms is to help the child use these new skills to manage emotion related to the end of treatment and to help the child and family see that they can use these new skills to mange stressors after treatment ends.

In rare cases, the child may experience a significant relapse of symptoms and problems during the end of treatment. In this case, the therapist should review the events leading to the relapse with the treatment team to determine whether the decision to end treatment was premature. The team should also be vigilant about whether there is any missing information that may have precipitated the decompensation, such as undisclosed environmental stressors or undisclosed episodes of emotional/behavioral dysregulation.

Three Steps to Bringing TST to a Meaningful Close

Saying goodbye is a topic that is bigger than this book. We offer here, however, a few thoughts on how to bring TST to a close—both for the family and the therapist. These thoughts are organized according to three basic steps:

1. Anticipate the goodbye early.
2. Acknowledge the meaning of the work.
3. Acknowledge the meaning of the relationship.

When considering each of the three steps, it is important to consider (1) the child's memory of the trauma and how it has affected him/her, and (2) the memory the child will have of the therapy and the therapeutic relationship and how it will sustain him/her. In many ways, the process of saying goodbye brings to the forefront exactly why therapy works: *It creates meaningful and sustaining memories that are exactly counter to the memories of trauma.*

Step 1: Anticipate the Goodbye Early

Description

As the relationship between the child, family, and TST clinician develops, strong attachments grow. It is extremely important for the clinician to be mindful of the strong attachment-related emotions that develop on the side of the child and family, and within the clinician him/herself. These emotions may powerfully evoke the earliest experiences and memories of attachments among all concerned (including the clinician). The degree to which these emotions and memories can be recognized early, the less likely they are to threaten the healthy ending of treatment where these emotions and memories are likely to be strongly elicited.

Trauma Memory

Loss for the traumatized child is usually precipitous. Suddenly the person on whom the child depends is gone. In cases where such a loss could be anticipated, no one took the time to prepare the child or to help him/her with feelings related to loss. Over time, the child learns that no one is dependable or trustworthy. The child expects that no one will treat his/her feelings with care.

TST Memory

The TST clinician is vigilant about the child's feelings related to loss and abandonment and is fully accountable for his/her role in caring for these feelings (TST Principle Five: Insist on accountability, particularly your own). This accountability begins with the initial treatment agreement, whereby the child and family are informed how long treatment is likely to last and the boundaries and limits of the clinician's role in helping the child and family. Nothing sets up a child who is vulnerable to abandonment more potently than false promises. As treatment progresses, the clinician should have a good understanding of the child and family's vulnerabilities to loss and abandonment. These should be proactively referenced during the course of treatment to help anticipate and manage feelings related to the end of treatment.

> The child and family's vulnerabilities to loss and abandonment should be proactively referenced during the course of treatment to help anticipate and manage feelings related to the end of treatment.

Step 2: Acknowledge the Meaning of the Work

Description

It is always a tremendous accomplishment when the child and family have reached the point of ending treatment. Usually, all concerned have worked very hard to reach this point. This type of achievement is often highly meaningful to the child, family, and clinician and should be acknowledged as clearly and as authentically as possible.

Trauma Memory

Many traumatized children learn that their efforts don't matter. This learning can originate at the time of the trauma, when all efforts to escape were ineffective and all words indicating *stop* were not attended. It may continue when the child's work at school or at home does not seem to matter to the adults in his/her life. Healthy development requires that the child have a basic sense of pride in his/her efforts to do good things. If this sense of pride is not acknowledged and mirrored by adults, it shrivels and dies. The repeated experience of unacknowledged pride creates memories and expectations within the traumatized child that he/she is ineffective and that nothing he/she does matters. The consequences of these memories were described in Chapter 3 as chronic adaptations to trauma, and can be expressed as chronic depression, helplessness, shame, or antisocial and self-destructive behavior.

TST Memory

The TST clinician is vigilant about acknowledging the child's efforts and good work. This acknowledgment is expressed throughout the treatment. The period leading to the end of treatment should be used to reflect on and review the child's effort and work. The child should be encouraged to feel proud of what he/she has accomplished. This sense of pride should be acknowledged, supported, and mirrored by the clinician. All of these interactions between child and clinician create powerful, meaningful, and sustaining memories that go exactly counter to the many of the memories related to the trauma, as detailed above.

Step 3: Acknowledge the Meaning of the Relationship

Description

The therapeutic relationship may be the most meaningful the child and/or family has ever experienced. The notion of "signals of care," described in Chapter 5, essentially concerns how the meaning of therapeutic relationships can directly counter the meaning of traumatic relationships for all concerned.

Trauma Memory

Children who have experienced interpersonal trauma have memories of relationships riddled with conflict, strife, betrayal, violence, loss, and abandonment. There are a great many consequences to these memories. Perhaps at a most basic level these memories indicate to the child that he/she is unloved and unlovable, uncared for and unworthy of care. The consequences of these memories and expectations, among other things, are lifelong difficulties with relationships and a low sense of self-esteem. These difficulties were described in Chapter 3 chronic adaptations to trauma, and can be expressed as the avoidance of all relationships, the failure of self-protection within relationships, or patterns of strife, conflict, and violence within relationships.

TST Memory

As described in Chapter 5, the TST clinician takes great care to acknowledge the meaning of the therapeutic relationship. The work of TST is a highly interpersonal process and is built on a foundation of a safe, trustworthy, and accountable therapeutic relationship. The TST clinician acknowledges the meaning of the therapeutic relationship frequently in the course of treatment. As treatment moves toward a close, the meaning of the relationship is acknowledged and discussed explicitly. This may be the child's first experience of an adult who expresses care, concern, and empathy.

Here is a story of a 9-year-old boy who was ending treatment.

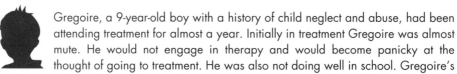 Gregoire, a 9-year-old boy with a history of child neglect and abuse, had been attending treatment for almost a year. Initially in treatment Gregoire was almost mute. He would not engage in therapy and would become panicky at the thought of going to treatment. He was also not doing well in school. Gregoire's teacher noted that he was frequently "in his own world" and she could not get him to "snap out of it." Gregoire's trauma history included experiences of being beaten by his birth mother's boyfriend and witnessing violence toward his mother. He was taken out of her custody by the state child welfare authorities. His mother abandoned him at age 5, when she moved to another state with a new boyfriend.

Following the initial assessment, the TST clinician helped the members of Gregoire's social environment (adoptive mother, teacher, etc.) to see how *new* relationships, particularly with adults, can evoke memories of trauma and abandonment. The TST clinician, with knowledge of the moment-by-moment process by which Gregoire would freeze and go "into his own world," offered practical solutions for helping in this process. This strategy was very successful. In the process of forming a safe, trustworthy relationship, filled with the "signals of care" described in Chapter 5, Gregoire began to look forward to his therapy sessions and would gradually be less anxious and would engage more in treatment. After 1 year of treatment, the TST clinician, teacher, and adoptive mother noted, with great hope, that his anxiety was gone, and he was much more successful in school.

The Process of Ending Treatment

At the beginning of treatment, the TST clinician discussed with Gregoire and his adoptive mother that therapy would need to end at some point over the next year or so. Six months into treatment she reintroduced the notion of therapy ending some point over the next 6–8 months, and had a frank discussion of what this might mean. Gregoire and the TST clinician talked about how much they would miss each other and how important their work was together.

The TST clinician used specific examples of the great work that Gregoire was doing and the things she liked most about him. She also highlighted that their work together would not end for a number of months. Over the next few sessions she noted that Gregoire did not seem as engaged as usual and was somewhat more anxious; however, within 2 weeks Gregoire appeared back to his usual self. Every month or so, the therapist would briefly anticipate feelings around termination with Gregoire. Finally, 1 year into therapy, the TST clinician believed that most of the goals of treatment had been accomplished and she initiated the discussion of planning for termination of treatment.

The first day she brought it up, Gregoire wanted to play "doctor." He was the "doctor," and made the therapist, who was the "patient," wait for a long period of time in the waiting room. He finally was able to see the patient, and examined her heart. He stated that her heart was very ill and that she would need to come back. Although Gregoire appeared to be a little more anxious than usual, he continued to be well engaged in therapy; however, he did not want to talk about its ending and just wanted to play. This same theme was replayed for several weeks. Finally, on one of the last days of treatment, Gregoire examined the patient's (therapist's) heart one last time. He then picked up a plastic chainsaw from the shelf and proceeded to "operate" on her heart.

"There," Gregoire said, "I've fixed your heart. Now you are all better, and you can't come to see me anymore." This lead to a discussion with Gregoire and his adoptive mother about the importance of their work together being "life saving" and that because of Gregoire's very hard work, he was able to accomplish things that he never thought possible. The last session included a review of Gregoire's many accomplishments with both the TST clinician and his adoptive mother expressing how proud they were of Gregoire. Gregoire had prepared a "goodbye" card for his therapist and said that "even though it is not Valentine's Day, I wanted to draw you a heart and say how much you have helped mine." The therapist also had a gift prepared for Gregoire. It was a small, inexpensive heart-shaped locket. She had a Polaroid camera and took a photograph of the two of them together. Gregoire and his therapist cut and pasted this photograph into his new locket before they said goodbye.

Comment

The TST clinician closely followed the three steps to bringing TST to a meaningful close. She understood some of the particular difficulties that Gregoire would have about saying goodbye, given his trauma history. She anticipated this "goodbye" very early in the treatment and built a language for the two of them about saying goodbye. Furthermore, she frequently would acknowledge the meaning of both the work and the relationship throughout treatment. The clinician's degree of care toward the three steps to bringing TST to a close, in very important ways, helped Gregoire to extract the most meaningful experience possible around saying goodbye. Given the history of abandonment from his mother, this would create memories that can sustain him through the hardest of times in the future because they are exactly contrary to his experiences and memories that lead to his need for treatment.

Gregoire's play with his therapist very eloquently shows the sad tradeoff of the therapeutic relationship. The "doctor" (therapist) had made Gregoire share his heart and helped him to feel better, but the cost of getting better is that Gregoire could no longer see his therapist. Gregoire poignantly expresses is readiness for therapy to end during his play sequence, but he is immeasurably helped in this process by a clinician who has consistently acknowledged the meanings of the work and the relationship. The ritual of play, regarding the mending of his broken heart, and the exchange of "heart" gifts at treatment's end, encapsulates in the best way how the meaning-making module can help a child transcend traumatic experiences.

What About You (Yes, YOU)?!

Helping a child to reach the point of treatment's conclusion is no small task. In fact, you should feel considerably proud for having influenced a child's development and future in such an important way. It should be a time of celebration between you and the child/family and between you and your team. The end of a treatment should be marked, noted, celebrated, and remembered. It is not only the child who needs to have these types of memories to keep going.

Remember . . . you have left a child with a better system.

Conclusions

Leaving a Better System

 You are not obligated to complete the work, nor are you free to abandon it. (Ethics of the Fathers 5:3)

We do not believe in finished products. The work of helping traumatized children requires, on the part of everyone, a continual struggle to make things better and better. This book is the result of an 8-year effort to develop a treatment that will work. We hope, however, that our book is only the first version of a process that is continually improved in response to people's experiences. Similarly, when we leave a traumatized child at what we call the end of therapy, we do not really believe he/she is "better" or "cured" or whichever professional term is used to make us feel better. The best we can hope for is to leave the child and the family with tools they will use to meet their challenges throughout their lives. An ancient Jewish tradition, quoted above, teaches that the profound business of making the world a better place is never ending and requires courage, humility, and, especially, tenacity. You will never finish, but you can also never give up. . . .

This is the business of TST and what our tenth principle, *leaving a better system*, is all about.

What does *leaving a better system* really mean? First let's consider the conventional way of determining treatment success.

How Is Treatment Effectiveness Defined?

 Hoagwood, Jensen, Petti, and Burns (1996) suggested that effectiveness of a treatment can be measured across five different domains:

- Symptoms
- Functioning
- Client perspectives
- Environments
- Systems

All of these domains are interrelated to some extent. Change in one can lead to change in another. Ideally, of course, we'd like to see change across all of them as a result of implementing TST. Sometimes, however, things don't happen all at once. Change in a system might take place, but the effect on symptoms might lag behind. The child's functioning might shoot up, but the parents' perspective hasn't caught up to the news ("Who says therapy works . . . he just got better on his own!"). So how do you know if *TST* "worked"?

To answer that question, we need to consider how implementing TST might lead to change and improvement across these domains and how to measure that improvement in a messy world.

Symptoms

 Measuring changes in symptoms seems easy enough. We give the client a questionnaire when he/she starts treatment and one when he/she finishes treatment, and the scores go down. Right?

Usually, yes. But there are some complicating factors to keep in mind.

Although we'd love to see symptoms disappear, sometimes only a *decrease* in symptoms is worth recognizing as a success. Maybe the child is no longer suicidal and sleeps better—but he/she still has a little bit of trouble concentrating. This is still a huge accomplishment! We always need to keep in mind where we started when measuring how far we've come.

> We always need to keep in mind where we started when measuring how far we've come.

Symptoms can also wax and wane. New developmental milestones in life and new social circumstances can lead to a resurgence in symptoms. That doesn't mean all is lost! Sometimes children can't do all of the cognitive processing they need to do at a younger age; as they develop and grow, cognitive skills can be brought to bear on understanding what happened to them. Around the end of treatment, families may worry about what to do if symptoms recur after the treatment ends. It can be helpful to remind families that symptoms may come and go. Remember that (1) symptoms after treatment are less likely to be as intense as they were before treatment, and (2) the family now knows how to recognize them and to engage services to help treat them.

TST specifically targets symptoms of emotion dysregulation. These symptoms can be expected to decrease under TST and are, by definition, part of what should improve as the child moves up the TST Assessment Grid.

Functioning

Sometimes it can be easy to confuse symptoms and functioning, which are often related, but don't necessarily go hand in hand. In fact, some research has shown that kids can have really high levels of symptoms but go through life functioning at a very high level—graduating from high school, going to college, making friends. And sometimes even with relatively low levels of symptoms we see big problems in functioning.

Functioning means being able to do what day-to-day life requires of you. It means getting yourself up in the morning, going to school and doing schoolwork, having relationships with people, and generally being able to be a part of the society in which we all live. Sometimes kids can function well in some contexts (e.g., a structured classroom) but not in others (e.g., an unstructured summer camp). Although we'd like every child to be able to function across all sorts of contexts, that may be an unrealistic goal for some. Sometimes helping to create an environment in which the child can function best is a more realistic goal, and one to be celebrated when it is achieved.

> Sometimes helping to create an environment in which the child can function best is a more realistic goal, and one to be celebrated when it is achieved.

TST focuses on two ways of improving child functioning: (1) by helping to create an environment that maximizes the child's chances of functioning well, and (2) by diminishing symptoms of emotion dysregulation that can interfere with functioning. We expect a child's functioning to improve over the course of treatment.

Client Perspectives

Is the parent happy with the outcome? Is the child? If a child's symptoms and functioning have improved, chances are good that the parent and child will feel good about the outcomes. There are other dimensions of success, however, that are also important to consider. For instance, has the child developed a trusting relationship with his/her providers so that he/she would be likely to reengage in treatment if she needed to later? Does the child think that the problem he/she wanted fixed was addressed? Within TST, the ready–set–go module lays the groundwork to make sure that this particular outcome is achieved. If the parent's source of pain was acknowledged up front and included in the treatment plan, then chances are good that the results he/she sees at the end of treatment will seem (and be) related to the problem he/she really wanted fixed. Sometimes, of course, there are problems that can't be fixed—but at least we can acknowledge what the parent wants to change and be transparent about why we've all worked on the areas addressed. Hopefully, a child's and parent's perspective at the end of treatment will reflect this transparency and good-faith effort to change what the parent and child really wanted to see change (not just what we, as therapists, wanted to change).

Environments

One of the elements of TST that sets it apart from other treatments is that we focus on changing environments as a way of changing a child's trauma-related symptoms. Again, by definition, a child who is making progress through the TST Assessment Grid is moving into a stabler environment. "The environment," of course, is not monolithic—there are many different elements that comprise a child's environment, and TST focuses its change efforts on just those aspects of the environment that are most closely linked to the child's emotion dysregulation. So change in the environment is expected in TST, and it is expected to occur in very specific ways.

Systems

TST is dedicated to changing systems: to changing the trauma system of an individual child, and to changing the system of care that surrounds the child.

 TST is dedicated to changing systems: to changing the trauma system of an individual child, and to changing the system of care that surrounds the child. Successful change of systems requires many steps. It starts with an agency deciding to take a look at the way services are put together and whether this could be done in a more concerted way. TST offers a very specific model of how to do that. From there, TST can be the catalyst for changes in many different systems—not just the agency, but also the different systems that a child and his/her clinician come into contact with along the way. Ultimately, TST is about leaving a better system.

Checking in on the Kids

Looking at treatment effectiveness in the way described above is very important. Ultimately, however, treatment effectiveness translates into how a treatment produced something meaningful to an individual child and family. You might be wondering whatever happened to all those kids we introduced in the course of this book. What did *leaving a better system* mean for them?

Remember Gerald who began our book?

 Gerald is now 15. His dad is still in jail, but Gerald is able to talk about him without becoming upset. In fact, in his meaning-making sessions he talked a lot about how he wanted to be a father someday and that he was going to "do it differently." Gerald's mother continues to struggle with depression but is actively seeking treatment and has begun to talk about how her own traumatic reactions from the domestic violence she experienced sometimes made it hard to parent Gerald and his brother in the way that she wanted to. Gerald's older brother was arrested and placed in Department of Youth Services (DYS) custody, and at the mom's request the TST team has been working with DYS providers to create a discharge plan that will help him access trauma treatment services. And Gerald? Gerald just completed a successful year in a specialized classroom. He passed all of his courses and did particularly well in his student leadership class. His concentration has improved and he is able to focus relatively well in the structured classroom. He no longer expresses any suicidal ideation and, in fact, does not seem to experience any symptoms of depression. Although he still sometimes thinks about what happened in the past, he says that it no longer "takes over."

And remember Denise from Chapters 2, 7, and 8?

 Denise's TST treatment team felt strongly that unless some of the key environmental stressors were removed, Denise was going to continue to have trouble. In fact, they felt that one of the most important things they could do to help Denise would be to get her a bedroom door. In response to services advocacy and writing letters clearly noting the link between the substandard housing and Denise's health problem, the recalcitrant landlord finally had a door installed. Meanwhile, the treatment team provided Denise's mom with a lot of education around trauma and domestic violence and how the ongoing abusive relationship with her boyfriend might be contributing to problems for everyone in the family. Things got worse before they got better, and Denise's mom threatened to "pick my boyfriend over my daughter if I have to," but after working closely with the SOS team, she admitted that she was staying with her boyfriend because she was afraid to leave. With the help of the team she broke off the relationship and filed a restraining order. And Denise? Denise began to feel markedly safer at home, and her nightmares stopped. She still is reminded of her abuser by some men she sees around town, but she says "I just make myself look at him again and say to myself, 'He can't hurt me, that's not the same guy.' " She is now finishing her GED and applying to the local community college.

And Robert, from Chapter 3?

 When Robert first started TST, the primary environmental threat—his stepfather—was already out of the picture. But Robert was having such trouble regulating that almost anything seemed to trigger him, including typical playground teasing. Robert, his mom, and his TST treatment team spent a lot of time and energy working on emotion regulation skills. Psychopharmacology helped to dampen Robert's arousal, but he still became dysregulated at school. He moved to a more structured classroom, where he was able to successfully complete the year without any suspensions. He is starting now in a mainstream classroom, and his mother reports that with the exception of gym class (which gets a little rambunctious), he hasn't had any problems. She told the TST team that she had already been to the school to talk about having him moved to a smaller gym class—in her words, "I know he can do it! He just needs the right setting until *he* knows he can do it."

No child's journey through TST looks quite the same. These are the stories based on a few of the children with whom we've worked. We hope that you'll have your own stories—because more than any outcome study, more than any balanced budget sheet, more than any symptom reduction score, it's these stories that tell us that what we're doing is working. It's these kids and their little—and big—successes, that keep us going. It's these kids who helped us develop TST. *They* are the ones who have really left a better system.

Appendix

TST TREATMENT PLANNING FORM

CHILD NAME _____ DOB _____ RECORD # _____ DATE _____

1. Indicate the "players" on the team

The Team	Name	Ways to reach	Signature
Child or adolescent			
Family			
Therapist			
SOS clinician			
SOS clinician			
Legal advocate			
Psychiatric consultant			
Others*			

*Godparents, involved neighbors, extended family, mentors, social service providers, pediatricians, religious leaders.

2. Indicate scores on relevant instruments

	TR HX	TSS SX	E Reg	B Reg	Soc Env	Str	Fn
CANS-TEA							
UCLA PTSD-RI							
TSCC							
CBCL			Int:	Ext:		Comp.	

3. Indicate the recommended treatment phase

	Stable	Distressed	Threatening
Regulated	Transcending Phase 5	Understanding Phase 4	Enduring Phase 3
Dysregulation of Emotion	Understanding Phase 4	Enduring Phase 3	Stabilizing Phase 2
Dysregulation of Behavior	Enduring Phase 3	Stabilizing Phase 2	Surviving Phase 1

(continued)

309

4. Indicate the recommended treatment modules

	Surviving	Stabilizing	Enduring	Understanding	Transcending
Stabilization on site (SOS)	***	***	—	—	—
Services advocacy	***	**	*	*	*
Psychopharmacology	**	**	**	*	*
Emotional regulation	*	**	***	—	—
Cognitive processing	—	—	—	***	—
Meaning making	—	—	—	—	***

Note. *** = essential; ** = often helpful; * = occasionally helpful; — = not used or contraindicated

5a. Identify the TST Priority Problems

TST Priority Problems:

1. Identify patterns of links between social–environmental stressor and emotional/behavioral dysregulation.
2. Prioritize those patterns that most interfere with the child's functioning. (Use point 5b to help decide on the level of priority. It is very important to note that point 5b offers only rough guidelines and should not override clinical discretion.)

Priority Problem 1	Priority Problem 2
Priority Problem 3	Priority Problem 4

5b. Guidelines for assigning priority to a problem identified in point 5a

1. Problems that jeopardize physical safety (e.g., suicide, violence, child abuse).
2. Problems that jeopardize engagement in treatment.
3. Problems that jeopardize home placement.
4. Problems that jeopardize school placement.
5. Problems that jeopardize healthy development (e.g., drug abuse, antisocial behavior, sexual activity, eating disturbances).
6. Problems that cause significant distress to the child or to family members.
7. Problems that can be solved relatively easily and are highly meaningful to the child or family members.

(continued)

6. Identify the solutions to TST Priority Problems

Who/what does solution address?	PP #	Description of solution	Person responsible	When noted	When resolved
Child (indicate skill module and/or psychopharmacology)					
Social environment					
Caregiver (e.g., emotional and/or substance abuse, monitoring/ supervision, knowledge, family violence)					
Siblings					
Housing					
Resources					
School					
Appropriateness of placement					
Neighborhood					
Peers					
Other					

Barriers (Describe practical barriers that may interfere with solving priority problems; describe strategies to surmount barriers.)

Description:	Strategy:			

Strengths (Describe strengths of child/assets in social environment that may be engaged to help with solutions to priority problems.)

Description:	Strategy:			

WEELY TST CHECK-IN

Emotional and Behavioral Dysregulation

How bad, sad, hurt, angry, guilty, or scared have I been **feeling** in the last week?	How much has my **behavior** toward myself or others been harmful, destructive, aggressive, or risky in the last week?

9 — As much as I can imagine   Why: _____

7 — A lot   _____

5 — Some   _____

3 — A little bit   _____

1 — Not at all   _____

_____

9 — As much as I can imagine   Why: _____

7 — A lot   _____

5 — Some   _____

3 — A little bit   _____

1 — Not at all   _____

_____

Environmental Stability

In the last week, how much have I been **reminded** of bad things that have happened to me?	In the last week, how much did I feel like people around me (my caregivers, teachers, social workers, etc.) were able to **protect** me from experiencing or being reminded of bad things, or **help** me in dealing with my emotions when I was reminded?

9 — As much as I can imagine   Why: _____

7 — A lot   _____

5 — Some   _____

3 — A little bit   _____

1 — Not at all   _____

_____

9 — As much as I can imagine   Why: _____

7 — A lot   _____

5 — Some   _____

3 — A little bit   _____

1 — Not at all   _____

_____

TST TREATMENT FIDELITY FORM

Date:	**Sources of Information (check all that apply)**
Participant ID#:	
Participant Name (if appropriate):	Clinician self-report:
Initials of Rater:	Clinician interview:
Initials of Co-Rater(s):	Supervisor report:
Initials of Primary Clinician:	Team meeting:
Initials of Team Leader:	Chart review:
	Other (specify):

Instructions

The following items assess how closely activities within TST interventions correspond to the 10 TST Treatment Principles as detailed in Chapter 6 in this volume. The rater should be familiar with this volume (and particularly with Chapter 6) when making these ratings. Each of the following items describes a different TST principle and the core construct addressed by the principle. The rater should look for evidence from a variety of sources (team meeting, chart review, clinical supervision sessions, etc.) to determine if there was fidelity to the respective treatment principle. This form should be used to note whether this evidence was "present," "absent," or "insufficient."

Principle 1: Fix a Broken System

CORE CONSTRUCT: The clinician (or clinical team) assesses the stability of the child's social environment, the capacity of the child to regulate his or her emotions and behavior, and the interaction between them (the trauma system). The clinician integrates this information into a concise list of 1–4 treatment goals ("TST Priority Problems"), and all interventions are devoted to addressing these TST Priority Problems. Evidence for fidelity to this principle includes the following:

Evidence	Present	Absent	Insufficient
1. Assessment activities explicitly reference the degree of emotional/behavioral dysregulation, the degree of environmental instability, and the link between them (e.g., use of TST Assessment Grid, identification of TST Priority Problems).			
2. Intervention activities explicitly reference the degree of emotional/behavioral dysregulation, the degree of environmental instability and the link between them (e.g., TST Priority Solutions are clearly linked to TST Priority Problems).			
3. Team discussion references the degree of emotional/behavioral dysregulation, the degree of environmental instability, and the link between them.			

(continued)

Principle 2: Put Safety First

CORE CONSTRUCT: The clinician (or clinical team) is attuned to the signs of a threatening social environment and proactively adjusts the TST treatment plan based on an ongoing safety assessment that occurs throughout treatment.

Evidence	Present	Absent	Insufficient
1. Information about safety is explicitly assessed.			
2. This information is explicitly used for treatment planning.			
3. Safety concerns are reassessed throughout treatment and treatment plans adjusted based on new information.			

Principle 3: Focused Plans That Are Based on Facts

CORE CONSTRUCT: The clinician (or clinical team) bases all clinical decisions on objective evidence gathered from clinical interviews, collateral contacts, and structured clinical assessments (e.g., self-report questionnaires). Clinical decision making targets the trauma system, as defined in Chapters 7 and 8, and is summarized in the TST Treatment Plan. Evidence for fidelity to this principle includes the following:

Evidence	Present	Absent	Insufficient
1. Moment-by-moment analysis is used to gather information regarding the child's emotional/behavioral dysregulation.			
2. The social environment is surveyed to identify possible stressful stimuli that may elicit this dysregulation.			
3. The TST Assessment Grid is completed using the clinical information gathered under steps #1 and #2.			
4. TST Priority Problems are identified by the clear links between stressful stimuli and dysregulated responses.			
5. TST Priority Solutions are drafted to intervene between these identified stimulus/response links.			
6. Problems and solutions are prioritized according to the format noted in Chapter 8.			
7. Information related to treatment planning is supplemented by relevant instruments and tools (e.g., Legal Services Screener, Emotional Regulation Guide, Weekly TST Check-in).			
8. Information related to treatment planning is supplemented by relevant collateral contacts (e.g., teachers, social service workers, youth service workers, extended-family members).			

(continued)

Principle 4: Don't "Go" Before You Are "Ready"

CORE CONSTRUCT: The clinician (or clinical team) enters the process of engaging the family in the TST Treatment Plan before providing focused interventions. Evidence of fidelity to this principle includes the following:

Evidence	Present	Absent	Insufficient
1. Prior to the initiation of treatment, the initial TST Assessment and treatment planning process are completed.			
2. This process includes the family members' perspectives on problems ("sources of pain") and solutions that they have considered.			
3. A treatment alliance is built around how the TST Priority Problems and Solutions may plausibly offer family members relief from this "source of pain." The treatment alliance should include a shared understanding about child traumatic stress and what will be required of the family should they choose to engage in treatment.			
4. Prior to the initiation of treatment, a family collaborative meeting is held where initial ideas regarding TST Priority Problems and Solutions are shared and discussed with the family. The final treatment plan is based on the agreement between the team and the family about how problems will be addressed in treatment.			
5. Prior to the initiation of treatment, the clinician, team members, and family work to surmount practical barriers to treatment engagement.			

Principle 5: Put Scarce Resources Where They'll Work

CORE CONSTRUCT: The TST Treatment Team strategically focuses on a limited set of highly specific priority problems and allocates their limited intervention resources toward the highest priority problems. Evidence of adherence to this principle includes the following:

Evidence	Present	Absent	Insufficient
1. Team discussion includes the reality of the team's limited intervention resources for the population they are serving as a whole.			
2. Team discussion includes allocation of these scarce resources for the highest priority problems of the families served by the team.			

(continued)

Principle 6: Insist on Accountability, Particularly Your Own

CORE CONSTRUCT: The clinician (or clinical team) ensures that all members of the treatment team are held fully accountable for agreements made within TST treatment. Evidence of fidelity to this treatment principle includes the following:

Evidence	Present	Absent	Insufficient
1. Treatment agreements are recorded and "signed off" by the responsible party on the TST Treatment Planning Form.			
2. The TST Treatment Planning Form is used in each treatment session to "check in" about whether agreements were kept.			
3. In cases where treatment agreements are not kept, this is addressed proactively. Reasons for not keeping agreements are discussed. Barriers are addressed. Renegotiation of the TST Treatment Plan is considered based on the reality of agreements not kept.			
4. Circumstances where a member of the TST Treatment Team did not keep an agreement are addressed in the same way as when a child or family member did not keep an agreement. The TST Treatment Team member is expected to apologize when appropriate.			

Principle 7: Align with Reality

CORE CONSTRUCT: The clinician (or clinical team) continually engages in the process of understanding the clinical realities of a case (e.g., a compromised caregiver, a child's being unable to achieve sufficient regulation to participate in desired activities) and makes every effort to distinguish the child's, caregivers', and their own wishes from this clinical reality. Evidence of fidelity to this principle includes the following:

Evidence	Present	Absent	Insufficient
1. Team meetings and clinical supervision sessions include critical review of such questions as "What is true?", "What is real?", "Do we have all the facts?", "Do we have the most accurate information?"			
2. Difficult decisions regarding a case are explicitly weighed against the wish to "preserve the alliance" with the family. Clinicians and team members openly discuss the tension between "alliance-preserving" wishes and clinical realities so that care is not compromised.			

Principle 8: Take Care of Yourself and Your Team

CORE CONSTRUCT: The clinician (or clinical team) delivers care mindful of the difficulties of the work and appropriately include self-care and social support in clinical decision making. Evidence of fidelity to this principle includes the following:

(continued)

Evidence	Present	Absent	Insufficient
1. Team discussion includes opportunities to address team members' reactions to their work.			
2. Team discussion includes levity, humor, and efforts to boost morale.			
3. Team leaders regularly underscore that team members should "never worry alone."			

Principle 9: Build from Strength

CORE CONSTRUCT: The clinician (or clinical team) assesses the strengths within the child, family, and social environment and organizes treatment plans around these preexisting strengths. Evidence of fidelity to this principle includes the following:

Evidence	Present	Absent	Insufficient
1. The assessment includes documentation of strengths within the child and the social environment.			
2. Emotional regulation interventions include strategies that build from the way the child has successfully managed emotion in the past.			
3. Social environmental stability strategies identify and engage any member of the child's environment who can help him or her manage emotion (e.g., immediate or extended family members, neighbors, or professionals).			
4. Social environmental interventions integrate understandings of the family's specific way of managing emotion (e.g., cultural or religious rituals).			

Principle 10: Leave a Better System

CORE CONSTRUCT: The clinician (or clinical team) prepares the family for the end of treatment and builds skills or systems that can help the child and family after treatment ends. The team is also aware that their work can inform public policy regarding improved service systems for traumatized children. Evidence of fidelity to this principle includes the following:

Evidence	Present	Absent	Insufficient
1. The notion of the end of treatment is raised during the *Ready–Set–Go* process and continues to be raised throughout treatment, as clinically appropriate.			
2. Skill building for emotional regulation, cognitive processing, or meaning making includes strategies for continuing to build these skills after treatment ends.			
3. Efforts to stabilize the social environment and/or system of care integrate how these changes can continue after treatment ends.			
4. Team discussion includes possible public policy implications of the work and, perhaps, strategies for using the clinical experience to inform public policy.			

EMOTION REGULATION GUIDE (OR PUT YOUR OWN TITLE HERE)

BY:

FOR: (List everyone who should get a copy. Possibilities include you, your therapist, parent, teacher, psychiatrist, home-based SOS clinicians, and anyone else who you think knows you well and can help you when things get tough!)

Instructions for clinicians: Please complete this form with the child and family. This form should be used to guide treatment, as outlined in Chapter 14. It should also be used to help assess whether there is/was an episode of dysregulation. Remember that an episode of dysregulation occurs when the child has changes in the three A's (awareness, affect, and action) when presented with a stressor (reviewed in Chapters 3 and 7).

(continued)

Regulating Stage: "Being in Control and Feeling OK"

People spend most of their time in regulated states of emotion—or just generally feeling in control. This doesn't necessarily mean you feel *good* all the time—feeling sad, frustrated, or worried are all part of life, just as feeling joyful or hopeful or excited are part of life. But even if we aren't feeling good, we can still be in control, aware of what's going on around us, and able to do things such as problem solve to make the situation better. Here think about what it's like when you are *regulated*—that is, in control and feeling OK.

How I know when I'm in feeling OK and in control

Ask others:	*Ask myself:*
Affect:	**Affect:**
What expression does my face show?	How do I feel?
How do I say I feel?	What does my body feel like?
Awareness:	**Awareness:**
Do I seem spaced out or in my own world?	What's going on around me?
How well am I paying attention to things?	What am I thinking about?
Action:	**Action:** What do I feel like doing?
What do I do?	
What do I say?	

Maintenance activities: How to keep feeling OK and being in control

Things an adult can help me with:	*Things I can do on my own:*

(continued)

Reacting or "Revving" Stage: Getting Upset

Usually when we get upset there's something that we just saw, experienced, felt, or thought that reminded us of some feelings or memories. Sometimes we get reminded, or "triggered," and have some feelings but can keep on being in control. Other times when we get "triggered," we start to have changes in the three A's—affect, awareness, and action. Make a list here of the types of things that can trigger difficult feelings and thoughts for you.

Reminders/Stressors: What Makes Me Upset?

1.

2.

3.

4.

5.

How I know when I'm upset: The "three A's"

Ask others:	*Ask myself:*
Affect:	**Affect:**
What expression does my face show?	How do I feel?
How do I say I feel?	What does my body feel like?
Awareness:	**Awareness:**
Do I seem spaced out or in my own world?	What's going on around me?
How well am I paying attention to things?	What am I thinking about?
Action:	**Action:** What do I feel like doing?
What do I do?	
What do I say?	

Interventions for the revving phase: How to get back to feeling OK

Things an adult can help me with:	*Things I can do on my own:*

(continued)

Reexperiencing Stage: Feeling and Being Out of Control

Sometimes after we are reminded, or triggered, our feelings keep growing and it becomes harder and harder to stay in control. Sometimes we just can't stop thinking of very upsetting things, or we feel like bad things are happening again. Other times we might forget where we are, who we are, or what we're doing. Sometimes things that wouldn't usually make us upset suddenly seem very frightening or make it really hard to stay in control. Write a list of those things . . .

Reminders/stressors: What leads to me being out of control?

```
1.
2.
3.
4.
5.
```

How I know when I'm reexperiencing: The "three A's"

Ask others:	*Ask myself:*
Affect:	**Affect:**
What expression does my face show?	How do I feel?
How do I say I feel?	What does my body feel like?
Awareness:	**Awareness:**
Do I seem spaced out or in my own world?	What's going on around me?
How well am I paying attention to things?	What am I thinking about?
Action:	**Action:** What do I feel like doing?
What do I do?	
What do I say?	

Interventions for the reexperiencing phase: How to stay safe

Things an <u>adult can help me with</u>:	*Things I can <u>do on my own</u>:*

(continued)

Reconstitution Stage: Getting Back in Control

No matter how bad things get, we eventually get back to feeling OK again. Sometimes right after we've been reminded or reexperiencing, though, things can still feel a little different from usual. We might still be thinking about what just happened or feeling badly about some action we did. This is an important time to do things that help keep you feeling OK.

How I know when I'm starting to be back in control again: The "three A's"

Ask others:	*Ask myself:*
Affect:	**Affect:**
What expression does my face show?	How do I feel?
How do I say I feel?	What does my body feel like?
Awareness:	**Awareness:**
Do I seem spaced out or in my own world?	What's going on around me?
How well am I paying attention to things?	What am I thinking about?
Action:	**Action:** What do I feel like doing?
What do I do?	
What do I say?	

Maintenance and repair activities: Things I can do to keep myself in control and to fix problems I contributed to

Things an <u>adult can help me with</u>:	*Things I can <u>do on my own</u>:*

(continued)

(FOR THE THERAPIST)
EVIDENCE OF DYSREGULATION

Definition of the emotionally dysregulated child

Child displays all of the following:

- Changes in awareness, affect, *and* action when faced with a stress provocation.
- An episode of dysregulation at least once monthly that interferes with functioning.
- Problems in functioning: There must be some evidence that the dysregulation episode caused a problem with the child's school, family, or peer relationships; this problem can either be related to the dysregulation episode itself or to feelings or behaviors related to the anticipation of a dysregulation episode.

Child does *not* display:

- Dangerous behavior **when stressed** (e.g., self-destructive, aggressive, substance-abusing, excessive eating, or sexual behavior).

Definition of the behaviorally dysregulated child

Child displays all of the following:

- Changes in awareness, affect, *and* action when faced with a stress provocation.
- An episode of dysregulation at least once monthly that interferes with functioning.
- **Dangerous behavior when stressed** (e.g., self-destructive, aggressive, substance-abusing, excessive eating, or sexual behavior).
- Problems in functioning: There must be some evidence that the dysregulation episode caused a problem with the child's school, family, or peer relationships; this problem can either be related to the dysregulation episode itself or to feelings or behaviors related to the anticipation of a dysregulation episode.

If child is EMOTIONALLY DYSREGULATED, use ER guide pages for *regulated*, *revving*, and *reconstituting*.

If child is BEHAVIORALLY DYSREGULATED, use all of the above PLUS *reexperiencing*.

Questions to ask to help assess changes in the three A's:

Awareness (consciousness)	Affect (emotion)	Action (behavior)
What were you noticing? Did what you noticed seem different? (*attention*)	What were you feeling? Did your feelings change?	What did you do? Did your behavior change?
Was it harder to pay attention to what was going on around you? (*attention*)	How strong were the feelings? Were they more intense, less intense, or about the same as before? Did you feel angrier? Did you feel sadder? Did you feel more scared? Did you have less of any of these feelings?	Sometimes kids do things that aren't very safe when they feel the way you described, such as throw things, or hit someone/something, or run away. I'm wondering if you felt like doing any of these things. What did you do?
What do you remember about what happened? Do you have trouble remembering what happened? (*attention*)		
Did it feel like something that happened before was happening again? (*orientation*)	Sometimes feelings seem really big and strong, or really far away and hardly there. Sometimes they're in the middle of those two extremes. What were your feelings like?	Did you yell or cry or feel like doing either or both of those things?
How long was this going on? Was it harder to keep track of time? (*orientation*)	Was it harder to control any of these feelings?	What did people around you say about what you were doing? Did people notice that you seemed different?
Where did this take place? Did you forget where you were? (*orientation*)	Did you have trouble feeling anything at all?	Did you feel like hurting yourself? Did you try?
Did it seem like you were back at the time or place of the bad thing that happened to you? (*orientation*)	Often people have more than one feeling at the same time. Did you have any other feelings? Tell me about those feelings.	What did you do that made you feel better? What did other people do to make you feel better? What do you think would have helped?
What did your body feel like? Did your body feel different? (*sense of self*)		Did you use drugs or alcohol?
Did it seem like you were younger (or older)? (*sense of self*)		Sometimes kids do things sexually when they feel really upset, such as touching other kids in private places or saying sexual things. Do you ever feel like doing those things? Did you do anything like that?
Did you feel like you were a different person? (*sense of self*)		What about eating? Tell me what your eating was like during that time. Did you eat something or get rid of what you ate?

COGNITIVE COPING LOG

Child _____

Caregiver _____ Therapist _____

Date _____

WHAT happened to make me feel or act upset:

RECOUNTING: WHAT I was thinking, feeling, and doing at the time

What I Was Thinking	*What I Was Feeling*	*What I Was Doing*

REFLECTING: What could I have thought, felt, and done instead?

What I Could Have Thought	*What I Would Have Felt*	*What I Would Have Done*

REWARDING: How can I reward myself after completing this worksheet?

SYSTEMS ADVOCACY SCREENER

1. ECONOMIC AND INCOME SUPPORT		
Do you ever have problems making ends meet?	Y	N
If YES:		
• Have you had a job in the past year?	Y	N
• Do you receive any government benefits?	Y	N
• Do you or your child have a physical or mental condition that restricts your ability to work?	Y	N
• Do you have citizenship, a green card, or a work visa?	Y	N
2. HOUSING		
Are you concerned about conditions, safety, or overcrowding at home?	Y	N
If YES:		
• Are you homeless or doubled up?	Y	N
• Do you live in public housing or Section 8 housing?	Y	N
• Are you concerned about conditions in your home?	Y	N
• Are you facing an impending eviction?	Y	N
• Do you need a housing transfer within public housing?	Y	N
• Are you behind in rent or utilities payments?	Y	N
3. HUNGER		
Do you ever have difficulty getting food for your family?	Y	N
If YES:		
• Are you receiving public benefits?	Y	N
• Are you receiving food stamps?	Y	N
• Are you pregnant, postpartum, or breastfeeding?	Y	N
• Do you have a child under the age of 5?	Y	N
4. CHILD CARE VOUCHERS		
Do you need, or are you eligible for, assistance paying for child care?	Y	N
If YES:		
• Is your family income < 185% of the federal poverty level (e.g., family of four with income less than $33,400/year)?	Y	N
• Have you received TAFDC in the last 12 months?	Y	N
• Do you have a child under the age of 5?	Y	N

(continued)

5. EDUCATION		
Do you have any concerns about your child's learning or education?	Y	N
If YES, do you have concerns about:		
• School behavior and discipline?	Y	N
• Enrollment, transfer, or transportation?	Y	N
• Taking or passing school achievement tests?	Y	N
• Your child's health as it relates to school or education?	Y	N
6. FAMILY LAW		
Do you have questions about paternity, custody, or visitation?	Y	N
Have you ever had to file a restraining order?	Y	N
7. DISABILITY		
Does your child have a disability that interferes with school performance, your work, home or family life?	Y	N
8. IMMIGRATION		
Were you or your children born in a foreign country?	Y	N
If YES:		
• Do you have a work visa?	Y	N
• Do you have questions about citizenship?	Y	N
• What is your immigration status?		
• How long have you been in the United States?		
• What country are you from?		
• What applications have you filed for with the Immigration and Naturalization Service (INS)?		
• Why did you leave your country?		

GOAL-SETTING GUIDE

What would you like to do in the future? List as many answers to the questions below as you can, and see if it helps you answer the bigger question of what you'd like to do in the future. There are no right or wrong answers, and there's no goal too big or too small.

What I Am Good At:

What I Like to Do:

What I Want to Do in the Future:

What Steps I Need to Take to Get There:

References

Barlow, D. H., Allen, L., & Choate, M. L. (2005). *The unified protocol for treatment of the emotional disorders.* Unpublished manual, Boston University.

Beck, A. T., Rush, A. J., Shaw, B. F., & Emery, G. (1979). *Cognitive therapy of depression.* New York: Guilford Press.

Bremner, J. D., Randall, P., Scott, T. M., Bronen, R. A., Seibyl, J. P., Southwick, S. M., et al. (1995). MRI-based measurement of hippocampal volume in patients with combat-related posttraumatic stress disorder. *American Journal of Psychiatry, 152,* 973–981.

Bremner, J. D., Randall, P., Vermetten, E., Staib, L., Bronen, R. A., Mazure, C., et al. (1997). Magnetic resonance imaging-based measurements of hippocampal volume in posttraumatic stress disorder related to childhood physical and sexual abuse—a preliminary report. *Biological Psychiatry, 41,* 23–32.

Bronfenbrenner, U. (1979). *The ecology of human development.* Cambridge, MA: Harvard University Press.

Bronfenbrenner, U., & Ceci, S. J. (1994). Nature–nurture reconceptualized in developmental perspective: A bioecological model. *Psychological Review, 101*(4), 568–586.

Cicchetti, D., & Lynch, M. (1993). Toward an ecological/transactional model of community violence and child maltreatment: Consequences for children's development. *Psychiatry, 56,* 96–118.

Cloitre, M., Koenen, K. C., Cohen, L. R., & Han, H. (2002). Skills training in affective and interpersonal regulation followed by exposure: A phase-based treatment for PTSD related to childhood abuse. *Journal of Consulting and Clinical Psychology, 70,* 1067–1074.

Cohen, J. A., & Mannarino, A. P. (1996). A treatment outcome study for sexually abused pre-school children: Initial findings. *Journal of the American Academy of Child and Adolescent Psychiatry, 35,* 42–50.

Cohen, J. A., Mannarino, A. P., Berliner, L., & Deblinger, E. (2000). Trauma focused cognitive behavior therapy: An empirical update. *Journal of Interpersonal Violence, 15,* 1203–1223.

Cohen, J. A., Mannarino, A. P., & Deblinger, E. (2003). *Child and parent trauma-focused cognitive behavioral therapy treatment manual.* Philadelphia: Drexel University College of Medicine. (Available from authors)

Cohen, J. A., Manarino, A. P., Greenberg, T., Padlo, S., Shipley, C., Deblinger, E., et al. (2001). *Cognitive behavioral therapy for childhood traumatic grief in children treatment manual.* Pittsburgh, PA: Center for Traumatic Stress in Children and Adolescents, Allegheny General Hospital.

Damasio, A. (1999). *The feeling of what happens: Body and emotion in the making of consciousness.* Fort Worth, TX: Harcourt College.

DeBellis, M. D., Baum, A. S., & Birmaher, B. (1999). Developmental traumatology: I. Biological stress systems. *Biological Psychiatry, 45*(10), 1259–1270.

DeBellis, M. D., Keshavan, M. S., Clark, D. B., Casey, B. J., Giedd, J. N., Boring, A. M., et al. (1999). Developmental traumatology: Part II. Brain development. *Society of Biological Psychiatry, 45,* 1271–1284.

Deblinger, E., & Heflin, A. H. (1996). *Treating sexually abused children and their nonoffending parents: A cognitive behavioral approach.* Thousand Oaks, CA: Sage.

Deblinger, E., McLeer, S. V., & Henry, D. (1990). Cognitive behavioral treatment for sexually abused children suffering post-traumatic stress: Preliminary findings. *Journal of the American Academy of Child and Adolescent Psychiatry, 29,* 747–752.

Donnelly, D. A., & Murray, E. J. (1991). Cognitive and emotional changes in written essays and therapy interviews. *Journal of Social and Clinical Psychology, 10*(3), 334–350.

Esterling, B., L'Abate, L., & Murray, E. J.(1999). Empirical foundations for writing in prevention and psychotherapy: Mental and physical health outcomes. *Clinical Psychology Review, 19*(1), 79–96.

First, M. (2006). Stress-induced and fear circuitry disorders. Retrieved from http://dsm5.org/conference7/cfm

Fitzgerald, H. E., Lester, B. M., & Zuckerman, B. S. (1995). *Children of poverty: Research, health, and policy issues.* New York: Garland.

Foa, E. B., Rothbaum, B. O., Riggs, D. S., & Murdock, T. B. (1991). Treatment of posttraumatic stress disorder in rape victims: A comparison between cognitive behavioral procedures and counseling. *Journal of Consulting and Clinical Psychology, 59*, 715–723.

Frankl, V. E. (1963). *Man's search for meaning: An introduction to logotherapy* (I. Lasch, Trans.). Boston: Beacon Press.

Hanh, T. N. (1976). *The miracle of mindfulness: An introduction to the practice of meditation.* Boston: Beacon Press.

Harvey, M., Milner, A. D., & Roberts, R. C. (1995). Differential effects on line length on bisection judgements in hemispatial neglect. *Cortex, 31*(4), 711–722.

Henggeler, S. W., Schoenwald, S. K., Borduin, C. M., Rowland, M. D., & Cunningham, P. (1998). *Multisystemic treatment of antisocial behavior in children and adolescents.* New York: Guilford Press.

Henggeler, S. W., Schoenwald, S. K., & Pickrel, S. G. (1995). Multisystemic therapy: Bridging the gap between university and community-based treatment. *Journal of Consulting and Clinical Psychology, 63*, 709–717.

Hoagwood, K., Jensen, P. S., Petti, T., & Bums, B. J. (1996). Outcomes of mental health care for children and adolescents: I. A comprehensive conceptual model. *Journal of American Academy of Child and Adolescent Psychiatry, 35*(8), 1055–1063.

James, B. (1989). *Treating traumatized children: New insights and creative interventions.* New York: Free Press.

Kandel, E. R. (1998). A new intellectual framework for psychiatry. *American Journal of Psychiatry, 155*, 457–469.

Kassner, B., & Kharasch, S. (1999). *Prevalence of violence exposure in adolescents who present to an emergency room.* Unpublished manuscript.

Kazak, A. E., & Christakis, D. A. (1996). The intense stress of childhood cancer: A systems perspective. In C. R. Pfeffer (Ed.), *Severe stress and mental disturbance in children* (pp. 277–305). New York: Cornell University.

Kirsch, P., Esslinger, C., Chen, O., Mier, D., Lis, S., Siddhanti, S., et al. (2005). Oxytocin modulates neural circuitry for social cognition and fear in humans. *Journal of Neuroscience, 25*, 11489–11493.

Koenen, K. C., Moffitt, T. E., Caspi, A., Taylor, A., & Purcell, S. (2003). Domestic violence is associated with environmental suppression ofIQ in young children. *Development and Psychopathology, 15*, 297–311.

Kosten, T. R., Mason, J. W., Giller, E. L., Ostroff, R. B., & Harkness, L. (1987). Sustained urinary norepinepherine and epinepherine elevation in posttraumatic stress disorder. *Psychoneuroendocrinology, 12*, 13–20.

LeDoux, J. (1998). *The emotional brain: The mysterious underpinnings of emotional life.* New York: Simon & Schuster.

LeDoux, J. (2002). *Synaptic self: How our brains become who we are.* New York: Viking Press.

Lichtenberg, J. D., Lachmann, F. M., & Fosshage, J. L. (1992). *Self and motivational systems: Toward a theory of psychoanalytic technique.* Hillsdale, NJ: Analytic Press.

Liebschutz, J. M., Frayne, S. M., & Saxe, G, N. (Eds.). (2003). *Violence against women: A physician's guide to identification and management.* Philadelphia: American College of Physicians.

Linehan, M. M. (1993). *Cognitive-behavioral treatment of borderline personality disorder.* New York: Guilford Press.

March, J. S., Amaya-Jackson, L., Murray, M. C., & Schulte, A. (1998). Cognitive-behavioral psychotherapy for children and adolescents with posttraumatic stress disorder after a single-incident stressor. *Journal of the American Academy of Child and Adolescent Psychiatry, 37*, 585–593.

McEwen, B. S. (1994). Endocrine effects on the brain and their relationship to behavior. In J. G. Siegel, B. W. Agranoff, R. W. Albers, & P. B. Molinoff (Eds.), *Basic neurochemistry: Molecular, cellular, and medical aspects* (5th ed., pp. 1003–1023). New York: Raven Press.

National Research Council Institute of Medicine (2000). *From neurons to neighborhoods: The science of early childhood development.* Washington, DC: National Academy Press.

Panksepp, J. (1998). *Affective neuroscience: The foundations of human and animal emotions.* New York: Oxford University Press.

Pennebaker, J. W., & Francis, M. E. (1996). Cognitive, emotional and language processes in disclusure. *Cognition and Emotion, 10*(6), 601–626.

Perry, B. D., & Pollard, R. (1998). Homeostasis,

stress, trauma, and adaptation: A neurodevelopmental view of childhood trauma. *Child and Adolescent Psychiatric Clinics of North America, 7,* 33–51.

Perry, B. D., Pollard, R. A., Blakley, T. L., Baker, W. L., & Vigilante, D. (1995). Childhood trauma, the neurobiology of adaptation, and "use-dependent" development of the brain: How "states" become "traits." *Infant Mental Health Journal, 16,* 271–291.

Porges, S. W. (1995). Orienting in a defensive world: Mammalian modifications of our evolutionary heritage: A polyvagal theory. *Psychophysiology, 32*(4), 301–318.

Pumariega, A. J., & Winters, N. C. (Eds.). (2003). *The handbook of child and adolescent systems of care: The new community psychiatry.* San Francisco: Jossey-Bass.

Putnam, F. W. (1997). *Dissociation in children and adolescents: A developmental perspective.* New York: Guilford Press.

Pynoos, R. S., & Nader, K. (1988). Psychological first aid and treatment approach to children exposed to community violence: Research implications. *Journal of Traumatic Stress, 1*(4), 445–473.

Pynoos, R. S., Steinberg, A. M., & Wraith, R. (1995). A developmental model of childhood traumatic stress. In D. Cicchetti & D. J. Cohen (Eds.), *Developmental psychopathology, Vol. 2: Risk, disorder, and adaptation* (pp. 72–95). Oxford, UK: Wiley.

Rauch, S. L., Whalen, P. J., Shin, L. M., McInerney, S. C., Macklin, M. L., Lasko, N. B., et al. (2000). Exaggerated amygdala response to masked facial stimuli in posttraumatic stress disorder: A functional MRI study. *Biological Psychiatry, 47*(9), 769–776.

Resick, P. A., & Schnicke, M. K. (1992). Cognitive processing therapy for sexual assault victims. *Journal of Consulting and Clinical Psychology, 60,* 748–756.

Saltzman, W. R., Steinberg, A. M., Layne, C. M., Aisenberg, E., & Pynoos, R. S. (2001). A developmental approach to school-based treatment of adolescents exposed to trauma and traumatic loss. *Journal of Child and Adolescent Group Therapy, 11,* 43–56.

Saxe, G. N., Ellis, H., Fogler, J., Hansen, S., & Sorkin, B. (2005). Comprehensive care for traumatized children: An open trial examines treatment using trauma systems therapy. *Psychiatric Annals, 35,* 443–448.

Saxe, G. N., Liebschutz, J. M., Edwardson, E., & Frankl, R. (2003). Bearing witness: The effect of caring for survivors of violence on health care providers. In J. M. Liebschutz, S. M. Frayne, & G. N. Saxe (Eds.), *Violence against women: A physician's guide to identification and management.* Philadelphia: American College of Physicians.

Saxe, G. N., Stoddard, F., Hall, E., Chawla, N., Lopez, C., Sheridan, R., et al. (2005). Pathways to PTSD: Part I. Children with burns. *American Journal of Psychiatry, 162,* 1299–1304.

Schore, A. N. (1994). *Affect regulation and the origin of the self: The neurobiology of emotional development.* Hillsdale, NJ: Erlbaum.

Schore, A. N. (2003). *Affect regulation and the repair of the self.* New York: Norton.

Shin, L. M., Orr, S. P., Carson, M. A., Rauch, S. L., Macklin, M. L., Lasko, N. B., et al. (2004). Regional cerebral blood flow in the amygdala and medial prefrontal cortex during traumatic imagery in male and female Vietnam veterans with PTSD. *Archives of General Psychiatry, 61*(2), 168–176.

Southwick, S. M., Krystal, J. H., Morgan, A., Johnson, D., Nagy, L. M., Nicolaou, A., et al. (1993). Abnormal noradrenergic function in posttraumatic stress disorder. *Archives of General Psychiatry, 50,* 266–274.

Stroul, B. A., & Friedman, R. M. (1994). *A system of care for children with severe emotional disturbances.* Washington, DC: Georgetown University Child Development Center, National Technical Center for Children's Mental Health, Center for Child Health and Mental Health Policy.

Suárez, L. M., & Hourigan, S. E. (2006). *Weekly TST Check-In.* Boston: Center for Anxiety and Related Disorders, Boston University.

Taylor, L., Zuckerman, B., Harik, V., & Groves, B. (1994). Exposure to violence among inner city children. *Developmental and Behavioral Pediatrics, 15,* 120–123.

Terr, L. (1990). *Too scared to cry: Psychic trauma in childhood.* New York: Basic Books.

van der Kolk, B. A. (1994). The body keeps the score: Memory and the evolving psychobiology of PTSD. *Harvard Review of Psychiatry, 1,* 253–265.

van der Kolk, B. A., & Fisler, R. E. (1994). Child abuse and neglect and loss of self-regulation. *Bulletin of the Menninger Clinic, 58,* 145–168.

Yehuda, R., Southwick, S. M., Krystal, J. H., Bremner, D., Charney, D. S., & Mason J. W. (1993). Enhanced suppression of cortisol following dexamethasone in posttraumatic stress disorder. *American Journal of Psychiatry, 150,* 83–96.

Yehuda, R., Southwick, S. M., Nussbaum, G., Wahby, V., Giller, E. L., Jr., & Mason, J. W. (1990). Low urinary cortisol excretion in patients with posttraumatic stress disorder. *Journal of Nervous and Mental Disease, 178,* 366–369.

Index

Page numbers appearing in *italic* denote figures or tables.